Urologic Oncology

Cancer Treatment and Research

WILLIAM L MCGUIRE, *series editor*

Urologic Oncology

edited by

TIMOTHY L. RATLIFF

and

WILLIAM J. CATALONA

Washington University School of Medicine and The Jewish Hospital of St. Louis, Division of Urology, Department of Surgery, St. Louis, Missouri, U.S.A.

1984 **MARTINUS NIJHOFF PUBLISHERS**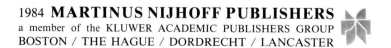
a member of the KLUWER ACADEMIC PUBLISHERS GROUP
BOSTON / THE HAGUE / DORDRECHT / LANCASTER

IV

Distributors

for the United States and Canada: Kluwer Boston, Inc., 190 Old Derby Street, Hingham, MA 02043, USA.
for all other countries: Kluwer Academic Publishers Group, Distribution Center, P.O.Box 322, 3300 AH Dordrecht, The Netherlands.

Library of Congress Cataloging in Publication Data

```
Main entry under title:

Urologic oncology.

   (Cancer treatment and research)
   Includes index.
   1. Genito-urinary organs--Cancer.  I. Catalona,
William J.  II. Ratliff, Timothy L.  III. Series.
[DNLM: 1. Urogenital neoplasms.  WJ 160 U788]
RC280.G4U77  1984         616.99'46         83-27482
ISBN 0-89838-628-4
```

ISBN 0-89838-628-4 (this volume)
ISBN 90-247-2406-0 (series)

PRINTED IN THE NETHERLANDS.

Contents

Cancer Treatment and Research

Foreword to the series

Where do you begin to look for a recent, authoritative article on the diagnosis or management of a particular malignancy? The few general oncology textbooks are generally out of date. Single papers in specialized journals are informative but seldom comprehensive; these are more often preliminary reports on a very limited number of patients. Certain general journals frequently publish good indepth reviews of cancer topics, and published symposium lectures are often the best overviews available. Unfortunately, these reviews and supplements appear sporadically, and the reader can never be sure when a topic of special interest will be covered.

Cancer Treatment and Research is a series of authoritative volumes which aim to meet this need. It is an attempt to establish a critical mass of oncology literature covering virtually all oncology topics, revised frequently to keep the coverage up to date, easily available on a single library shelf or by a single personal subscription.

We have approached the problem in the following fashion. First, by dividing the oncology literature into specific subdivisions such as lung cancer, genitourinary cancer, pediatric oncology, etc. Second, by asking eminent authorities in each of these areas to edit a volume on the specific topic on an annual or biannual basis. Each topic and tumor type is covered in a volume appearing frequently and predictably, discussing current diagnosis, staging, markers, all forms of treatment modalities, basic biology, and more.

In Cancer Treatment and Research, we have an outstanding group of editors, each having made a major commitment to bring to this new series the very best literature in his or her field. Martinus Nijhoff Publishers has made an equally major commitment to the rapid publication of high quality books, and world-wide distribution.

Where can you go to find quickly a recent authoritative article on any major oncology problem? We hope that Cancer Treatment and Research provides an answer.

WILLIAM L. MCGUIRE
Series Editor

Preface

The study of genitourinary tumors is an area of recent rapid growth both in the understanding of disease processes and in the development of new diagnostic and therapeutic modalities. During rapid growth phases within any field, it is desirable to reflect on the current 'state of the art'. It is difficult even for experts in reputed areas of advancement to distinguish true advances from false leads, but it is far more difficult yet for those whose expertise lies in other areas to evaluate important advances. Thus, an objective assessment of evolving areas of investigation in the form of a comprehensive review is of considerable value.

In this volume, we have attempted to provide the reader with an overview of some of the current areas of investigation in urologic oncology by experts in each area. There often is a tendency for invited papers in books of this nature to lack important critical peer review and therefore, suffer from a lack of objectivity. We have attempted to diminish this problem by the selection of two experts to discuss each subject. We believe that this format has improved the overall quality of the book for two reasons: 1) the knowledge of each contributor that his or her work would be reviewed by a peer encourages more rigorous scholarship, and 2) the fact that contributions by two experts, including the individual insights of each, provides a better perspective for the reader.

We gratefully acknowledge the efforts of each contributor. The strength and utility of this volume lies within the individual contributions. Also, we particularly wish to acknowledge the secretarial assistance of Kimberly Merritt and Christine Baumann whose efforts made completion of this volume possible.

List of Contributors

CATALONA, William J., M.D., Professor of Surgery, Division of Urology, Washington University School of Medicine, 4960 Audubon Avenue, and The Jewish Hospital of St. Louis, 216 South Kingshighway, St. Louis, MO 63110, USA.

CHODAK, Gerald W., M.D., Assistant Professor, Department of Surgery, Section of Urology, Box 403, 950 East 59th Street, Chicago, IL 60637, USA.

CHU, T. Ming, Ph.D., Professor and Director Diagnostic Immunology Research and Biochemistry Department, Roswell Park Memorial Institute, Department of Health, State of New York, 666 Elm Street, Buffalo, NY 14263, USA.

CHUNG, Leland W. K., Ph.D., Associate Professor of Pharmacology, University of Colorado, School of Pharmacy, Boulder, CO 80309, and Department of Pharmacology, University of Colorado Health Sciences Center, Denver, CO 80262, USA.

DRAGO, Joseph R., M.D., Associate Professor of Urology, Hershey Medical Center, 500 University Drive, Hershey, PA 17033, USA.

DEWOLF, William C., M.D., Assistant Professor of Surgery, Harvard Medical School, Beth Israel Hospital, 330 Brookline Avenue, Boston, MA 02215, USA.

ELDER, Jack S., M.D., Clinical Assistant Professor of Urology, Section of Urology, The Mason Clinic, University of Washington School of Medicine, Seattle, WA 98111-0900, USA.

FAIR, William R., M.D., A. Ernest and Jane G. Stein Professor and Chairman, Division of Urology, Washington University School of Medicine, 4960 Audubon Avenue, St. Louis, MO 63110, USA.

FLEISCHMANN, Jonathan, M.D., Resident in Urology, Washington University School of Medicine, 4960 Audubon Avenue, St. Louis, MO 63110, USA, and National Kidney Foundation Fellow.

FOLKMAN, Judah, M.D., Julia Dyckman Andrus Professor of Pediatric Surgery and Professor of Anatomy, Harvard Medical School/Childrens Hospital Medical Center and Director, Laboratory for Surgical Research, Childrens Hospital Medical Center, 300 Longwood Avenue, Boston, MA 02115, USA.

GROSSMAN, H. Barton, M.D., Assistant Professor, Department of Surgery, Section of Urology, University of Michigan Medical Center, Ann Arbor, MI 48109, USA.

HESTON, Warren D. W., Ph.D., Research Assistant Professor of Surgery (Urology), Washington University School of Medicine, 4960 Audubon Avenue, St. Louis, MO 63110, USA.

HRICAK, Hedvig, M.D., Associate Professor of Radiology and Urology, University of California, School of Medicine, San Francisco, CA 94143, USA.

JACOBS, Stephen C., M.D., Associate Professor of Urology, The Medical College of Wisconsin, Froedtert Memorial Lutheran Hospital, 9200 West Wisconsin Avenue, Milwaukee, WI 53226, USA.

JEWETT, Michael A. S., M.D., F.R.C.S. (C), Associate Professor, Department of Surgery (Urology), University of Toronto, Jones Building, Suite 206, The Wellesley Hospital, 160 Wellesley Street East, Toronto, Ontario M4Y 1J3, Canada.

KELLEY, David R., M.D., Resident in Urology, Washington University School of Medicine, 4960 Audubon Avenue, St. Louis, MO 63110, USA.

KRIM, Mathilde, Ph.D., Head, Interferon Laboratory, Memorial Sloan-Kettering Cancer Center, 1275 York Avenue, New York, NY 10021, USA.

LAMM, Donald L., M.D., Associate Professor, Division of Urology, University of Texas Medical School Health Science Center, 7703 Floyd Curl Drive and Chief of Urology, Audie Murphy Veterans Administration Hospital, 7400 Merton Minter, San Antonio, TX 78284, USA.

LIEBER, Michael M., M.D., Consultant in Urology and Cell Biology; Director, Urology Research Laboratories, Mayo Clinic; Associate Professor Urology, Mayo Medical School, Rochester, MN 55905, USA.

NARAYAN, Perinchery, M.D., Instructor in Surgery, Harvard Medical School, Beth Israel Hospital, 330 Brookline Avenue, Boston, MA 02215, USA.

NEWHOUSE, Jeffrey H., M.D., Associate Professor of Radiology, Columbia Presbyterian Medical Center, 622 West 168th Street, New York, NY 10032, USA.

NOVICK, Andrew C., M.D., Head, Section of Renal Transplantation, Department of Urology, The Cleveland Clinic Foundation, 9500 Euclid Avenue, Cleveland, OH 44106, USA.

POLLACK, Marilyn S., Ph.D., Head, HLA Serology Laboratory, Memorial Sloan-Kettering Institute for Cancer Research, 1275 York Avenue, New York, NY 10021, USA.

RATLIFF, Timothy L., Ph.D., Research Assistant Professor of Surgery (Urology), Washington University School of Medicine at The Jewish Hospital of St. Louis, 216 South Kingshighway, St. Louis, MO 63110, USA.

ROCCO, Audrey K., University of Colorado, School of Pharmacy, Boulder, CO 80309, USA.

ROWLAND, Randall G., M.D., Ph.D., Associate Professor, Department of Urology, Indiana University School of Medicine, Emerson Hall 246, 545 Barnhill Drive, Indianapolis, IN 46223, USA.

SAGALOWSKY, Arthur I., M.D., Assistant Professor Urology, Southwestern Medical School, The University of Texas Health Science Center at Dallas, 5323 Harry Hines Blvd., Dallas, TX 75235, USA.

SHAPIRO, Amos, M.D., Associate Professor of Urology, Hadassah University Hospital, Kiryat Hadassah, il-90, 120 Jerusalem, Israel.

SMITH, Joseph A. Jr., M.D., Associate Professor of Surgery, Division of Urology, University of Utah Medical Center, 50 North Medical Drive, Salt Lake City, UT 84132, USA.

SPEERS, Wendell C., M.D., Assistant Professor of Pathology, Department of Pathology B216, University of Colorado Health Sciences Center, 4200 East Ninth Avenue, Denver, CO 80262, USA.

THOMPSON, Timothy C., University of Colorado, School of Pharmacy, Boulder, CO 80309, USA.

TRACHTENBERG, John, M.D., F.R.C.S. (C), Assistant Professor of Surgery, Division of Urology, The Toronto General Hospital, 101 College Street, Eaton 9-240, Toronto, Ontario, Canada.

TRAISH, Abdulmaged M., M.D., Departments of Biochemistry and Urology, Boston University School of Medicine, Boston, MA 02108, USA.

WILLIAMS, Richard D., M.D., Associate Professor of Urology, Chief of Urologic Oncology, University of California, School of Medicine, and Chief of Urology, Veterans Administration Medical Center, San Francisco, CA 94143, USA.

WOTIZ, Herbert H., Ph.D., Professor of Biochemistry, Boston University Medical Center, 80 East Concord Street, Boston, MA 02118, USA.

1. Tumor Angiogenesis: Importance in Tumor Detection and Growth

GERALD W. CHODAK *

1. INTRODUCTION

Tumor angiogenesis has been defined as the growth of new capillary blood vessels in response to a tumor stimulus. This process is caused by a diffusable tumor product(s) and is directly responsible for enabling tumors to enlarge in size. Over the last ten years, significant progress has been made toward understanding the mechanism of this response. In addition, there now appears to be a potential for exploiting this understanding in order to assist with the diagnosis and possibly the treatment of solid tumors. This chapter will present an overview of the current knowledge in this field and the potential direction for this area in the near future.

2. THE AVASCULAR PHASE OF TUMOR GROWTH

The development of a solid tumor begins as an avascular collection of densely packed tumor cells. The developing mass of cells survives by obtaining nutrients and releasing waste products by simple diffusion with the extracellular fluid. The mechanics of the diffusion process limit the size of the tumor mass to a spheroid of approximately 1–2 mm in diameter. If no other changes occurred, tumors would be incapable of enlarging beyond this finite size. This has been called the avascular phase of tumor growth [15]. Brem et al. [5] illustrated this by injecting a suspension of cells from a rabbit V2 carcinoma into the vitreous of experimental rabbits. After one week they noted that spheroidal nodules had developed but these consistently remained finite in size. This pattern was maintained until the cells

* Gerald W. Chodak is an American Urological Association Scholar, an American Cancer Society Junior Faculty Clinical Scholar and a Gould Scholar.

T. L. Ratliff and W. J. Catalona (eds), Urologic Oncology. ISBN 0-89838-628-4.
© *1984. Martinus Nijhoff Publishers, Boston. Printed in the Netherlands.*

reached the retinal surface at which time neovascularization occurred and the tumors enlarged in size.

Gimbrone et al. [19] used the anterior chamber of the rabbit to similarly demonstrate the size limitation imposed on a tumor in the absence of angiogenesis. In these experiments, tumor cells were injected into the anterior chamber of the rabbit eye. Tumor spheroids were formed but they failed to grow larger than 1 mm in diameter. The mass of cells remained constant with a similar number of cells dying and being produced. If a spheroid was placed in contact with the iris, then tumor volume rapidly increased as vascularization commenced.

In an in vitro experiment, Folkman and Hochberg [16] implanted mouse melanoma cells into soft agar. Following 6 days of incubation, a spheroidal colony was formed with a diameter of approximately 0.1 mm. Colonies were then transferred to new agar where they grew to a realtively constant diameter and then remained dormant for several months. At that time proliferating cells near the outer edge were balanced by dying cells near the center.

Each of these models support the concept that tumor size must remain finite unless neovascularization occurs. Once new capillaries reach the tumor mass a new pattern of growth is possible.

3. THE VASCULAR PHASE OF TUMOR GROWTH

When solid tumors are placed within a few millimeters of blood vessels, new capillary growth does not occur for approximately 24 h [24]. Once new capillaries penetrate the avascular mass, exponential growth begins. Gimbrone and Gullino [18] found that following implantation of a tumor fragment into a rabbit corneal pocket, new blood vessels grew at a constant rate from the edge of the limbus toward the tumor. Once the capillaries penetrated the mass there was a 16 000-fold increase in tumor volume within 2 weeks.

4. MECHANISM OF TUMOR-INDUCED ANGIOGENESIS

Algire et al. were the first to observe that tumors could stimulate new capillary production by the host [1]. They inserted transparent chambers into mice skin flaps and implanted mouse tumors onto the vessel surface. They observed new capillary sprouts as early as the third day after tumor implantation.

In 1968, Greenblatt and Shubik [20] were the first to demonstrate that the new capillaries induced by tumors were the result of a diffusable substance. They implanted a tumor on one side of a 0.45 micron Millipore filter which separated the tumor from direct contact with the blood vessels of the hamster cheek pouch. This still resulted in new capillary growth. Using an in vitro model, Klagsbrun et al. [23] collected media from several animal tumor cell lines and also filtered the media through a 0.45 micron filter to remove all cellular material. They then used the chorioallantoic membrane (CAM) of the chick embryo to test for angiogenesis activity and found that the lyophilized conditioned media from some confluent tumor cell lines could induce new capillary growth. Conditioned media from human tumor cells have similarly been shown to induce angiogenesis [21, 28, 34].

As more information is obtained, it appears that the growth of new capillaries is a complex process consisting of several events. Ausprunk and Folkman [2] implanted tumors into the rabbit cornea and used electron microscopy to demonstrate that tumor angiogenesis involved both the migration and proliferation of capillary endothelial cells. They found that an early event is migration of endothelial cells through the intercellular gaps toward the angiogenic stimulus. Using tritiated thymidine incorporation they found that endothelial cell proliferation occurred at the tips of the spreading vessels. This process occurred in the absence of an inflammatory cell infiltrate. Later, Zetter [37] developed an in vitro bioassay to quantitate the migration of capillary endothelial cells and found that crude tumor angiogenesis factor (TAF) could stimulate migration as well as proliferation of these cells.

Another early event in the formation of new capillaries is the accumulation of mast cells in the region of the angiogenic stimulus. Kessler et al. [22] measured the mast cell density on the chick chorioallantoic membrane after implanting crude preparations of TAF derived from an animal tumor grown in vitro. Within 24 h after implantation and before new capillaries developed, the mast cell concentration was significantly increased. In order to determine whether these cells were responsible for new capillary growth, they implanted one million mast cells on to the CAM of the chick embryo. These cells were unable to stimulate angiogenesis. They concluded that mast cells were a necessary condition for angiogenesis although by themselves they were insufficient to produce this response.

The role that mast cells played was later elucidated by Azizkhan et al. [3]. They used the in vitro assay developed by Zetter [37] which measured the motility of cloned capillary endothelial cells. After demonstrating that mast cell-conditioned media could stimulate capillary endothelial cell migration, they tested various mast cell products and other glycosaminoglycans for their ability to stimulate endothelial cell migration. Only heparin was able to stimulate migration and this response was similar to that caused by a tumor cell extract. Further proof was provided by the loss of migration stimulatory activity when heparin was degraded by heparinase or combined with protamine sulfate prior to testing in the assay. These experiments provided evidence that both a tumor cell and a mast cell product were similar in being able to stimulate capillary cell migration. They differed, however, in that only the tumor cell product could also stimulate capillary proliferation. Heparin thus appears to assist in the angiogenic response. It may also play a role in this response by affecting the basement membrane surrounding capillaries. Sakamoto et al. [32] have shown that heparin enhances collaginase production and activity in vitro.

Other substances which appear to be involved in the angiogenic response are prostaglandins of the E series. Ben Ezra [4] incorporated prostaglandin E1, E2, I2, or F2 alpha into ethylene vinyl acetate copolymers which provide for a relatively constant rate of release. The polymers were implanted into the rabbit cornea and observed for new capillary growth. Only prostaglandin E1 and E2 were able to induce a response and prostaglandin E1 was found to be significantly more active than E2. In both cases a mild inflammatory cell infiltrate accompanied the response.

In a similar study performed with lower doses of prostaglandins, Ziche et al. [39] demonstrated that PGE1 was able to stimulate angiogenesis in the rabbit cornea in the absence of any inflammatory cell infiltrate. Furthermore, they showed that prostaglandins were necessary for a tumor-induced angiogenic response by preventing vascularization in the cornea of rabbits treated 3 times daily with oral indomethicin.

Form et al. [17] also demonstrated the angiogenic activity of PGE2 by implanting prostaglandin-containing pellets onto the CAM of the chick embryo. In their study, however, no histology was performed; thus making it possible that this response was really secondary to inflammation.

Another substance which plays a role in the angiogenic response is copper. McAuslan [29] found elevated amounts of copper in an extract from parotid glands that caused angiogenesis. He then incorporated different metal salts into polymers which were implanted into the rabbit cornea; only the copper-containing salts induced a neovascular response. His supposition was that copper attracted leukocytes, although he again provided no histological evidence to support this idea. McAuslan and Reilly also demonstrated that copper could stimulate bovine aortic endothelium to migrate in vitro [30]. As previously discussed, endothelial cell migration is one of the events necessary for the formation of new capillaries. This observation implicates copper as playing a role in the angiogenic response.

Based on this observation, Ziche et al. [39] measured the amount of copper and other ions in the rabbit cornea in response to an angiogenic stimulus. They found that only copper was increased just prior to new vessel formation. In addition, when they fed rabbits a diet deficient in copper, angiogenesis was inhibited. To further demonstrate that copper was important, they studied a group of copper-deficient rabbits that were unable to develop an angiogenic response. At that point the animals were placed on a normal diet for 3 weeks at which time a normal angiogenesis response could be elicited. As a result of these findings they also tested the copper-carrying protein, ceruloplasmin, for angiogenesis activity. This protein was incorporated into slow release polymers and again implanted into the rabbit cornea. This resulted in an angiogenic response in 70% of the corneal implants. In an interesting experiment that demonstrated the relationship between copper and prostaglandins in angiogenesis, Ziche et al. [39] implanted ceruloplasmin containing polymers into the cornea of rabbits treated with the prostaglandin inhibitor, indomethicin. These animals failed to develop an angiogenic response suggesting that prostaglandin production is probably an earlier event than copper mobilization.

In summary, the events that now appear to be necessary for tumor-induced angiogenesis include capillary endothelial cell migration and proliferation, prostaglandins of the E series, copper and ceruloplasmin, mast cells and heparin. The unfolding mechanism appears to involve a number of events which occur in a defined sequence. Further elucidation of this mechanism will probably be available by the time this book has been completed.

5. DETECTION OF TUMORS BASED ON THE ANGIOGENIC RESPONSE

An abundance of tumor markers have been tested for their ability to indicate the presence of a tumor. They usually consist of enzymes or antigens whose function, if any, is not known. Tumor angiogenesis factor appears to be unique in having a defined role in the growth of solid tumors. There is increasing evidence that tumor angiogenesis factor may be useful as a marker for the detection of solid tumors. Furthermore, there is also evidence that the expression of angiogenesis activity may be used to identify potentially malignant lesions. In one of the first studies which suggested that angiogenesis activity might indicate malignant transformation, Gimbrone and Gullino [18] implanted murine mammary glands onto the rabbit iris and found that a high frequency of hyperplastic alveolar nodules had angiogenesis activity. This is known to be a lesion with a high frequency of neoplastic transformation. Brem et al. [8] used the same assay to test human breast biopqies and mastectomy specimens for angiogenesis activity. They found that normal breast lobules and benign lesions, such as fibrocystic disease and fibroadenomas rarely could stimulate neovascularization but implants containing carcinoma in situ and invasive carcinoma could induce a response. They, too, found that approximately 30% of the implnats containing hyperplastic lobules could stimulate angiogenesis. Thus, the presence of angiogenesis distinguished between benign and malignant tissue. They suggested that the acquisition of angiogenesis activity might indicate that a tissue has progressed further toward a malignant state and perhaps this finding in a biopsy could identify which patients are at high risk for developing a breast tumor.

In another study, Brem et al. [7] tested murine breast tissue following treatment of the animals with two breast carcinogens which initially induce a benign papilloma. If these lesions were serially transplanted into syngeneic mice, tumors ultimately appeared after a variable latent period. Even though there was no histologic evidence of a tumor, almost all the implants could induce new blood vessels when implanted onto the rabbit iris. These results again supported the hypothesis that angiogenesis activity could be used to indicate which tissue had a potential for becoming malignant.

Chodak et al. have shown that angiogenesis could be a distinguishing factor between benign and malignant bladder tissue from humans [9] and other mammals [11]. In one study, bladder biopsies were obtained from humans with various diseases and implanted onto the rabbit iris. In four days almost all the biopsies containing transitional cell carcinoma were able to stimulate angiogenesis, while very few of the biopsies containing normal or benign tissue had this effect. In this study, angiogenesis was also detected in atypical hyperplasia, a known premalignant lesion, in specimens containing inflammatory cells, and in half the implants containing cystitis cystica. When the implants were incubated with human anti-lymphocyte serum just prior to implantation, angiogenesis was inhibited in the specimens with inflammatory cell infiltrates, but not in those containing transitional cell carcinoma or cystitis cystica. In the past, cystitis cystica has been considered to be a premalignant lesion. These results suggest that similar to the experimental breast studies, some of the bladder biopsies that contained cystitis cystica have acquired one of the requirements necessary for malignant transformation and have therefore progressed further toward a malignant state.

In another study [11] benign hyperplasia of the urothelium was produced by administering cyclophosphamide intravenously to rabbits. The animals were sacrificed and the bladder was cut into 1 mm fragments which were then placed on the rabbit iris. After 4 days no angiogenesis occurred whereas mouse bladder tumors stimulated new capillary growth within 4 days.

In a more recent study, Ziche and Gullino [38] established an important relationship between the timing of angiogenesis in relation to oncogenesis. They tested fibroblasts and human mammary cells grown in vitro for their ability to induce new capillary formation in the rabbit cornea. In both cases the early cell passages lacked both angiogenesis activity and tumorigenesis activity. As the cells were passaged, angiogenesis was eventually acquired in a significant number of implants; the ability to develop a tumor, however, was lacking. As passage of the cells continued, oncogenesis also coccurred. This study gives further support to the idea that angiogenesis is an early event which occurs prior to malignant transformation but which indicates that malignant transformation will follow. The major problem, however, is to determine the length of the time interval between the acquisition of angiogenesis activity and the transformation to a malignant state.

Although angiogenesis activity can distinguish between a malignant and benign tissue and may suggest a potential for malignant transformation, it is unlikely that in the near future actual biopsies could be tested for angiogenesis activity on a wide scale. An intriguing alternative, however, is to test body fluids for the presence of this activity. It is readily evident that the factor, or factors responsible for producing this response is(are) released from tumor cells. Therefore it would be reasonable to expect that any body fluid which is in contact with a tumor should contain the angiogenic activity.

Tapper et al. [35] first demonstrated this idea by lyophilizing a small volume of aqueous humor obtained from patients undergoing ophthalmologic surgery and testing for angiogenesis activity on the chorioallantoic membrane of the chick embryo. They found that 78 % of the specimens obtained from patients with malignant eye tumors stimulated new capillaries, but only 6 % of the specimens from patients with benign disease had this effect.

Based on this study and the demonstration that transitional cell carcinoma contained angiogenesis activity, Chodak et al. [10] collected urine samples from patients with a variety of diseases. Each sample was dialyzed and concentrated and then tested in an in vitro assay which measured capillary endothelial cell migration. As previously discussed, this is one of the events that occurs during new capillary formation. The investigators found that patients with biopsy-proved transitional cell carcinoma had significantly more endothelial cell migration stimulating activity than did several other groups; patients with a recent or past history of transitional cell tumor, patients with benign urologic or non-urologic diseases and normal controls. In addition, when patients with a tumor underwent surgical removal, the level of activity declined significantly after surgery. Furthermore, in a small group of patients who had several urine samples collected over an extended period of time, the level of activity appeared to correlate with the presence or absence of a tumor. Thus, this study further substantiates the potential use of the angiogenic response as a marker which could be used for detecting early or recurrent malignant disease. One question not yet answered is whether any factors related to angiogenesis are passed into the urine when a tumor is in the body but not in the urinary tract.

In another study which tested a human body fluid, Lopez-Pousa et al. [27] demonstrated that cerebrospinal fluid from patients with primary tumors of the central nervous system contained angiogenesis activity. They lyophilized small aliquots of this fluid obtained from patients with a variety of diseases and implanted the specimens onto the CAM of the chick embryo. Although only 4% of control specimens stimulated angiogenesis, 35% of specimens obtained from patients with tumors not metastatic to the CNS still had angiogenesis activity. One interpretation of this result is that tumors in any part of the body may release angiogenesis factors which equilibrate with the extra-cellular fluid. This might make it possible to test body fluids for tumors which are located elsewhere in the body. Further testing will be necessary to substantiate this concept.

In summary, there appears to be a substantial potential for using angiogenesis as a tumor marker for following the course of a tumor and perhaps even suggesting when a high malignant potential exists. Unfortunately, most of the currently available tests are cumbersome, time consuming and only moderately sensitive. As further progress is made toward isolation and purification of an angiogenic factor, eventually it may be possible to develop a radioimmunoassay which circumvents these problems.

6. INHIBITION OF TUMOR ANGIOGENESIS

As previously discussed, tumor growth can be divided into a vascular and avascular phase. The observation that tumor growth is limited until vascularization occurs suggests a potential control point for neoplastic disease; if angiogenesis could be inhibited or reversed, then a new method of treatment for solid tumors could be developed.

The first real evidence that neovascularization could be inhibited was provided by Eisenstein et al. [13]. They observed that various tissues placed onto the CAM of the chick embryo resulted in rapid invasion of vascularized mesenchyme by host tissue. The only tissue which failed to become vascularized was hyaline cartilage. Sorgante et al. [33] demonstrated that extraction of cartilage with low concentrations of guanidine HCl resulted in increased invasion of cartilage by host blood vessels. They suggested that a protease inhibitor was responsible for inhibiting new capillary growth. Eisenstein et al. [12] later tested this extract for its ability to affect the growth of bovine aortic endothelial cells in vitro. The material extracted from cartilage resulted in a significant inhibition of cell growth.

Expanding on this concept, Brem and Folkman [6] demonstrated that cartilage could also inhibit tumor-induced angiogenesis. They implanted crude extracts from a Walker carcinosarcoma onto the CAM of the chick embryo. Approximately 1–2 mm away, they placed 1 mm fragments of cartilage derived from neonatal rabbit scapula. Angiogenesis was induced around the tumor extract except in the region of the cartilage fragment. In a related experiment, fragments of the same cartilage were placed in between the limbus of the rabbit eye and a corneal implant of V2 carcinoma. If the cartilage was boiled prior to implantation into the corneal pocket, then new capillaries grew toward the tumor in a normal fashion. Once penetrating the tumor, the size greatly increased. In the animals with active cartilage, however, new capillary growth was significantly inhibited. In some cases capillaries grew and then regressed. The prevention of angiogenesis resulted in marked impairment of tumor growth. This was the first time that a substance from normal tissue could inhibit tumor-induced neovascularization.

Langer et al. [25] further purified this cartilage-derived angiogenesis inhibitor and found that the active fractions had high trypsin inhibitory activity. Affinity chromatography with trypsin-sepharose was used as part of the purification process. They lyophilized each of the fractions collected and incorporated them into ethylene vinyl acetate copolymers. The polymer and a fragment of a rabbit V2 carcinoma were placed in a rabbit corneal pocket with the pellet in between the limbus and the tumor. Over a 9 week period, negligible blood vessel growth occurred in the animals with active inhibitor. In contrast, new blood vessel growth continued in the controls and in the animals with the non-active fractions. The most active fraction had a molecular weight of approximately 16 000 daltons.

As more partially purified inhibitor was obtained, it became possible to test the effect of systemically administered cartilage-derived inhibitor. Langer et al. [26] implanted a rabbit V2 carcinoma into the rabbit cornea and a mouse melanoma tumor into the mouse cornea. Three days after new capillary growth began, the carotid artery of these animals was infused with either Ringer's lactate, trasylol, or the cartilage-derived angiogenesis inhibitor. During the infusion of the angiogenesis inhibitor, tumor growth and capillary growth were both prevented in each experimental model. After 7 days, the animals were sacrificed and the tumors weighed. There was a 40-fold reduction in tumor weight in the animals receiving the cartilage-derived inhibitor as compared to each of the control groups. Work is presently in progress to improve the purification of this substance.

In order to determine whether the inhibitor was possibly inhibiting the growth rate of the malignant cells, it was incubated with melanoma cells or V2 carcinoma cells grown in vitro. At concentrations of inhibitor up to 1 mg per ml there was no reduction in the growth rate. These results further support the idea that the inhibitor is acting solely on the tumor-induced capillaries.

One interesting aspect of the capillaries induced by tumors is their apparent need for continued stimulation. Falterman et al. [14] made this observation when they induced new capillaries in the rabbit cornea by implanting slow release pellets of crude TAF obtained from a Walker carcinosarcoma that had been grown in tissue culture. The eyes were observed until the proliferating capillaries reached the edge of the implanted polymer and then the polymers were removed. Over the next several weeks, the newly formed vessels began to regress until they almost completely disappeared. This observation is significant because it suggests that 'anti-angiogenesis' has the potential of not only inhibiting further tumor growth but also causing tumor regression as tumor-induced capillaries recede.

An obvious method for attempting to inhibit angiogenesis is to produce an antibody against an angiogenic factor. Phillips and Kumar [31] raised an antiserum against TAF extracted from rat Walker 256 carcinoma. The activity of the antiserum was demonstrated by Ouchterlony gel diffusion and immunoelectrophoresis. Inhibition of angiogenesis activity was assessed by combining crude TAF and antiserum directly on the chick embryo CAM. They observed that angiogenesis was inhibited in the eggs receiving both TAF and antiserum but not in those eggs receiving normal serum. If the antiserum was first absorbed with the TAF and then placed on the CAM, the inhibitory activity was lost. These results suggest an important area for additional work as purification of an angiogenic factor is completed.

In the most recent attempt to inhibit angiogenesis, Taylor and Folkman [36] used protamine sulfate in several assay systems. This drug was selected because of the previous observation that heparin was the mast cell product that assisted in the angiogeneic response by stimulating capillary endothelial cell migration. They hypothesized that protamine sulfate would combine with the heparin and thereby neutralize its role in the growth of new capillaries.

The first evidence for an effect came from work on the chick embryo CAM. They observed that if heparin was added to a crude TAF extract placed on the CAM then angiogenesis occurred more quickly and required less TAF. Protamine sulfate was able to inhibit this enhancing effect of heparin. They also observed that larger amounts of protamine sulfate could prevent all angiogenesis induced by the tumor extract.

The effect of protamine was also demonstrated by incorporation a drug into slow release polymers and implanting the polymer into the rabbit cornea between the edge of the limbus and a V2 carcinoma. New vessel growth was almost completely inhibited by the protamine as compared to controls. If the pellets were removed then new capillary growth resumed. Additional experiments revealed that protamine sulfate could not only inhibit tumor-induced angiogenesis but also the vessels normally induced by inflammation or the immune response.

The most dramatic effect occurred when protamine was administered systemically to mice that had received an intravenous injection of either mouse melanoma cells or Lewis lung tumor cells. The mice received either of two different doses of protamine sulfate twice daily as a subcutaneous injection. Treatment with protamine resulted in a 77–92% inhibition of mean volume of lung metastases as compared to the saline-treated animals. In these experiments, treatment with protamine was begun 24 h after tumor inoculation. In order to reduce toxicity, only one dose was administered on the first day of treatment. An important observation was that the protamine did not prevent the implantation of tumor cells into the lung but it did significantly inhibit neovascularization.

Similar experiments were conducted in a rat tumor model. Walker 256 carcinoma cells were injected intravenously and the animals were similarly treated with subcutaneous protamine. The animals receiving protamine had a 97% reduction in the mean tumor volume of lung metastases.

Treatment of subcutaneous tumors was less successful. Although one of the melanoma tumors had decreased growth in response to the protamine, two other tumors were not inhibited. Unfortunately, significant toxicity results from high doses of protamine making it difficult to determine the maximum effect of this drug. Perhaps a continuous infusion of protamine might maximize the tolerable dose of the drug while also augmenting its effect.

Although most of these attempts to interfere with tumor-induced angiogenesis are still in preliminary stages, they do establish that 'anti-angiogenesis' is a viable concept which warrants extensive investigation. As the mechanism of angiogenesis is further elucidated other angiogenesis inhibitors will probably be developed which may eventually play an important role in the treatment of solid tumors.

7. SUMMARY

In this chapter an overview has been presented of the expanding field of tumor-induced angiogenesis. The stimulation of new capillaries is a vital step in the grwoth of solid tumors. As can be seen from the studies that have been reviewed, this process is now being exploited for both the diagnosis and treatment of solid tumors. Although current methods of detecting angiogenesis activity primarily involve bioassays which are not currently amenable to widespread clinical use, they nevertheless provide the tools that may be used to develop improved methods of detection. In the area of tumor therapy continued progress toward understanding the mechanism of this response will suggest other drugs that may be used to interfere with angiogenesis and thus affect tumor growth. This area is still in its infancy and it is likely that rapid developments will be forthcoming in the near future which have important clinical implications for uro-oncologists as well as other cancer specialties.

REFERENCES

1. Algire GH, Chalkley HW, Legallais FY, Park HD: Vascular reactions of normal and malignant tissues in vivo. I. Vascular reactions of mice to wounds and to normal and neoplastic transplants. J Natl Cancer Inst 6:73, 1945.
2. Ausprunk DH, Folkman J: Migration and proliferation of endothelial cells in preformed and newly formed blood vessels during tumor angiogenesis. Microvas Res 14:53, 1977.
3. Azizkhan RG, Azizkhan JC, Zetter BR, Folkman J: Mast cell heparin stimulates migration of capillary endothelial cells in vitro. J Exp Med 152:931, 1980.
4. Ben Ezra D: Neovasculogenic ability of prostaglandins, growth factors, and synthetic chemoattractants. Am J Ophthalmol. 86:455, 1978.
5. Brem S, Brem H, Folkman J, Finkelstein, Patz A: Prolonged tumor dormancy by prevention of neovascularization in the vitreous. Can Res 36:2807, 1976.
6. Brem H, Folkman J: Inhibition of tumor angiogenesis mediated by cartilage. J Exp Med 141:427, 1975.
7. Brem SS, Gullino PM, Medina D: Angiogenesis: a marker for neoplastic transformation of mammary papillary hyperplasia. Science 199:880, 1977.
8. Bremm SS, Jensen HM, Gullino PM: Angiogenesis as a marker of preneoplastic lesions of the human breast. Cancer 41:239, 1978.
9. Chodak GW, Haudenschild C, Gittes RF, Folkman J: Angiogenic activity as a marker of neoplastic and preneoplastic lesions of the human bladder. Ann Surg 192:762, 1980.
10. Chodak GW, Scheiner CJ, Zetter BR: Urine from patiens with transitional-cell carcinoma stimulates migration of capillary endothelial cells. New Engl J Med 305:869, 1981.
11. Chodak GW, Summerhays L, Folkman J: Angiogenesis assay of benign and malignant mammalian urothelium. Surg Forum 31:587, 1980.
12. Eisenstein R, Kuettner KE, Neapolitan C, Soble LW, Sorgente N: The resistance of certain tissues to invasion. III. Cartilage extracts inhibit the growth of fibroblasts and endothelial cells in culture. Am J Pathol 81:337, 1975.
13. Eisenstein R, Sorgente N, Soble LW, Miller A, Kuettner KE: The resistance of certain tissues to invasion. Penetrability of explanted tissues by vascularized mesenchyme. Am J Pathol 73:765, 1973.
14. Falterman KW, Ausprunk DH, Klein MD: Role of tumor angiogenesis factor in maintenance of tumor-induced vessels. Surg Forum 27:157, 1976.
15. Folkman J, Cotran R: Relation of vascular proliferation to tumor growth. Int Rev Exp Pathol 16:207, 1976.
16. Folkman J, Hochberg M: Self-regulation of growth in three dimensions. J Exp Med 138:745, 1973.
17. Form DM, Sidky YA, Kubai L, Auerbach R: PGE2-induced angiogenesis. Prostaglandins and cancer: In: First International Conference. New York: Alan R. Liss Inc, p 685, 1982.

18. Gimbrone MA, Jr, Gullino P: Neovascularization induced by intraocular xenografts of normal, preneoplastic and neoplastic mouse mammary tissues. J Natl Cancer Inst 56:305, 1976.

19. Gimbrone MA, Jr, Leapman SB, Cotran RS et al: Tumor dormancy in vivo by prevention of neovascularization. J Exp Med 136:261, 1072.

20. Greenblatt M, Shubik P: Tumor angiogenesis: transfilter diffusion studies in the hamster by the transparent chamber technique. J Natl Cancer Inst 41:111, 1968.

21. Kelly PJ, Suddith RL, Hutchison HT et al: Endothelial growth factor present in tissue culture of CNS tumors. J Neurosurg 44:342, 1976.

22. Kessler DA, Langer RS, Pless NA, Folkman J: Mast cells and tumor angiogenesis. Int J Cancer 18:703, 1976.

23. Klagsbrun M, Knighton D, Folkman J: Tumor angiogenesis activity in cells grown in tissue culture. Cancer Res 36:110, 1976.

24. Knighton D, Ausprunk D, Tapper D, Folkman J: Avascular and vascular phases of tumour growth in the chick embryo. Br J Cancer 35:347, 1977.

25. Langer R, Brem H, Falterman K et al: Isolation of a cartilage factor that inhibits tumor neovascularization. Science 193:70, 1976.

26. Langer R, Conn H, Vacanti J et al: Control of tumor growth in animals by infusion of an angiogenesis inhibitor. Proc Natl Acad Sci USA 77:4331, 1980.

27. Lopez-Pousa S, Ferrier L, Vich JM, Domenech-Mateu J: Angiogenic activity in CSF in human malignancies. Experientia 37:413, 1981.

28. Matsuno H: Tumor angiogenesis factor (TAF) in cultured cells derived from central nervous system tumors in humans. Neurol Med Chir (Tokyo) 21:765, 1981.

29. McAuslan BR: A new theory of neovascularisation based on identification of an angiogenic factor and its effect on cultured endothelial cells. In: Control Mechanisms in Animal Cells, Jimenez de Asua et al. L. (eds.) New York: Raven Press, p 285, 1980.

30. McAuslan BR, Reily W: Endothelial cell phagokinesis in response to specific metal ions. Exp Cell Res 130:147, 1980.

31. Phillips P, Kumar S: Tumour angiogenesis factor (TAF) and its neutralisation by a xenogeneic antiserum. Int J Cancer 23:82, 1979.

32. Sakamoto S, Goldhaber P, Glimcher MJ: Mouse bone collagenase: the effect of heparin on the amount of enzyme released in tissue culture and on the activity of the enzyme. Calif Tissue Res 12:247, 1973.

33. Sorgante N, Kuettner KE, Soble LW, Eisenstein R: The resistance of certain tissues to invasion. II. Evidence for extractable factors in cartilage which inhibit invasion by vascularized mesenchyme. Lab Invest 32:217, 1975.

34. Suddith RL, Kelly PJ, Hutchison HT et al: In vitro demonstration of endothelial proliferative factor produced by neural cell lines. Science 190:682, 1975.

35. Tapper D, Langer R, Bellows AR, Folkman J: Angiogenesis capacity as a diagnostic marker for human eye tumors. Surgery 86:36, 1979.

36. Taylor S, Folkman J: Protamine is an inhibitor of angiogenesis. Nature 297:27, 1982.

37. Zetter BR: Migration of capillary endothelial cells is stimulated by tumour derived factors. Nature 285:41, 1980.

38. Ziche M, Gullino PM: Angiogenesis and neoplastic progression in vitro. J Natl Cancer Inst 69:483, 1982.

39. Ziche M, Jones J, Gullino P: Role of prostaglandin El and copper in angiogenesis. J Natl Cancer Inst 69:475, 1982.

Editorial Comment

JUDAH FOLKMAN

Dr Gerald Chodak has summarized some of the progress in the study of angiogenesis that has occurred over the past decade. Until the late 1960s, the mechanism of the growth of capillary blood vessels was of little or no interest to either biological scientists or clinicians. This neglect was based partly on the lack of suitable techniques to study angiogenesis. It was also not generally recognized that angiogenesis per se could play an essential role in common pathological processes such as tumor growth. Except for the work of Algire in the 1940s [1] and Greenblatt and Shubik in 1968 [2], capillary growth was thought by many workers to be a non-specific side effect of necrotic tumor or of its metabolic products. While the phenomenon of capillary growth occurs in a sequence of multiple steps analogous to blood coagulation, the connection between angiogenesis and disease was not as apparent as was the relation between blood coagulation and its disorders.

However by the early 1970s there was sufficient experimental evidence, mainly from tumors grown in isolated, perfused organs [3], to advance the hypothesis that tumors might be 'angiogenesis-dependent' [4, 5]. A corollary of this hypothesis was that inhibition of angiogenesis, 'anti-angiogenesis', might some day be used therapeutically [6].

Further experimental evidence for these ideas stimulated renewed interest in studying the mechanism of capillary growth. Four new techniques for the study of angiogenesis were developed: (i) from tumors implanted in the rabbit cornea, it became possible for the first time to make linear measurements of capillary growth [7]; (ii) the chorioallantoic membrane of the chick embryo assay became useful for testing many angiogenic substances without the interference of immune reactions [8]; (iii) implantable polymers of ethylene-vinyl acetate permitted sustained release of macromolecules [9]; and (iv) cloned capillary endothelial cells provided in vitro assays for study of the components of angiogenesis [10].

As these methods were used by us and by other investigators, a broader perspective of the role of angiogenesis in certain normal and pathological processes began to develop. With the cornea technique, Auerbach [11] demonstrated that sensitized lymphocytes could also induce angiogenesis. Polverini et al. [12] showed that macrophages could induce angiogenesis; and Hunt and Knighton and their colleagues [13] isolated a macrophage angiogenesis factor and also proved that its production increased under hypoxic conditions [14]. An essential role for angiogenesis in wound healing has emerged from these macrophage studies. Eisenstein et al. [15, 16], and subsequently Brem and Folkman [17] used the chick embryo and the rabbit cornea to show that an angiogenesis inhibitor was present in cartilage. The rabbit eye was used by Gullino and his associates [18] to show that angiogenesis is a pre-neoplastic marker. They introduced the novel concept that at a certain stage during the multistep transformation from a normal cell to a malignant one, angiogenesis activity is either turned on or turned up to such an extent that it can be readily detected in currently available assays.

Gullino's group also showed that once tumor cells begin to release angiogenic activity, they do so indefinitely, and apparently maximally [19]. This more or less permanent production of angiogenic activity by neoplastic cells may turn out to be an essential difference between tumor angiogenesis and angiogenesis induced by non-neoplastic or normal cells. Where the macrophage can turn off or turn down its angiogenic activity as tissue oxygen tension rises, once tumor cells have begun to release angiogenic activity, they continue to do so independently of local conditions.

This unique property of tumors is the basis of Dr Chodak's important work, clearly described in his review. His experiments demonstrate that normal urothelium has a level of angiogenic activity so low as to be essentially undetectable by current assays. However, angiogenic activity is consistently high and easily detectable in pre-neoplastic or neoplastic urothelium. These experiments led Chodak et al. to look for angiogenic activity in the urine of patients with bladder cancer [20]. They used an in vitro assay of capillary endothelial cell migration for the purpose of rapid screening [21]. While not a direct measure of angiogenic activity, induced endothelial migration is a component of the process of capillary growth and is highly correlated with angiogenesis. Most angiogenic factors so far isolated can stimulate migration of capillary endothelial cells in vitro.

The nature of angiogenic activity is less well understood. The methods so useful for expanding our knowledge about the biology of angiogenesis, have not been sufficiently sensitive or rapid for easy biochemical study. Nevertheless, considerable progress has been made by Schor et al. [22], Fenselau et al. [23], Weiss et al. [24], and Gross et al. [25] in terms of angiogenic factors from tumors, and by Knighton et al. [26], and Wissler and Renner [27] in terms of angiogenic factors from macrophages and lymphocytes; and by D'Amore and Glaser and their colleagues [28] in purifying a retinal angiogenesis factor. Although none of these factors has been completely purified, the first complete purification will no doubt facilitate progress with the others.

From the biochemical standpoint, greater progress has been made in identifying compounds that are angiogenesis inhibitors. Protamine, as discussed by Dr Chodak, was found to be an angiogenesis inhibitor during a detailed study of the sequential steps of capillary growth and the host factors that modify it [29]. With protamine it was possible to hold pulmonary metastases in an avascular phase, but it was not possible to eradicate them, nor to regress primary tumors because of the toxicity of high doses of protamine. However, more recently it has been shown that a fragment of heparin which by itself is non-anticoagulant, when administered with cortisone results in potent angiogenesis inhibition. With this combination, it is possible to cause tumor regression and prevent metastases in some experimental tumor systems [30].

When will this new knowledge about angiogenesis become useful in clinical practice? It is too early to say. However, Dr Chodak's work has certainly pointed the way. He has shown the potential diagnostic value of angiogenesis as a preneoplastic marker. As the urologist now uses evidence of local angiogenesis around a suspected bladder tumor to guide him during cystoscopy, he may someday use a simplified test for angiogenesis. Such a test of urine angiogenic activity might alert him to recurrence of tumor, or for that matter, to the presence of a premalignant lesion. While all of this is speculative, it must be remembered that only a few years ago the existence of angiogenesis inhibitors was also speculative.

REFERENCES

1. Algire GJ: J Natl Cancer Inst 4:13-20, 1943.
2. Greenblatt M, Shubik P: J Natl Cancer Inst 41:111-124, 1968.

3. Folkman J: In: Carcinoma of the Colon and Antecedent Epithelium, Burdette WJ (ed). Springfield: C.C. Thomas, pp 113-127, 1970.
4. Folkman J: In: Advances in Cancer Research, Klein G, Weinhouse S (eds). New York: Academic Press, 331-358, 1947.
5. Folkman J, Cotran RS: In: International Review of Experimental Pathology, Richter GW, (ed). New York: Academic Press, pp 207-248, 1976.
6. Folkman J: Ann Surg 175:409-416, 1972.
7. Gimbrone MA Jr, Leapman S, Cotran RS, Folkman J: JNCI. 52:413-427, 1974.
8. Klagsbrun M, Knighton D, Folkman J: Cancer Res 36:110-114, 1976.
9. Langer R, Folkman J: Nature 263:797-800, 1976.
10. Folkman J, Haudenschild CC, Zetter B: Proc Natl Acad Sci USA 76:5217-5221, 1979.
11. Auerbach R: Lymphokines 4:69-88, 1981.
12. Polverini PJ, Cotran RS, Gimbrone MJ Jr, Unanue ER: Nature 269:804-806, 1977.
13. Banda MJ, Knighton DR, Hunt TK, Werb Z: Proc Natl Acad Sci USA 79:7773-7777, 1982.
14. Knighton DR, Hunt TK, Scheuenstuht H. Halliday H: Science 221:1283-1285, 1983.
15. Eisenstein R, Sorgente N, Soble LW, Miller A, Kuettner KE: AM J Pathol 73:765-774, 1973.
16. Eisenstein R, Kuettner K, Neapolitan C, Soble LW, Sorgente N: Am J Pathol 81:337-347, 1975.
17. Brem H, Folkman J: J Exp Med 141:427-439, 1975.
18. Brem SS, Jensen HM, Gullino PM: Cancer 41:239-244, 1978.
19. Ziche M, Gullino PM: J Natl Cancer Inst 69:483-487, 1982.
20. Chodak GW, Scheiner CJ, Zetter BR: New Engl J Med 305:869-874, 1971.
21. Zetter BR: Nature 285:41-43, 1981.
22. Schor AM, Kumar S, Phillips PJ: Int J Cancer 25:773, 1980.
23. Fenselau A, Watt S, Mello RJ: J Biol Chem 256:9605, 1981.
24. Weiss JB, Brown RA, Kumar S, Phillips P: Br J Cancer 40:498, 1979.
25. Gross JL, Moscatelli D, Jaffe EA, Rifkin DB: J Cell Biol 95:974-981, 1982.
26. Knighton DR, Hunt TK, Thakral KK, Goodson WH III: Ann Surg 196:379-388, 1982.
27. Wissler JH, Renner H: Immunobiol 14:438, 1982.
28. D'Amore PA, Glaser BM, Brunson SK, Fenselau AH: Proc Natl Acad Sci USA 78:3068-3072, 1981.
29. Taylor S, Folkman J: Nature 297:307-312, 1982.
30. Folkman J, Langer R, Linhardt RJ, Haudenschild C, Taylor S: Science 221:719-725, 1983.

2. Role of Androgen Receptors in Stromal–Epithelial Interactions in Prostatic Cancer

LELAND W. K. CHUNG, TIMOTHY C. THOMPSON and AUDREY K. ROCCO

1. INTRODUCTION

Since the demonstration in 1941 by Huggins and Hodges on the endocrine dependency of neoplastic human prostate [1], this relationship has formed the foundation for investigations into the mechanism(s) of steroid hormone action on hormone-responsive target tissues. The discovery of the high affinity and limited capacity of estrogen receptors in immature rat uterus by Jensen [2] has firmly established the initial steps of steroid hormone and target tissue interactions. The rigid structural requirements of steroid hormones, their specific binding to cytoplasmic receptor proteins to form receptor protein complexes, and their ability to elicit specific biological responses have been documented at molecular [3, 4], genetic [5, 6], and developmental [7, 8] levels. Similar receptor proteins for androgens [9, 10], estrogens [11, 12], and/or progestins [13] have been demonstrated to exist in the prostate gland of virtually all species studied.

The concept of endocrine dependency underlies the attempt to correlate the levels of steroid receptors in various subcellular compartments, such as cytosol, nuclear, and residual fractions, with the clinical responsiveness of patients with prostatic [14, 15], breast [16, 17], or endometrial [18] cancer. These attempts have met with variable success. A number of recent publications have been devoted to discussion of steroid receptors and their potential as a means of predicting the responsiveness of prostatic cancer patients to endocrine therapy [14, 19–21].

The purposes of the present review are three-fold. First, we will consider technical problems in and current solutions for the determination of the levels of steroid receptors in prostatic tissues. Basic understanding of methodology is critical for assessment of laboratory data. Second, we will review recent published data on the levels of androgen receptors in normal human prostate and human prostatic cancer. The relevance of androgen receptors

T. L. Ratliff and W. J. Catalona (eds), Urologic Oncology. ISBN 0-89838-628-4.
© 1984. Martinus Nijhoff Publishers, Boston. Printed in the Netherlands.

in transplantable rat prostatic cancers will also be reviewed to provide further insight into the possible relationship between levels of androgen receptors and the hormone-dependent status of these tumors. Finally, we will discuss the role of androgen receptors in an experimental model based on the concept of tissue interaction to determine the involvement of stromal and/or epithelial androgen receptors in the overall gene expression of the prostate gland. Because the prostate gland is androgen-dependent, the measurement of the levels of androgen receptors simultaneous with the expression of specific androgen-induced gene product(s) either by the stromal and/or epithelial compartment [22] is assumed to correlate closely with the hormone-dependent status of prostatic tissues. This concept may lead to future development of new diagnostic and prognostic tools which can be used for predicting the clinical course of patients with prostatic cancer.

2. TECHNICAL CONSIDERATIONS

Unlike the significant correlation observed between estrogen receptors and hormonal responsiveness of human breast cancer, a similar correlation between androgen receptors and prostatic cancer in men has not yet been firmly established. The lack of a correlation between androgen receptors and prostatic cancer may be due in part to difficulties encountered in the measurement of androgen receptors in tissues. Table 1 lists a number of problems incurred in the measurement of androgen receptors in prostatic tissues and the resolutions currently available; each problem is discussed briefly in this section.

(a) Naturally occurring androgens such as testosterone and dihydrotesterone are known to bind the sex steroid binding globulins and (b) are metabolized during prolonged incubation with tissue cytosols. These problems are resolved by using the synthetic androgen analogue R1881 (methyltrienolone or 17β-hydroxy-17α-methylestra-4,9,11-trien-3-one). (c) R1881, however, also binds to progesterone receptors in human prostatic tissues. This binding can be efficiently masked by the addition of a high concentration of the unlabeled synthetic progesterone analogue R5020 or the unlabeled synthetic glucocorticoid triamcinolone acetonide, which displaces only the binding of R1881 to progesterone receptors without perturbing R1881 binding to androgen receptors. (d) Many methods have been employed for the separation of free and bound steroid ligands. These include the use of dextran-coated charcoal to remove the free steroids, the use of protamine sulfate or hydroxyapatite to precipitate the bound receptor complexes, or the use of density gradient or gel filtration methods to separate the ligand-bound complexes from unbound steroid ligands, based on their molecular sizes and shapes. (e) To properly differentiate occupied and unoccupied androgen receptors, pretreatment of the cytosol with dextran-coated charcoal has been reported to increase levels of assayable androgen binding proteins of a non-receptor nature [30]. Elevation of temperature during receptor analysis has been applied successfully in differentiating occupied and unoccupied estrogen receptors, and has been claimed to achieve the same result in the analysis of androgen receptors [32]. However, because of the susceptibility of androgen receptors to temperature inactivation, it remains controversial whether elevation of temperature for androgen receptor analysis may be the method of choice for differentiating

Table 1. Technical considerations of androgen receptor analysis.

Problems	Resolutions
(a) Non-specific binding to sex steroids binding globulins	Use synthetic androgen R1881 [23]
(b) Metabolism during receptor analysis	Use synthetic androgen R1881 [23]
(c) R1881 binding to progesterone receptor	Mask such binding by the addition of unlabeled triamcinolone acetonide or R5020, a synthetic progesterone analogue [24, 25]
(d) Separation of free and bound steroids	Dextran-coated charcoal [26]; protamine sulfate [27]; hydroxyapatite [28]; sucrose density gradient [9]; gel filtration [29]
(e) Differentiation between occupied and non-occupied receptors	Elevation of temperature [23, 31, 32]; mersalyl acid, a mercurial reagent [33]
(f) Stabilization of receptor from degradation during isolation and storage	Low temperatures [31]; vertical rotor centrifugation [34]; addition of sodium molybdate [35]; addition of protease inhibitor, such as phenylmethylsulfonyl floride (PMSF) [36]
(g) Increase sensitivity of receptor assay	Microassay with triplicate samples [42]; agar gel electrophoresis [15]; isoelectric focusing [43]; high performance liquid chromatography [44]
(h) Physical-chemical characterization of receptors	Gel infiltration [29]; density gradient centrifugation [9]; photoaffinity labeling [45]
(i) Functionality of receptors in tissues	Histochemistry [49]; autoradiography [7]; subcellular fractionation [20, 36]; gene expression of specific proteins [50, 51]

occupied and unoccupied androgen receptors. Recently, Traish et al. [33] demonstrated that the use of mersalyl acid, a mercurial reagent, can remove the steroid ligands from occupied androgen receptors at 0 °C in one hr. Thus, after mersalyl acid treatment of tissue samples, the levels of total (occupied + unoccupied) androgen receptors can be measured. This new procedure has not been used to measure androgen receptors in human prostatic specimens. (f) Because androgen receptors are labile, a number of methods, including the storage of tissues under low temperatures, rapid separation of steroid receptor complexes from unbound steroids by density gradient centrifugation utilizing vertical rotors [34], homogenization of the tissues in the presence of steroid ligand, addition of sodium molybdate [35], or inclusion of the protease inhibitor phenylmethylsulfonyl floride [36] in the homogenizing medium, have been used to circumvent this problem. These procedures all increase androgen receptor levels in tissues. The inclusion of sodium molybdate in the homogenizing medium has complex effects, such as direct interaction with steroid receptors [37], stabilization of steroid receptors from proteolytic action [38], preventing the transformation of steroid receptor complexes to their chromatin-bound form [39], and extraction of additional nuclear steroid receptors from liver [40] and prostatic [41] nuclei. (g) Because the quantities of human prostatic biopsy material generally are limited, attempts have been made to increase the sensitivity and reliability of receptor analysis. Hicks and Walsh [42] have developed dextran-coated charcoal methods for the assay of triplicate prostatic cytosol samples at one saturating ligand concentration. De Voogt and Dingjan [15] have used agar-gel electrophoretic procedures for receptor analysis. Wrange et al. [43] and Pousette et al. [44] developed a thin-layer polyacrylamide gel isoelectric focusing and high performance liquid chromatographic systems, which have resulted in reliable determinations of the levels of androgen receptors in needle aspiration biopsies of human prostate. Finally, the physicochemical (h) and the functional properties (i) of androgen receptors also have been the subject of extensive investigation. A number of publications have been devoted to characterizing androgen receptors in normal [9, 45, 46] and neoplastic [47, 48] male accessory sex organs. The development of a photoaffinity steroid ligand by Chang et al. [45] can potentially enhance the sensitivity and avidity of androgen binding to receptors. Future correlations between the presence of androgen receptors and the hormonal responsiveness of the prostate gland thus may be achievable by closely monitoring the localization of androgen receptors in different cell and subcellular compartments [7, 20, 36, 49].

3. ANDROGEN RECEPTOR CONTENTS IN NORMAL AND CANCEROUS HUMAN PROSTATIC TISSUES

Table 2 lists several recent studies on the androgen receptor levels in normal and cancerous (untreated and hormonally or chemically treated) human prostatic tissues. In general, androgen receptor levels determined by conventional methods, i.e., ligand exchange assay at $0-4\,°C$ for $16-24$ hr followed by either dextran-coated charcoal treatment to remove the unbound steroid ligand or hydroxyapatite or protamine sulfate treatment to remove the bound steroid receptor complexes, resulted in a wide range of variation between tissue samples and laboratories where assays were performed. In addition, a correlation between tissue androgen receptor content and clinical responsiveness of patients to endocrine therapy was not determined in most of the cases studied.

Problems in the analytical technique may account for the variable results (Table 1). Alternatively, the variations may reflect constitutive differences among heterogenous tumor cell populations [52]. In one study, Pertschuk et al. [49] demonstrated excellent correlation between androgen receptors analyzed by biochemical and histochemical methods in human prostatic cancer tissue. This finding suggests that the biochemical analysis of androgen receptors is not the result of selecting receptor populations from specific cell types but rather represents the true androgen receptor levels at the cellular level. In this study, it was demonstrated further that both biochemical and histological analyses of androgen receptors failed to correlate with the tumor grades and the pathological stages of the prostatic cancer [49].

Another potential source of variation in the quantitation of androgen receptor contents in prostatic tissues is attributed to the endocrine status of the prostatic cancer. For example, prostatic androgen receptors increased following estrogen treatment [11]. Estrogen also is known to increase the circulating sex steroid binding globulin (SSBG), which lowers the unbound

Table 2. Androgen receptor contents in normal and cancerous human prostate gland.

Condition [*]	Ligand used	Androgen receptor contents [**]		Comments
		ARc	ARn	
Snochowski et al. (1977) [31]				
CA (2)	R1881	20 (13.6–26.3) [a]		Correlation between ARc and responsiveness to endocrine therapy was not determined
De Voogt and Dingjan (1978) [15]				
CA-untreated (19)	DHT	49 ± 13 (0–205) [a] 184 ± 105 (0–1621) [a]		Good correlation between combined ARc and cytosolic estrogen receptors and responsiveness to endocrine therapy was observed
Lieskovsky and Bruchovsky (1979) [57]				
Normal (5)	DHT		1000 ± 200 [b]	Correlation between ARn and responsiveness to endocrine therapy was not determined
CA (5)			1900 ± 200 [b]	
Ekman et al. (1979) [14]				
CA (11)	R1881	26.6 (7.7–73.8) [a]		ARc correlated well with responsiveness to endocrine therapy
Walsh and Hicks (1979) [58]				
CA (11 for ARc and 20 for ARn)	R1881	29 ± 26 (2–91) [a]	904 ± 667 (0–2300) [c]	Correlation between AR and responsiveness to endocrine therapy was not determined
Kreig et al. (1980) [59]				
Normal (7)	DHT	none 30.9 (6–93.5) [a]		Correlation between ARc and responsiveness to endocrine therapy was not determined

Table 2 (continued).

Condition *	Ligand used	Androgen receptor contents **		Comments
		ARc	ARn	
Ghanadian and Auf (1980) [60]	R1881			Correlation between AR and responsiveness to endocrine therapy was not determined
CA-untreated (16)		90.7 ± 19.5 (22–288)[a]	367 ± 123 (44–1123)[d]	
CA-treated (5)		72.9 ± 20.5 (23–333)[a]	232 ± 30.6 (25–566)[d]	
Traish et al. (1981) [30]	R1881			Pretreatment of cytosol with dextran-coated charcoal increased non-receptor binding; correlation between ARc or non-receptor binding and responsiveness to endocrine therapy was not determined
CA (25)		38.6 ± 16.6 (0–78)[a]		
Barrack et al. (1983) [20]	R1881			ARn was comparable between normal and CA tissues, but % salt-extractable ARn was significantly elevated in CA tissues; correlation between ARc or ARn and responsiveness to endocrine therapy was not determined
Normal (7)		387 ± 26[e]	327 ± 27[e]	
CA (11)		364 ± 26[e]	355 ± 23[e]	

* Prostatic tissues were obtained from normal subjects and cancer (CA) patients with (CA-treated) or without (CA-untreated) prior endocrine or chemotherapy. Numbers in parentheses indicate total number of cases studied.

** Data are expressed as averages $\pm$ SEM (range); [a] fmole/mg cytosolic protein; [b] molecules/nucleus; [c] mole/g tissue; [d] fmole/mg nuclear protein; [e] fmole/mg DNA.

Abbreviations: ARc, cytoplasmic androgen receptors; ARn, nuclear androgen receptors; R1881, methyltrienolone; DHT, dihydrotestosterone.

fraction of endogenous sex steroids. This increased SSBG may result in an overestimation of androgen receptors in tissues. A further source of variation is the extent of the effect of radiation and chemotherapy on the level of androgen receptors in prostatic cancer specimens. The effect(s) of these parameters has not been determined. Thus, it is reasonable to assume that prior therapeutic regimens may also contribute to variations in the tissue levels of androgen receptors.

4. ANDROGEN RECEPTORS IN NORMAL AND CANCEROUS RAT PROSTATIC
   TISSUES

Because of the inherent limitations of studying steroid receptors in human prostatic cancer, attention in recent years has focused on rat prostatic cancer models in order to gain further insight into the relationship between steroid receptors and the biological potential of the prostatic cancer. Four transplantable rat prostatic cancer models have been established using Dunning, Nb, ACI or Pollard tumors. These rat prostatic tumor models circumvent the difficulties of human prostatic cancer in that abundant amounts of tissues with known morphological and biochemical homogeneity can be obtained and measurements of the levels of androgen receptors can be performed repeatedly in the same tumor specimen with matched controls. The availability of subclones of the initiatl prostatic tumors which are androgen dependent and independent provides a unique opportunity for developing methods of differentiating tumors of different hormonal dependency [41, 48, 53, 54, 55]. Although species differences in the relationship between androgen receptors and the hormonal dependency of prostatic cancer may exist, animal models provide a rational basis for an understanding of the complexities of human prostatic cancer.

By far the best studied steroid receptor system is that composed of Dunning tumor. Lea and French [47] characterized the androgen receptors in Dunning R-3327 tumor and found these receptors have the same physiochemical properties (sedimentation coefficient, Stokes radius, steroid specificity, affinity and capacity) as those of normal rat prostate. Markland et al. [48] correlated the histological grades of Dunning tumors with their androgen and estrogen receptor contents. Heston et al. [56] reported that the hormone-dependent Dunning tumor which recurs after castration acquires progesterone receptors which were not detectable in the primary tumor.

In an attempt to compare the levels of androgen receptors in normal and cancerous rat prostatic tissues, we have performed a number of experiments to measure cytosolic and nuclear-extractable androgen receptor contents in hormone-dependent, hormone-independent (or autonomous) and anaplastic

Table 3. Scatchard analyses of soluble androgen receptor in normal and neoplastic prostatic tissues: effects of sodium molybdate.

Source of tissue[a]	N[b]	−MoO$_4$			+MoO$_4$		
		K_d (nM)	B_{max}[c] (fmol/mg protein)	(fmol/mg DNA)	K_d (nM)	B_{max}[c] (fmol/mg protein)	(fmol/mg DNA)
I. Nb rats							
VP	4	0.27 ± 0.05	8.5 ± 2.3	251.8 ± 51.5	0.05 ± 0.003 *	59.1 ± 11.8 *	189.8 ± 449.3 *
DLP	4	0.50 ± 0.18	1.8 ± 0.8	41.4 ± 17.0	0.13 ± 0.01	8.8 ± 1.0 *	210.9 ± 13.0 **
HDT	5	0.48 ± 0.05	14.5 ± 2.6	164.6 ± 41.5	0.13 ± 0.02 **	23.3 ± 3.1 **	260.0 ± 48.8 ***
AT	4	0.57 ± 0.18	1.4 ± 0.5	11.2 ± 4.8	0.60 ± 0.30	5.2 ± 1.2 *	42.6 ± 14.8 *
II. Copenhagen rats							
VP	1	0.46	22.0	289.9	0.32	48.1	510.7
DLP	1	7.6	8.0	80	6.4	29.0	316.0
HDT	4	0.33 ± 0.17	12.1 ± 4.1	149.4 ± 49.9	0.16 ± 0.04	22.1 ± 4.8 *	255.4 ± 48.4 *
HIT	4	0.36 ± 0.04	29.7 ± 5.7	208.6 ± 44.3	0.25 ± 0.10	53.8 ± 14.3	372.7 ± 77.3 *
AT	4	0.81 ± 0.10	3.3 ± 0.5	18.8 ± 2.8	0.32 ± 0.04 *	4.0 ± 1.0	22.9 ± 5.2

* = $p < 0.05$;   ** = $p < 0.01$;   *** = $p < 0.001$.

[a] VP, ventral prostate; DLP, dorsolateral prostate; HDT, hormone-dependent Dunning tumor; HIT, hormone-independent Dunning tumor; AT, anaplastic Dunning tumor; HDT, hormone-dependent Nb tumor; and AT autonomous Nb tumor.

[b] N represents the total number of experiments per group. Each experiment involved the use of 2 to 5 tumors or normal prostate glands which were combined and homogenized in TEDG buffer either with or without 10 mM Na$_2$MoO$_4$.

[c] Protein contents were determined in the soluble fractions assayed, whereas DNA contents were determined in pooled tissue samples which were assayed separately. Data are presented either as single determinations or as averages ± SEM of 4 to 5 determinations.

Dunning and Nb prostatic tumors in the presence or absence of an established stabilizing reagent, sodium molybdate [Table 3, Ref. 41]. In these studies, we observed that the basal levels of cytosolic androgen receptor activities as measured by ligand exchange assay correlated well with the hormonal dependency status of the Nb tumor, but failed to correlate with that of the Dunning tumor. Sodium molybdate increased the total number of cytosolic androgen receptors in all normal and neoplastic prostatic tissues studied except that of the Dunning anaplastic tumor. Significant changes of the dissociation constant (K_d) also were observed in some prostatic tissues by the inclusion of sodium molybdate in the homogenizing medium; the effects on the K_d by sodium molybdate depends on the type of tumor, the strain of the rat and the hormonal dependency status of the animals [41, 61; also see Table 3]. Sodium molybdate also appears to have a dual effect on androgen receptors; i.e., this compound directly interacts with cytosolic androgen receptors and alters the B_{max} and K_d androgen binding, as well as extracts additional nuclear androgen receptors from prostatic nuclei. Sodi-

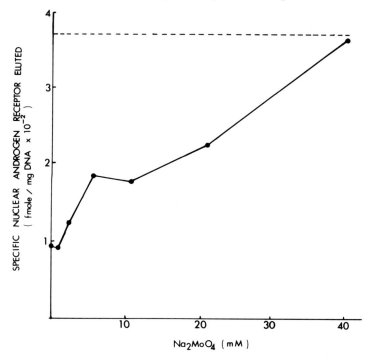

Figure 1. Concentration-dependent extraction of nuclear androgen receptors from prostatic nuclei by sodium molybdate. Ventral prostates isolated from Wistar rats were minced and incubated with [³H]-R1881 at 37 °C for one hour. Prostatic nuclei were isolated and extracted with TEDG buffer containing varying concentrations of sodium molobydate (up to 40 mM). ●–●–● represents the amount of nuclear androgen receptors extracted and – – – – represents the amount of nuclear androgen receptors extracted with TEDG buffer containing 0.4 M KCl [41].

um molybdate extracts androgen receptors from prostatic nuclei in a concentration-dependent manner (Figure 1); significant ($p<0.05$) extraction of nuclear androgen receptors was noted in our studies when crude nuclear pellets were extracted by a homogenizing buffer containing 10 mM sodium molybdate (171.2 ± 57.2 fmole/mg DNA as compared to 115.3 ± 51.5 fmole/mg DNA extracted by homogenizing buffer only; mean $\pm$ SEM). Extracted nuclear androgen receptors appear to be associated with intranuclear matrices, because sodium molybdate extracted the same amount of androgen receptors from triton-washed and unwashed prostatic nuclei [41]. The amount (but not the percent) of sodium molybdate-extractable nuclear androgen receptors correlated well with the hormonal dependency status of both Dunning and Nb tumors (Table 4). Finally, sodium molybdate-extracted nuclear androgen receptors sedimented identically as 0.4 M KCl-extracted nuclear androgen receptors on sucrose density gradients under high salt conditions. The receptors appeared as a single 4S protein complex [41].

These results support the concept that the nuclear rather than cytoplasmic androgen receptor contents correlate with the degree of endocrine dependency of rat prostatic tumors. In these studies, nuclear androgen receptors were determined by a new translocation and extraction procedure recently developed by Traish et al. [33]. Several advantages were noted in this new procedure over the conventional ligand exchange method: (1) The nuclear androgen receptors assayed were translocated from the cytoplasm, thus they represent the 'functional' pool of the receptor population. (2) The ligand exchange method underestimates the level of cytosolic androgen receptors by a factor of 2 when compared to translocation and extraction procedures [41]. This may be due to a more efficient transport of steroid receptor complexes to prostatic nuclei and the stabilization of steroid receptors in the presence of the steroid ligand during in vitro incubation. Similar results on the quantitation of glucocorticoid receptor contents in human leukocytes obtained from patients with various forms of leukemia were reported by Iacobelli et al. [62]. These authors detected a 2- to 3-fold higher level of cytosolic glucocorticoid receptors in human leukocytes by whole cell assay than by ligand exchange assay. (3) A lower background of non-specific binding ($<25\%$) is detected by the translocation and extraction procedure than by ligand exchange method ($>50\%$). The lower background occurs as a result of a much lower non-specific binding that appears on sucrose density gradients in regions outside of the true receptor binding areas (<4 S region) under high salt conditions [41]. (4) Similar to that demonstrated by glucocorticoid receptor studies [62], the application of translocation and extraction methods using intact cells results in a faster and more complete equilibrium between ligand and receptors than the conventional ligand exchange

Table 4. Androgen receptor content in soluble and residual fractions of nuclear extract from normal prostates and prostatic tumors.

Source of tissue	Androgen receptor content [a]	
	Soluble	Residual
	(fmol/mg DNA)	
Nb rats [b]		
VP		
Cytosol (2)	75	—
TEDG extract (3)	75 ± 9	1199 ± 707
0.4 M KCl extract (3)	595 ± 68	276 ± 121
40 mM Na_2MoO_4 extract (5)	360 ± 42	751 ± 267
DLP		
Cytosol (2)	6	—
TEDG extract (3)	16 ± 1	173 ± 109
0.4 M KCl extract (3)	73 ± 23	112 ± 42
40 mM Na_2MoO_4 extract (5)	65 ± 12	91 ± 17
HDT-129		
Cytosol (3)	9 ± 5	—
TEDG extract (3)	2 ± 1	102 ± 47
0.4 M KCl extract (3)	17 ± 3	74 ± 43
40 mM Na_2MoO_4 extract (8)	13 ± 2	45 ± 18
Autonomous		
Cytosol (3)	4 ± 3	—
TEDG extract (4)	1 ± .3	11 ± 7
0.4 mM KCl extract (4)	2 ± .3	15 ± 7
40 mM Na_2MoO_4 extract (7)	2 ± .2	22 ± 7
Copenhagen rats		
HDT		
Cytosol (3)	28 ± 22	—
TEDG extract (3)	3 ± 1	60 ± 21
0.4 M KCl extract (3)	20 ± 8	42 ± 8
40 mM Na_2MoO_4 extract (7)	18 ± 4	56 ± 5
HIT		
Cytosol (3)	1 ± 1	—
TEDG extract (5)	1 ± .3	22 ± 14
0.4 M KCl extract (5)	9 ± 3	14 ± 11
40 mM Na_2MoO_4 extract (7)	7 ± 1	14 ± 8

[a] 0.6 g of rat prostatic tissues were incubated with [^{3}H]-R1881 (20 nM) in the presence or absence of unlabeled R1881 (1 μM) in 2 ml of Dulbecco's modified Eagle's medium at 37 °C for 2 hr in a tissue culture incubator. Crude nuclear pellets and prostatic cytosols were isolated and the content of androgen receptor in buffer (TEDG) or salt (0.4 KCl or 0.04 M Na_2MoO_4)-extracted fractions was determined by the method of Traish et al. [30, 33]. Data represent the average or average ± SEM of 2 to 8 determinations.

[b] VP, ventral prostate; DPL, dorsolateral prostate. Numbers in parentheses = total number of experiments.

method. (5) The levels of androgen receptors assayed by translocation and extraction procedures in vitro are 'physiological', because tissues assayed prior to nuclear isolation are capable of maintaining their normal morphology and biochemical functions when grafted under the renal capsules of syngeneic hosts [8]. The positive correlation obtained between the quantity of salt-extractable nuclear androgen receptors and the hormonal dependency status of the Dunning and Nb tumors by in vitro ligand translocation and extraction assay has not been tested in human prostatic tissue specimens.

5. ROLE OF ANDROGEN RECEPTORS IN STROMAL – EPITHELIAL INTERACTIONS

In general, biochemical analyses of androgen receptors in prostatic tissues have failed to distinguish receptor populations in either stromal and/or epithelial compartments. Experimental evidence using tissue recombinant techniques has demonstrated clearly the importance of embryonic prostatic mesenchyme in regulating epithelial growth and differentiation [63, 64]. To

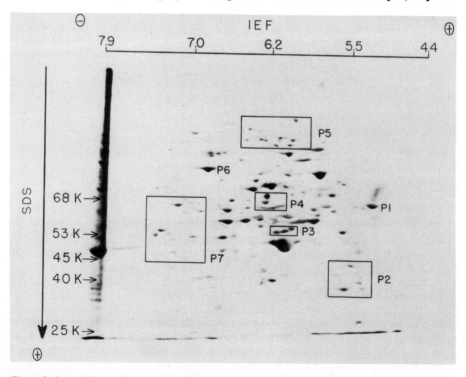

Figure 2. Autoradiographic protein profiles of mouse prostate. Mouse prostate was prelabeled in vitro with [^{35}S]-methionine and total tissue proteins were separated by two-dimensional polyacrylamide gel electrophoresis. The electrophoretogram was exposed to an X-ray film. P1 to P7 designates areas of mouse prostatic-specific proteins.

understand the role of androgen receptors in stromal or epithelial compartments during tissue interactions, we recently have analyzed androgen receptor activities in tissue recombinants composed of fetal rat urogential sinus mesenchyme (UGM) and adult bladder epithelium isolated from testicular feminized (Tfm/y) mice. This model system has been demonstrated by us to express prostatic morphology and functional activities [63, 64]. Furthermore, fetal UGM isolated only from the wild-type but not from the Tfm/y mouse is capable of inducing the expression of prostatic morphology and biochemical functions by the responding competent bladder epithelium. These results provide experimental evidence in support of the role of androgen receptors in the mesenchyme (stroma) which mediate androgen-induced morphogenesis and expression of functional activities. Total tissue protein profiles in control and recombinant tissues previously labeled with [35S]-methionine in vitro show that tissue recombinants express specific protein identities when analyzed by two-dimensional polyacrylamide gel electrophoresis in seven areas of the electrophoretogram (designated as R_1 to R_7). The identities are similar to those of the host prostate gland and differ from those of the host bladder (Figures 2 to 4).

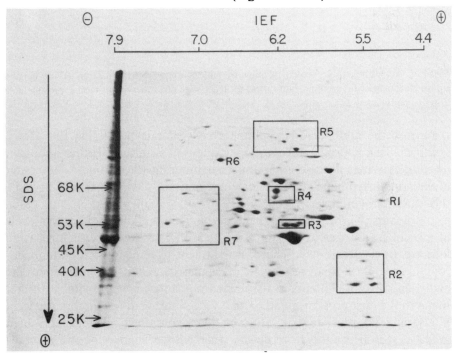

Figure 3. Autoradiographic protein profiles of tissue recombinants composed of UGM and adult bladder epithelium isolated from Tfm/y mice. R1 to R7 designates areas of mouse tissue recombinant-specific proteins. Note the similarity between these proteins and the P1 to P7 proteins.

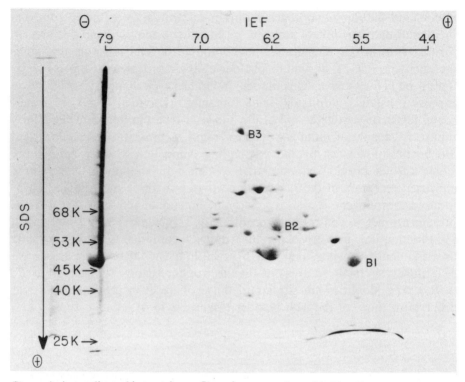

Figure 4. Autoradiographic protein profiles of mouse urinary bladder. B1 to B3 designates mouse bladder-specific proteins. Note these proteins were not observed in mouse prostate and tissue recombinants.

Because the adult bladder epithelial cells of rats possessing the Tfm/y syndrome lack androgen receptors, the question is raised whether androgen receptor activities in the epithelium are required for the ultimate expression of the protein synthetic activities detected in tissue recombinants. To pursue this question, androgen receptor activities were measured in the tissue recombinants (UGM_{rat} + adult bladder epithelium (Tfm/y)). First the levels of cytosolic androgen receptors were measured by ligand exchange assay followed by dextran-coated charcoal treatment to remove the unbound steroid ligand. Data analyzed by the Scatchard method indicated that the androgen receptor contents in tissue recombinants were comparable to that found in the host prostate gland, with a value intermediate to those found in mouse and rat prostate [65]. Host bladders contained no detectable high affinity cytosolic androgen receptors when assayed under the same conditions. Second, sucrose density gradient analyses of cytosolic androgen receptors under low salt conditions revealed a distinct 8S androgen receptor complex in the tissue recombinants [65]. Similar receptor protein profiles were detected in the host prostate but were absent from the host bladder. Finally, salt-extractable nuclear androgen receptors analyzed by the translocation and extraction procedure showed that tissue recombinants contained amounts of salt-extractable nuclear androgen receptors equivalent to those found in the host prostate gland [65]. Host bladder analyzed under the same conditions failed to show any significant levels of androgen receptors. Thus, androgen receptor activities assayed by all three methods are consistent with the suggestion of the presence of a high affinity, limited capacity, 8S androgen receptor protein complex in the cytosol of tissue recombinants. These cytosolic androgen receptors can be translocated into salt-extractable nuclear androgen receptor fractions and presumably are responsible for the expression of prostate-like protein synthetic activities detected in tissue recombinants (Figures 2 to 4).

Recently, Shannon and Cunha [66] analyzed androgen binding activities in these tissue recombinants by autoradiography and showed that the radioactive ligand-binding complexes were heavily concentrated in the stromal component of the recombinants; epithelial acini were devoid of silver grains. These results, combined with the results of biochemical analyses of the levels of androgen receptors in the tissue recombinants, suggest that the androgen-induced expression of protein synthetic activities in tissue recombinants can occur in the absence of androgen receptors in the epithelium. The suggestion has led to the proposal of a new mechanism of androgen action in the prostate gland, in which androgenic steroid interacts with its receptors in the stroma which regulate the functional activities of the epithelium through certain putative stromal growth factors [67].

Although the roles of embryonic UGM in the regulation of prostatic growth have been described [63, 64], little attention has been focused on the importance of embryonic urogenital sinus epithelium (UGE) in regulating the expression of UGM. Recently, we have obtained data to suggest that the expression of stromal growth inductive activity is tightly regulated by the adjacent epithelium. Rocco et al. [68] showed that UGM_{rat} (UGM isolated from rat) induced 2- to 4-fold more growth when associated with UGE_{mouse} (UGE isolated from mouse) than UGE_{rat} and grown in adult athymic male hosts. This difference is not attributable to a host factor(s) because homotypic recombinants composed of $UGM_{rat} + UGE_{rat}$ grew to an equivalent size in adult male syngeneic and athymic hosts. Because both types of tissue recombinants utilize UGM_{rat} as the growth inductor, with the only difference between these recombinants being the associated UGE (UGE_{rat} vs UGE_{mouse}), it therefore is concluded that UGE may regulate the expression of UGM. The regulation between UGM and UGE may be analogous to the paracrine system where adjacent cells are closely interacting [69].

The importance of UGE in regulating the expression of UGM has also been demonstrated in another model system where marked (10- to 60-fold increase in DNA content) overgrowth of the adult prostate in situ can be elicited by direct implantation of intact fetal urogenital sinus (UGS) or UGM but not UGE into the prostate [70–72]. In this new mouse model of prostatic hyperplasia, UGS-induced adult prostatic overgrowth is 2- to 4-fold greater than UGM. The growth is due to the proliferation of adult prostatic cells by close tissue interaction between fetal UGS or UGM and adult prostate as determined by the isoenzymic patterns in the resultant chimeric tissues [68]. Since UGE alone has no growth-promoting effects, it is possible that UGE may participate indirectly in the growth of the adult prostate by mechanisms such as regulation of the gene expression of UGM.

There are numerous examples in the literature to suggest that the indirect action of steroid hormones on epithelial gene expression is a rule rather than an exception during normal development of male and female reproductive tracts [7]. Androgen and estrogen receptors as measured by autoradiography are found in the mesenchymal compartment during early development but appear in both mesenchymal and epithelial compartments during later development [67]. Similar regulatory roles of mesenchyme in developing lung [73] and the differential localization of corticosteroid receptors in embryonic mesenchyme, as determined by autoradiography [74] during early lung development, all support the possibility that androgen may exert an indirect action on the growth and differentiation of the prostate gland. Parallel to these indirect actions of sex steroids and corticosteroid on the development of reproductive tracts and the lung, the indirect action of estrogens on the growth of MCF-7 cells, a human breast cancer cell line, has been documented [75].

6. SIGNIFICANCE OF ANDROGEN RECEPTORS IN STROMAL – EPITHELIAL INTERACTIONS IN PROSTATIC CANCER GROWTH AND DIFFERENTIATION

Although mechanisms of cancer development are complex, it has been firmly established that cancer cells are derived from normal cells as a result of genetic and/or epigenetic phenomena [76]. The continuing proliferation and differentiation of cancer cells depend on the selective advantages of cancer cells within their microenvironment. The importance of cellular interactions and cancer growth and differentiation has been the subject of several recent reviews [77–79].

In this review, we emphasize the importance of stromal – epithelial interactions in androgen-regulated prostatic growth. From tissue recombination studies, we concluded that androgen receptors in the stromal compartment are the primary target for androgenic steroids which are required for eliciting prostatic morphogenesis and expression of functional activities. This conclusion is based on the experimental observation that fetal UGM isolated from wild-type (androgen receptor positive) mice exerts its directive influence on adult bladder epithelium isolated either from wild-type or Tfm/y mice (androgen receptor negative) to express typical prostatic morphology and prostate-like protein synthetic activities.

The role of epithelium in stromal – epithelial interactions is less well defined. Although there is no experimental evidence to support the concept that fetal UGE exerts a directive influence on prostatic growth and differentiation, fetal UGE may play important modulatory roles in the gene expression of adjacent stroma. The possible role of androgen receptors in the epithelial compartment for its modulatory function has not been determined.

Another aspect of androgen receptors worthy of consideration is their subcellular localization. Within a given cell type, it has been demonstrated that salt-resistant steroid receptors associated with nuclear matrices may be the primary effector that regulates the actual growth of rat uterus [80] and rat prostate glands [81]. Therefore, it can be assumed that the coupling of the measurement of androgen receptors in a specific cell type or subcellular compartment with the actual expression of specific gene products [50, 51] may yield new development in the future that may eventually be of predictive value in the hormonal responsiveness of prostatic cancer.

7. SUMMARY

The present review emphasizes that (1) the level of androgen receptors, particularly in the nuclear compartment, may correlate with endocrine responsiveness by the rat prostatic cancer, (2) further refinement in the methods for determining the levels of androgen receptors in the human prostate gland is necessary to reduce the variability and enhance the reliability of laboratory determinations, thus allowing more definitive correlations to be made between endocrine responsiveness and the clinical progression of the disease, and (3) the results of experiments utilizing tissue recombination techniques have shown that the presence of androgen receptors in the epithelium may not be obligatory for androgen action. Alternatively, androgen receptors in the stroma may be important in regulating their adjacent epithelial growth and differentiation via certain putative stromal growth factors. Analysis of the growth of the prostate gland in heterospecific recombinants and in the overgrowth of adult prostate gland in the in situ model reveals that epithelium may govern the expression of stroma and hence the growth potential of the prostate gland.

34

The role of stromal – epithelial interactions in prostatic cancer growth and differentiation, and the association of androgen receptors with certain cell or subcellular sites need to be investigated in depth in the prostate gland. The understanding of regulation of the growth, metastasis, and differentiation of prostatic cancer at cellular and molecular levels will provide a rational basis for developing new methods which may have prognostic values in prostatic cancer. It may also serve as the basis for developing new therapeutic agents for the management of both prostatic cancer and benign prostatic hyperplasia in man.

REFERENCES

1. Huggins C, Hodges CV: Studies on prostatic cancer. I. Effect of castration, of estrogen and androgen injection on serum phosphatases in metastatic carcinoma of the prostate. Cancer Res 1:293-297, 1941.
2. Jensen EV: Proc 4th Intern Congr Biochem, Vienna. Oxford: Pergamon, Vol 15, p 444, 1958.
3. Jensen EV, DeSombre ER: Estrogens and progestins. In: Biochemical Action of Hormones, Litwack G (ed). New York and London: Academic Press, pp 215-256, 1972.
4. Mainwairing WIP, King RJB: Steroid Cell Interactions. London: Butterworths Co Ltd, pp 1-101, 1974.
5. Guerrero L, Gautier T, Peterson RE: Steroid 5α-reductase deficiency in man: An inherited form of male pseudohermaphroditism. Science 186:1213-1215, 1974.
6. Ohno S, Christian L, Attardi BJ, Kan J: Modification of expression of the testicular feminization (Tfm) gene of the mouse by a 'controlling agent' gene. Nature 245:92, 1973.
7. Stumpf WE, Narbaitz R, Sar M: Estrogen receptors in the fetal mouse. J Steroid Biochem 12:55-64, 1980.
8. Chung LWK, Anderson NG, Neubauer BL, Cunha GR, Thompson TC, Rocco AK: Tissue interactions in prostate development: Roles of sex steroids. In: The Prostatic Cell: Structure and Function, Part A, Murphy GP, Sandberg AA, Karr JP (eds). New York: Alan R Liss, Inc, pp 177-203, 1981.
9. Fang S, Liao S: Androgen receptors: Steroid and tissue specific retention of a 17β-hydroxy-5α-androstan-3-one-protein complex by the cell nuclei of ventral prostate. J Biol Chem 246:16-24, 1971.
10. Menon M, Tananis CE, Hicks L, Hawkins EF, McLoughlin MG, Walsh PC: Characterization of binding of a potent synthetic androgen, methyltrienolone, to human tissues. J Clin Invest 61:150-162, 1978.
11. Bouton MM, Pornin C, Grandadam JA: Estrogen regulation of rat prostate androgen receptor. J Steroid Biochem 15:403-408, 1981.
12. Hawkins EF, Nijs M, Brassine C: Steroid receptors in the human prostate. II. Some properties of the estrophilic molecule of benign prostatic hypertrophy. Biochem Biophys Res Commun 70:854, 1976.
13. Gustafsson JA, Ekman P, Pousette A, Snochowski M, Hogberg B: Demonstration of a progestin receptor in human benign prostatic hyperplasia and prostatic carcinoma. Invest Urol 15:361-366, 1978.
14. Ekman P, Snochowski M, Zetterberg A, Hogberg B, Gustafsson, JA: Steroid receptor content in human prostatic carcinoma and response to endocrine therapy. Cancer 44:1173-1181, 1979.

15. De Voogt HJ, Dingjan P: Steroid receptors in human prostatic cancer: A preliminary evaluation. Urol Res 6:151-158, 1978.
16. Jensen EV, Block BE, Smith S, Kyser K, DeSombre ER: Estrogen receptors and breast cancer response to adrenalectomy. NCI Monograph: Prediction of Responses in Cancer Therapy 34:55-61, 1971.
17. Horwitz KB, McGuire WL, Peirson OH: Predicting responses in human breast cancer: A hypothesis. Science 189:726-727, 1975.
18. King RJB, Townsend PT, Siddle N, Whitehead MI, Taylor RW: Regulation of estrogen and progesterone receptor levels in epithelium and stroma from pre- and postmenopausal endometria. J Steroid Biochem 16:21-29, 1982.
19. Robel P: Sex steroid hormone receptors and human prostatic hyperplasia and carcinoma. Annals of Clin Res 12:216-222, 1980.
20. Barrack ER, Bujnovszky P, Walsh PC: Subcellular distribution of androgen receptors in human normal, benign hyperplastic, and malignant prostatic tissues: Characterization of nuclear salt-resistant receptors. Cancer Res (in press).
21. Trachtenberg J, Walsh PC: Correlation of prostatic nuclear androgen receptor content with duration of response and survival following hormonal therapy in advanced prostatic cancer. J Urol 127:466-471, 1982.
22. Lea OA, Petrusz P, French F: Prostatein: A major secretory protein of the rat ventral prostate. J Biol Chem 254:6196-6202, 1979.
23. Bonne C, Raynaud JP: Assay of androgen binding sites by exchange with methyltrienolone (R1881). Steroids 27:497-507, 1976.
24. Asselin J, Labrie F, Gourdeau Y, Bonne C, Raynaud JP: Binding of ^{3}H-methyltrienolone (R1881) in rat prostate and human benign prostatic hypertrophy (BPH). Steroids 28:449-459, 1976.
25. Zava DT, Landrum B, Horwitz KB, McGuire, WL: Androgen receptor assay with ^{3}H-methyltrienolone (R1881) in the presence of progesterone receptors. Endocrinology 104:1007-1012, 1979.
26. Korenman SG, Dukes BA: Specific estrogen binding by cytoplasm of human breast carcinoma. J Clin Endocrinol Metab 30:639-645, 1970.
27. Blondeau JP, Corpechot C, le Goascogne C, Baulieu EE, Robel P: Androgen receptors in the rat ventral prostate and their hormonal control. Vit Hormon 33:319-344, 1975.
28. Williams D, Gorski J: Equilibrium binding of estradiol by uterine cell suspensions and whole uteri in vitro. Biochemistry 13:5537-5542, 1974.
29. Rennie P, Burchovsky N: Studies on the relationship between androgen receptors and the transport of androgens in rat prostate. J Biol Chem 248:3288-3297, 1973.
30. Traish AM, Muller RE, Burns ME, Wotiz HH: Steroid binding proteins in rat and human prostate. In: The Prostatic Cell: Structure and Function, Part A, Murphy GP, Sandberg AA, Karr JP (eds). New York: Alan R Liss, Inc, pp 417-434, 1981.
31. Snochowski M, Pousette A, Ekman P, Bression D, Andersson L, Hogberg B, Gustafsson JA: Characterization and measurement of the androgen receptor in human benign prostatic hyperplasia and prostatic carcinoma. J Clin Endocrinol Metab 45:920-930, 1977.
32. Olsson CA, White RD, Goldstein I, Traish AM, Muller RE, Wotiz HH: A preliminary report on the measurement of cytostolic and nuclear prostatic tissue steroid receptors. In: Progress in Clinical and Biological Research, Murphy GP, Sandberg AA (eds). New York: Alan R Liss, Vol 33, pp 209-221, 1979.
33. Traish AM, Muller RE, Wotiz HH: A new procedure for the quantitation of nuclear and cytoplasmic androgen receptors. J Biol Chem 256:12028-12033, 1981.
34. Robel P: Sex Steroid hormone receptors and human prostatic hyperplasia of Carcinoma. Annals of Clin Res 12:216-222, 1980.

35. Nielson CJ, Sando JJ, Vogel WM, Pratt WB: Glucocorticoid receptor inactivation under cell-free conditions. J Biol Chem 252:7568-7578, 1977.
36. Wilson EM, French FS: Effects of protease and protease inhibitors on 4.5 S and 8.0 S androgen receptor. J Biol Chem 254:6210-6219, 1979.
37. Miller LK, Tuazon FB, Niu EM, Sherman MR: Human breast tumor estrogen receptor: Effect of molybdate and electrophoretic analyses. Endocrinology 108:1369-1378, 1981.
38. Bevins CL, Bashirelahi N: Stabilization of 8 S progesterone receptor from human prostate in the presence of molybdate ion. Cancer Res 40:2234-2239, 1980.
39. Leech KL, Dahmer MK, Hammond ND, Sando JJ, Pratt WB: Molybdate inhibition of glucocorticoid receptor inactivation and transformation. J Biol Chem 254:11884-11890, 1979.
40. Murakami N, Quattrociocchi TM, Healy SP, Moudgil VK: Effects of sodium tungstate on the nuclear uptake of glucocorticoid receptor complex from rat liver. Arch Biochem Biophys 214:326-334, 1982.
41. Thompson TC, Chung LWK: Extraction of nuclear androgen receptors by sodium molybdate from normal rat prostates and prostatic tumors. Cancer Res (March 1984).
42. Hicks LL, Walsh PC: A microassay for the measurement of androgen receptors in human prostatic tissue. Steroid 33:389-406, 1979.
43. Wrange O, Nordenskjold B, Gustafsson JA: Cytosol estradiol receptor in human mammary carcinoma: An assay based on isoelectric focusing in polyacrylamide gel. Anal Biochem 85:461-475, 1978.
44. Pousette A, Borgstrom E, Hogberg B, Gustafsson JA: Analysis of the androgen receptor in needle biopsies from human prostatic tissue. In: The Prostatic Cell: Structure and Function, Part B, Murphy GP, Sandberg AA, Karr JP (eds). New York: Alan R Liss, Inc, pp 299-311, 1981.
45. Chang CH, Rowley DR, Lobl TJ, Tindall DJ: Purification and characterization of androgen receptor from steer seminal vesicle. Biochemistry 21:4102-4109, 1982.
46. Wilson EM, French FS: Binding properties of androgen receptors. J Biol Chem 251:5620-5629, 1976.
47. Lea OA, French FS: Androgen receptor protein in the androgen-dependent Dunning R-3327 prostate carcinoma. Cancer Res 41:619-623, 1981.
48. Markland FS, Chopp RT, Cosgrove MD, Howard EB: Characterization of steroid hormone receptors in the Dunning R-3327 rat prostatic adenocarcinoma. Cancer Res 38:2818-2826, 1978.
49. Pertschuk LP, Rosenthal HE, Macchia RJ, Eisenberg KB, Feldman JG, Wax SH, Kim DS, Whitemore WF, Abrahams JI, Gaetjens E, Wise GJ, Herr HW, Karr JP, Murphy GP, Sandberg AA: Correlation of histochemical and biochemical analyses of androgen binding in prostatic cancer: Relation to therapeutic response. Cancer 49:984-993, 1982.
50. Wilson EM, Viskochil DH, Bartlett RJ, Lea OA, Noyes CM, Petrusz P, Stafford DW, French FS: Model systems for studies on androgen-dependent gene expression in the rat prostate. In: The Prostatic Cell: Structure and Function, Part A, Murphy GP, Sandberg AA, Karr JP (eds). New York: Alan R Liss, Inc, pp 351-380, 1981.
51. Parker MG, White R, Williams JG: Cloning and characterization of androgen-dependent m-RNA from rat ventral prostate. J Biol Chem 255:6996-7001, 1980.
52. Isaacs J: Mechanisms for and implications of the development of heterogeneity of androgen sensitivity in prostatic cancer. In: Tumor Cell Heterogeneity, Owens AH, Coffey DS, Bayein SB (eds). New York: Acad Press, pp 99-111, 1982.
53. Chung LWK, Breitweiser K: Comparison of soluble protein kinases from normal rat prostates and prostatic (Dunning) tumors. Cancer Res 43:3297-3304, 1983.
54. Isaacs JT, Isaacs WB, Coffey DS: Models for development of non-receptor methods for

distinguishing androgen-sensitive and -insensitive prostatic tumors. Cancer Res 39:2652-2659, 1979.

55. Isaacs JT, Heston WDW, Weissman RM, Coffey DS: Animal models of the hormone-sensitive and -insensitive prostatic adenocarcinomas, Dunning R-3327H, R-3327-HI, and R-3327-AT. Cancer Res 38:4353-4359, 1978.

56. Heston WDW, Menon M, Tananis C, Walsh PC: Androgen, estrogen and progesterone receptors of the R-3327H Copenhagen rat prostatic tumor. Cancer Lett 6:45-50, 1979.

57. Lieskovsky G, Burchovsky N: Assay of nuclear androgen receptor in human prostate. J Urol 121:51-58, 1979.

58. Walsh PC, Hicks LL: Characterization and measurement of androgen receptors in human prostate tissue. In: Prostate Cancer and Hormone Receptors, Murphy GP, Sandberg AA (eds). New York: Alan R Liss, Inc, pp 51-63, 1979.

59. Krieg M, Bartsch W, Voigt KD: Binding, metabolism and tissue level of androgens in human prostatic carcinoma, benign prostatic hyperplasia and normal prostate. In: Steroid Receptors, Metabolism and Prostatic Cancer, Schroder FH, De Voogt HJ (eds). Excerpta Medica, pp 102-109, 1980.

60. Ghanadian R, Auf G: Receptor proteins for androgens in benign prostatic hypertrophy and carcinoma of the prostate. In: Steroid Receptors, Metabolism and Prostatic Cancer, Schroder FH, De Voogt HJ (eds). Exerpta Medica, pp 110-125, 1980.

61. Gaubert CM, Tremblay RR, Dube JY: Effect of sodium molybdate on cytosolic androgen receptors in rat prostate. J Steroid Biochem 13:931-937, 1980.

62. Iacobelli S, Natoli V, Longo P, Ranelletti FO, De Rossi G, Pasqualetti D, Mandelli F, Mastrangelo R: Glucocorticoid receptor determinations in leukemia patients using cytosol and whole cell assays. Cancer Res 41:3979-3984, 1981.

63. Chung LWK, Cunha GR: Stromal-epithelial interactions. II. Regulation of prostatic growth by embryonic urogenital sinus mesenchyme. The Prostate 4:503-511, 1983.

64. Cunha GR, Chung LWK: Stromal-epithelial interactions. I. Induction of prostatic phenotype in urothelium of testicular feminized (Tfm/y) mice. J Steroid Biochem 14:1317-1321, 1981.

65. Thompson TC, Cunha GR, Chung LWK: Expression of androgen receptors in prostate-like structures derived from wild-type urogenital sinus mesenchyme and testicular-feminized (Tfm/y) bladder epithelium. Fed Proc 42:June 1983.

66. Shannon JT, Cunha GR: Characterization of androgen binding and DNA synthesis in prostate-like structures induced in the urothelium of testicular feminized (Tfm/y) mice. Biology of Reproduction, 1983 (in press).

67. Cunha GR, Chung LWK, Shannon JM, Taguchi O, Fujii H: Hormone-induced morphogenesis and growth: Role of mesenchymalepithelial interactions. Recent Progress in Hormone Res, 1983 (in press).

68. Rocco A, Matsuura J, Runner M, Chung L: Biochemical characterization of growth induction by fetal urogenital sinus: A new mouse model for studying prostatic hyperplasia. Fed Proc 42:1768, 1983.

69. Hakanson R, Sundler F: The design of the neuroendocrine system: A unifying concept and it consequence. Trends in Pharmacological Sciences 4:41-44, 1983.

70. Chung LWK, Matsuura J, Thompson TC, Chao RCFY: A new approach to regulation of prostatic growth: Interactions between embryonic urogenical sinuses and adult prostate in situ. Proc West Pharmacol Soc 25:141-145, 1982.

71. Chung LWK, Matsuura J, Miller GJ, Runner MN, Thompson TC: A new mouse model for prostatic hyperplasia: inductions of adult prostatic overgrowth by fetal urogenital sinus implants. In: New Approaches to the Study of Benign Prostatic Hyperplasia, Buhl A (ed). New York: Alan R Liss, 1983 (in press).

72. Chung LWK: Tissue interactions and prostatic growth. In: NICHD Testis Workshop, October 14-17, 1983 (in press).
73. Alescio T, di Michele M: Relationship of epithelial growth to mitotic rate in mouse embryonic lung developing in vitro. J Embryol Expt Morph 19:227-237, 1968.
74. Beer DG, Malkinson AM: Autoradiographic localization of [³H]-dexamethasone in lung. The Pharmacologist 25:107, 1983.
75. Shafie SM: Estrogen and the growth of breast cancer: New evidence suggests indirect action. Science 209:701-702, 1980.
76. Owens AH, Coffey DS, Baylin SB: Tumor Cell Heterogeneity, Bristol-Myers Cancer Symposium, Vol 4. New York: Acad Press, pp 1-494, 1983.
77. Feinberg AP, Coffey DS: Organ site specificity for cancer in chromosomal instability disorders. Cancer Res 42:3252-3254, 1982.
78. Mintz B: Genetic mosaicism and in vitro analysis of neoplasia and differentiation. In: Cell Differentiation and Neoplasia, Saunders GF (ed). New York: Raven Press, p 27, 1978.
79. Pierce GB, Wells RS: Embryonic microenvironment in the regulation of cancer cells. In: Tumor Cell Heterogeneity, Owens AH, Coffey DS, Baylin SB (eds). New York: Acad Press, pp 249-258, 1982.
80. Clark JH, Peck EJ, Jr: Nuclear retention of receptor oestrogen complex and nuclear acceptor sites. Nature (London) 260:635-637, 1976.
81. Barrack ER, Coffey DS: The specific binding of estrogens and androgens to the nuclear matrix of sex hormone responsive tissues. J Biol Chem 255:7265-7275, 1980.

Editorial Comment

ABDULMAGED M. TRAISH and HERBERT H. WOTIZ

1. INTRODUCTION

Binding of androgen to the cytoplasmic receptor proteins of target cells results in translocation of the activated hormone receptor complexes into the nucleus where further interactions with the chromatin induces gene expression [1–10]. Understanding the role of androgen receptors in mediating prostatic cell growth requires more precise knowledge of: hormone receptor interactions in the cytoplasm; receptor activation and transformation leading to nuclear translocation; distribution of hormone receptor complexes between cytoplasmic and nuclear compartments; residence of the hormone receptor complexes in the nucleus; and the biochemical nature of the interaction of these complexes with the gene.

In order to understand these reactions, one has to have quantitative and qualitative methods for characterization and measurement of hormone receptor complexes, so that changes in the physicochemical properties of these complexes can be related appropriately to the observed biological response.

The postulated involvement of androgen receptor complexes in controlling transcriptional and post-transcriptional processes requires quantitative assessment of steroid retention and distribution of the bound hormone receptor complexes among the subcellular fractions. While it is not difficult to measure unbound receptor sites in the cellular cytoplasm this is of relatively little consequence since in the normal animal and untreated patient, continuous exposure to endogenous androgens saturates most of the available receptor sites which, therefore, reside in the nucleus. Thus, biologically useful information requires the ability to measure both the occupied and unoccupied receptor sites in the various cell fractions. These measurements require complete exchange of endogenously bound ligand with a labeled ligand. Despite the reports of several such exchange assays none have proven satisfactory. Indeed, so uncertain are the methods described so far, that the generally accepted concept of cytoplasmic receptor depletion coupled to nuclear accumulation [7] has been questioned and thought not to occur in rat [11] or human prostates [12]. More importantly, correlation of human prostatic androgen receptor with tumor hormone sensitivity, similar to observations in human breast cancer, has yet to be established.

The principal difficulties encountered in developing a quantitative exchange assay reside in the extremely slow dissociation of endogenously bound dihydrotestosterone (DHT) from the complex at $0\,°C$ [13–15]. Thus exchange assays performed for 24 hr at $0\,°C$ [16–23] measure only a small fraction of the total receptors. For a quantitative exchange one may have to carry out such experiments for several days; unfortunately, such long incubation times result in proteolysis and alteration of the physicochemical properties of the receptor [24] with concomitant loss of binding sites.

Attempts to speed up ligand dissociation from the receptor by elevated temperature [25–30], while resulting in a significant accelleration of DHT dissociation leads to loss of binding activity (denaturation) [16, 17, 31]. Contribution from plasma and tissue binding proteins to total binding, as well as metabolism of DHT further complicate the development of exchange assay procedures.

Finally, a number of different methods with greatly varying efficiency for separation of bound hormone receptor complexes from free hormone have been applied to measurement of androgen receptor [32–34].

In this review we will discuss some of the advantages and disadvantages of the existing methodology used for receptor measurement and possible approaches for the development of new and, hopefully, more useful quantitative methods.

2. SEPARATION OF BOUND FROM FREE HORMONE

Specific binding of labeled ligands to receptor proteins can only be determined after removal of free (unbound) steroid and correction for non-specific binding. Since procedures used to separate bound from unbound steroids vary in their efficiency of separation, the amount of non-specific binding remaining may result in significant errors of estimation. A critical evaluation of these procedures is presented below.

2.1 *Dextran-coated charcoal (DCC)*

DCC is routinely used by some investigators for assay of steroid receptors [11–16], because it is rapid, inexpensive, and less cumbersome to use than other adsorbants. It has been reported, however [32, 35], that this method, when applied to measurement of androgen receptors, results in an underestimation of the binding protein. We have also found that non-specific binding frequently exceeds 50–70% of total binding when $[^3H]$-R1881 is used as ligand, making evaluation of specific binding more hazardous [25, 28, 32]. Attempts to improve this procedure have included addition of ethanol or γ-globulin [12, 27] to the incubation. Since DCC was shown to inactivate androgen receptors upon prolonged incubation [36] and to strip ligand from the receptor at high ionic strength [37, 38], this method remains unsatisfactory for quantitative measurement of androgen receptors. Thus, validation of this technique under strict conditions is required prior to its use.

2.2 *PROTAMINE SULFATE PRECIPITATION*

Steroid receptor measurement by precipitation with protamine sulfate to allow removal of free steroid by successive washing of the precipitate has been described [15, 26, 30, 33, 35]. This method, however, is far from quantitative [15, 33]. Furthermore, interaction of the receptor protein with this polycation depends strongly on the surface charge of the receptor. Thus, alteration in the receptor properties may result in inefficient precipitation. Thus, while procedures using protamine sulfate precipitation have been described by several investigators [15, 26, 33], it remains unclear under what conditions protamine sulfate precipitation is optimal for androgen receptor measurement.

2.3 *Ammonium sulfate precipitation*

This procedure has proven useful in the partial purification of steroid receptors [39, 40]; however, quantitative precipitation is dependent on the state of the receptor and the buffer composition used for receptor preparation [39–41]. For instance, in the presence of 10 mM molybdate, untransformed receptors precipitate at 50–55% saturation of ammonium sulfate, while transformed receptors precipitate at 30–35% saturation. We have confirmed these observations with rat ventral prostate androgen receptors [42]. One should emphasize that when ammonium sulfate precipitation is used for receptor measurement, it should first be evaluated under the conditions used and compared quantitatively to an alternate method.

2.4 Sucrose density gradient analysis

This method has been widely used for characterization of hormone receptor complexes [32–34]. It is not routinely used for receptor quantitation because ligand dissociation during long periods of centrifugation results in underestimation of the bound hormone. Furthermore, only a limited number of samples can be assayed simultaneously due to the expense of the equipment used and the complexicity of the procedure.

Nevertheless, the method remains valuable for qualitative characterization of receptor hormone complexes.

2.5 Gel filtration on Sephadex G-25

Separation of bound from free hormone has been achieved by gel filtration using Sephadex gels [13, 43–45]. Application of such procedures to analysis of multiple small samples has been reported [13, 44]. We have used this method for measurement of estrogen receptor in calf and rat uterine cytosol [44] and androgen receptor of rat prostate cytosol [13]. It was found to be reliable and can be routinely used. The method is rapid, simple and quantitative.

2.6 Hydroxylapatite (HAP)

HAP is frequently used [13, 32, 46, 47, 48] for measurement of steroid receptors in various tissue cytosols. The wide use of this method is attributed to several advantages: (i) steroid receptors are quantitatively (~90%) adsorbed to HAP; (ii) removal of free hormone can be easily achieved by washing with low concentrations of detergents to disrupt non-specific binding without desorbing hormone receptor complexes (since immobilization on HAP increases their stability in presence of such detergents); (iii) non-specific binding rarely exceeds 10–20% of total bound hormone; (iv) HAP can be used in batch-wise or column procedures allowing analysis of multiple samples; (v) the recovery of hormone receptor complexes by extraction of HAP-immobilized receptors with phosphate buffer allows further characterization of these complexes. Thus, this method is superior to the DCC procedure [13, 32, 46, 48].

2.7 Agar gel electrophoresis

This methodology is useful for characterization and separation of the androgen receptor from plasma and other binding proteins [49, 50], but it cannot be used for quantitative determination of receptor hormone complexes partly because receptor aggregation, instability, and hormone dissociation occur during electrophoresis. Furthermore, only a limited number of samples can be assayed at one time.

2.8 Hydrophobic chromatography

Sephadex LH 20 and lipidex-1000 gels have been used for the measurement of androgen receptors [51]. So far, this method has not been extensively evaluated, and can not be compared at the present time to the other methods discussed here.

3. SELECTION OF LIGAND

3.1 Metabolism of natural ligand

DHT is metabolized by prostatic tissue, to form the 3α or 3β, 17β-diols by the enzymes 3α or 3β-oxidoreductase [52, 53]. The metabolites produced have little or no affinity for the androgen receptor. Thus, measurement of androgen receptor with [^{3}H]-DHT may result in its underestimation. It remains to be verified, however, to what extent DHT is metabolized in the subcellular fractions. For instance, Wilson and French [14] showed, that only 10% of total DHT is metabolized at 0°C or 23°C, whereas Bonne and Raynaud [54] reported metabolism of DHT exceeding 60%. Indeed, several investigators have used [^{3}H]-DHT as ligand for measurement of bound receptors [13, 14, 15, 9, 26] and their data do not differ significantly from those in which the synthetic ligand R1881 [17, 35, 32] was used. Recently [13] we have compared the binding characteristics of [^{3}H]-DHT and [^{3}H]-R1881 in rat prostatic cytosol, prostatic tissue slices and after injection. Our findings suggest, in contrast to previous reports [25, 54], that [^{3}H]-DHT binding to the androgen receptor was consistently greater than [^{3}H]-R1881 at identical concentrations. If 60% of [^{3}]-DHT added to the incubation is metabolized to the androstanediols [54], then a lower number of binding sites should have been obtained with [^{3}H]-DHT compared to [^{3}H]-R1881. At least in rat ventral prostate this was not the case and in this tissue [^{3}H]-DHT can be safely used as binding ligand. The fact that [^{3}H]-R1881 dissociates faster than DHT from in vitro [13, 55] and in vivo [13] bound receptor complexes may result in an underestimation of total receptor content. Further, DHT metabolism by tissue extracts requires NAD generating systems; if they are not replenished DHT metabolism will cease. This may be the case in prostatic homogenate. Thus the choice of ligand remains unresolved and further studies are required to determine to what extent DHT is metabolized under receptor assay conditions.

3.2 DHT binding to plasma proteins

Human plasma contains a sex steroid binding protein (SSBG) that binds DHT with high affinity ($K_D = 10^{-9}$ M). Thus, assay of androgen receptors in tissue specimens is complicated through contamination of the tissue by plasma proteins during surgical removal. In contrast to measurement of rat prostatic androgen receptor with [^{3}H]-DHT, human prostatic androgen receptor will be significantly overestimated if DHT is used as a ligand without proper separation of SSBG from the receptor protein. Krieg et al. [49] have developed an agar gel electrophoretic procedure which distinguishes [^{3}H]-DHT bound to receptor from that bound to SSBG. This latter method is not quantitative and can not be used routinely for receptor measurement.

The advent of the synthetic ligand R1881 provided a solution to this particular problem, since it has low affinity for human plasma proteins [54]. The use of this ligand, however, is complicated by the fact that it binds progesterone [56, 57] and glucocorticoid receptors [58]. The latter difficulty is readily overcome by inclusion of an excess of triamcinolone acetonide, a synthetic glucocorticoid which binds progesterone and glucocorticoid but not androgen receptors. As discussed above [^{3}H]-R1881 offers a solution for some problems of receptor measurement but may not be the appropriate ligand for receptor characterization and studies of receptor dynamics [13, 59].

4. BINDING OF ANDROGENS TO A 'NON-RECEPTOR STEROID BINDING PROTEIN'

The presence of steroid binding proteins in rat prostatic cytosol has been demonstrated by several investigators [60–62]. We have reported the presence of a similar binding protein in human prostatic tissue cytosol [63, 64] which markedly increased ligand binding upon delipidation by charcoal treatment [63, 64]. DCC treatment of cytosols prior to exchange is often used to reduce the concentration of endogenous steroid normally found in rat and human tissue, since the endogenous hormone causes dilution of specific activity of the added ligand, making the assay more tenuous. Thus, exchange assay protocols that require treatment of cytosol with DCC prior to incubation with radioactive ligand will measure not only the androgen receptor but also the non-receptor steroid binding protein. In contrast, alternate procedures for removal of free steroid, such as gel filtration [13] and hydrophobic chromatography [51] do not promote binding of radioactive ligand to this non-receptor binding protein. It is, therefore, very important to verify that the exchanged binding sites exhibit the characteristics of the classical androgen receptors (i.e. high affinity, heat sensitivity, sedimentation characteristics). Further studies are obviously necessary to develop procedures that distinguish between the androgen receptor and the 'non-receptor steroid binding protein'.

5. PROBLEMS OF LIGAND EXCHANGE

5.1 Slow dissociation of DHT from the androgen receptor at low temperatures

A prerequisite to developing a procedure that insures complete exchange is essentially total displacement of endogenously bound DHT with radiolabeled ligand under conditions which maintain maximal receptor binding activity (stability).

It has been shown [13, 14, 15, 46] that at 0 °C [^{3}H]-DHT dissociates from in vitro and in vivo bound androgen receptor complexes very slowly with a half time variously reported as 55–160 hr.

This slow rate of dissociation requires that incubations with radiolabeled ligand last for several days to achieve complete exchange. Recent studies [46] have shown that prolonged incubation (72–96 hr) at 0 °C, while resulting in a significant recovery of androgen binding sites, is associated with marked loss of receptor due to instability. Only 50 % of the total androgen binding sites were recovered by these procedures.

In view of these observations it is difficult to reconcile the data reported for exchange assays carried out at 0 °C for 16–24 hr [16–22]. In our opinion these data represent non-quantitative measurements of androgen receptor. Therefore, it is essential to determine conditions at which endogenous DHT can be dissociated from the receptor in a reasonable period of time with minimum inactivation of binding sites.

5.2 Temperature and chemically induced inactivation of androgen binding sites

Attempts to accelerate DHT dissociation by incubation at elevated temperatures, while enhancing the dissociation of DHT, also produced significant losses of receptor binding capacity [16, 17, 31, 46]. Similarly NaSCN (0.4 M), which enhances the exchange of estrogen receptors at 4 °C, inactivates the androgen receptor under identical incubation conditions. It should also be pointed out that exchange assay data reported for measurement of androgen receptors by incubation at 15 °C for 16 hr are equally non-quantitative [25–30]. In many instances the proper receptor stability controls were not performed to assess the extent of binding site inactivation.

As shown recently by Hechter et al. [46] the exchange assay at 15 °C for 16 hr measures only a small fraction of the total receptors while prolonged incubations at 15 °C resulted in total inactivation of androgen receptors, even though the experiments were performed in the presence of sodium molybdate, a reagent known to stabilize steroid receptors [39, 40, 44, 65, 66, 67]. This failure of molybdate to stabilize androgen receptors at 15 °C is probably due to the fact that molybdate exerts its effect only on the in vitro, untransformed receptor complexes [39, 40, 44, 68]; thus, in vivo bound androgen hormone receptor complexes are likely to be transformed and molybdate offers no protection when heated at 15 °C for long periods of time.

Recognizing such difficulties Blondeau et al. [35, 69] have developed an indirect method for measurement of hormone receptor complexes in the cytosolic and nuclear fractions. This procedure measures the DHT extracted from tissue subcellular fractions by radioimmunoassay following removal of free and loosely bound steroid. The cytosolic receptor is precipitated with protamine sulfate and the remaining bound DHT reflects the DHT bound to androgen receptors. Unfortunately this method can not be applied to measurement of human prostatic androgen receptors because of the significant interference of plasma protein binding of androgen.

6. RECENT EXPERIMENTAL APPROACHES

In the continuous effort to develop a reliable and quantitative method for measurement of prostatic androgen receptor, we have attempted to use reagents that induce ligand dissociation under conditions where receptor properties remain unaltered. The observation of Coty [70] that organic mercurials dissociate progesterone and Vit D_3 receptor hormone complexes reversibly prompted us to use one of these reagents to develop an exchange assay for the androgen receptor. Mersalyl acid (0.3 mM) [32] dissociates 90% of [^{3}H]-R1881 bound in vitro to cytoplasmic or nuclear androgen receptor at 0 °C. The dissociation is rapid ($t\frac{1}{2} = 15$ min) and is reversible with excess thiol reagents. Other investigators [71] have shown the exchange of rat liver glucocorticoid receptors with 0.5 mM p-hydroxymercuribenzoate. DeLuca and his associates also used mersalyl to exchange in vivo bound Vit D_3 receptors [72].

Attempts to apply this newly developed exchange assay to rat and human androgen receptors bound in vivo met with little success. It was found that, in contrast to in vitro bound R1881 or DHT where 90% of bound ligand can be dissociated at 0.3 mM mersalyl, only 10–30% of in vivo bound ligand is dissociated under identical conditions [13]. This strongly suggests that in vivo and in vitro bound hormone receptor complexes differ in their interaction with mersalyl acid. Since mercurial reagents interact with SH groups of proteins one can postulate that upon binding of the steroid in vivo the hormone receptor complexes undergo structural or conformational changes rendering the critical SH groups inaccessible. Thus, one must conclude that while this reagent is useful in the dissociation of hormone bound in vitro [32, 35, 70–72], it is not useful for exchange of endogenously bound androgens.

These observations [13] and the reported differences in elution of in vivo and in vitro bound hormone receptor complexes from phosphocellulose [73] suggest that characterization of the in vivo bound receptor complexes is an important aspect of developing an exchange assay for the androgen receptor. We have undertaken such studies and the results have been reported [13]. It was found that in vivo bound [^{3}H]-DHT and [^{3}H]-R1881 dissociated from the cytoplasmic receptor at a much slower rate than in vitro bound hormone receptor complexes.

Thus, conditions developed for the exchange assay of in vitro labeled receptor can not be directly applied to in vivo bound receptor. Moreover, dissociation data obtained with [^{3}H]-R1881 can result in erroneous conclusions regarding receptor ligand exchange.

7. CONCLUSIONS

The development of a reproducible and quantitative exchange assay for the measurement of androgen receptors in the subcellular fractions of target cells will allow investigators to correlate steroid binding, subcellular distribution of hormone receptor complexes, and hormone receptor complex residency in the nuclei, with the biological response, similar to correlation made for estrogen receptors [74]. In the development of a quantitative exchange assay for the androgen receptor, the following requirements must be met: (i) the assay must be performed under conditions in which the receptor remains stable over the entire period of the procedure; (ii) dissociation of the endogenously bound DHT must be complete, and the rebinding of the radiolabeled ligand must be maximal within a reasonable period of time; (iii) specificity, accuracy, and precision of the procedure must be demonstrated.

So far these criteria have not been met in any of the published procedures [16-32], since none have been shown to measure total receptor content.

A necessary control, often ignored in performing exchange assay experiments, is the assessment of the total number of receptors originally present. One must compare the number of binding sites measured by direct binding of labeled ligand after injection of [^{3}H]-steroid to castrated animals or incubation with tissue slices at 37 °C in tissue culture medium or with a cell free system, with those measured by exchange after identical treatment, but with the same concentration of unlabeled ligand. Since the current methodology for measurement of androgen receptors is inadequate and the need for better methodology remains, one should explore methods developed for other steroid receptors and adapt them to the measurmeent of androgen receptor. For instance, Kim et al. [75] have shown that the anaesthetic drug tetracaine enhances the dissociation of estradiol from the estrogen receptor at 10 °C. Muller et al. [76] have shown that 1:2 cyclohexanedione increases the rate of estradiol dissociation from the estrogen receptor. Other reagents such as NaSCN and pyridoxal phosphate [77] have also been shown to speed the exchange of estrogen receptor. It may be possible to modify these procedures to allow adequate exchange assay of the androgen receptor.

ACKNOWLEDGEMENTS

This is as Publication #115 of the Hubert H. Humphrey Cancer Research Center of Boston University, Boston, Massachusetts.

This work was supported by research grants CA#28856 from the National Cancer Institute and from 'Aid for Cancer Research', Boston, Massachusetts.

REFERENCES

1. Liao S, Tymoczko JL, Castaneda E, Liang T: Androgen receptors and androgen-dependent initiation of protein synthesis in the prostate. Vit Hormon 33:297-317, 1975.
2. Mainwaring WI: The mechanism of action of androgens. Monographs on Endocrinology. New York: Springer-Verlag, 1977.
3. Davies P, Fahmy AR, Pierrepoint CG, Griffiths K: Hormone effects in vitro on prostatic ribonucleic acid polymerase. Biochem J 129:1167-1169, 1972.
4. Davies P, Griffths K: Stimulation in vitro of prostatic ribonucleic acid polymerase by 5α-dihydrotestosterone receptor complexes. Biochem Biophys Res Comm 53:373-382, 1973.
5. Fang S, Anderson KM, Liao S: Receptor proteins for androgens. On the role of specific proteins in retention of 17β-hydroxy-5α-androstan-3-one by the rat ventral prostate in vivo and in vitro. J Biol Chem 244:6584-6595, 1969.
6. Liao S, Fang S: Receptor proteins for androgens and the mode of action of androgens on gene transcription in ventral prostate. Vit, Hormon 27:17-91, 1969.
7. Mainwaring WI, Peterken BM: A reconstituted cell free system for the specific transfer of steroid receptor complexes into nuclear chromatin isolated from rat ventral prostate gland. Biochem J 125:285-295, 1971.
8. Rennie P, Bruchovsky N: In vitro and in vivo studies on the functional significance of androgen receptors in rat prostate. J Biol Chem 247:1546-1554, 1972.
9. Tveter K, Attramadal A: Selective uptake of radioactivity in rat ventral prostate following administration of testosterone 1-2 [^{3}H]. Acta Endrocrinol 59:218-225, 1968.

46

10. Aakvaag A, Tveter KJ, Unhjem O, Attramadal A: Receptors and binding of androgens in the prostate. J Steroid Biochem 3:375-384, 1972.
11. Boesel RW, Klipper RL, Shain SA: Androgen regulation of androgen receptor content and distribution in the ventral and dorsolateral prostate of aging AXC rats. Steroids 35:157-177, 1980.
12. Shain SA, Gorelic LS, Boesel RW, Radwin HM, Lamm DL: Human prostate androgen receptor quantitation: Effects of temperature on assay parameters. Cancer Res 42:4849-4854, 1982.
13. Traish AM, Muller RE, Wotiz HH: Differences in the physicochemical characteristics of in vivo and in vitro formed androgen receptor complexes. Endocrinology 114:(5), 1984.
14. Wilson EM, French FS: Binding properties of androgen receptors: Evidence of identical receptors in rat testis, epididymis and prostate. J Biol Chem 251:5620-5629, 1976.
15. Feit ET, Muldoon TG: Differences in androgen-binding properties of the low molecular forms of androgen receptor in rat ventral prostate cytosol. Endocrinology 112:592-600, 1983.
16. Barrack ER, Coffey DS: The specific binding of estrogens and androgens to the nuclear matrix of sex hormone responsive tissues. J Biol Chem 255:7265-7275, 1980.
17. Olsson CA, White RD, Goldstein I, Traish AM, Muller RE, Wotiz HH: A preliminary report on the measurement of cytosolic and nuclear prostatic tissue steroid receptors. In: Progress in Clinical and Biological Research, Murphy GP, Sandberg AA (eds). New York: Alan R Liss, Vol 33, pp 209-221, 1979.
18. Chang CH, Rowley DR, Lobl TJ, Tindall DJ: Purification and characterization of androgen receptor from steer seminal vesicle. Biochemistry 21:4102-4109, 1982.
19. Lieskovsky G, Bruchovsky N: Assay of nuclear androgen receptor in human prostate. J Urol 121:51-58, 1979.
20. Isomaa V, Pajunen AEI, Bardin CW, Jänne OA: Nuclear androgen receptors in the mouse kidney: Validation of new assay. Endocrinology 111:833-843, 1982.
21. Hicks LL, Walsh PC: A microassay for the measurement of androgen receptors in human prostatic tissue. Steroids 33:389-406, 1979.
22. Walsh PC, Hicks LL: Characterization and measurement of androgen receptors in human prostate tissue. In: Prostate Cancer and Hormone Receptors, Murphy GP, Sandberg AA (eds). New York: Alan R Liss, Inc, pp 51-63, 1979.
23. Trachtenberg J, Walsh PC: Correlation of prostatic nuclear androgen receptor content with duration of response and survival following hormonal therapy in advanced prostatic cancer. J Urol 127:466-471, 1982.
24. Wilson EM, French FS: Effects of protease and protease inhibitors on 4.5 S and 8.0 S androgen receptor. J Biol Chem 254:6210-6219, 1979.
25. Bonne C., Raynaud JP: Assay of androgen binding sites by exchange with methyltrienolone (R1881). Steroids 27:497-407, 1976.
26. Davies P, Thomas P, Griffiths K: Measurement of free and occupied cytoplasmic and nuclear androgen receptor sites in rat ventral prostate gland. J Endrocinol 74:393-404, 1977.
27. Shain SA, Boesel RW, Lamm D, Radwin HM: Characterization of unoccupied (R) and occupied (RA) androgen binding components of the hyperplastic human prostate. Steroids 31:541-556, 1978.
28. Ghanadian R, Auf G, Chaloner PJ, Chisholm GD: The use of methyltrienolone in the measurement of the free and bound cytoplasmic receptors for dihydrotestosterone in benign hypertrophied human prostate. J Steroid Biochem 9:325-330, 1978.
29. Tezon GG, Vazques MH, Blaquire A: Androgen-controlled subcellular distribution of its receptor in the rat epididymis: 5α-dihydrotestosterone-induced translocation is blocked by antiandrogens. Endocrinology 111:2039-2045, 1982.

30. Mobbs BG, Johnson EE, Connolly JG, Clark AF: Evaluation of the use of cyproterone acetate competition to distinguish between high affinity binding of [³H] dihydrotestosterone to human prostate cytosol receptors and to sex hormone binding globulin. J Steroid Biochem 8:943-949, 1977.

31. Snochowski M, Pousette A, Ekman P, Bression D, Andersson L, Hogberg B, Gustafsson JA: Characterization and measurement of the androgen receptor in human benign prostatic hyperplasia and prostatic carcinoma. J Clin Endocrinol Metab 45:920-930, 1977.

32. Traish AM, Muller RE, Wotiz HH: A new procedure for the quantitation of nuclear and cytoplasmic androgen receptors. J Biol Chem 256:12028-12033, 1981.

33. Menon M, Tananis CE, McLaughlin G, Lippman ME, Walsh PC: The measurement of androgen receptors in human prostatic tissue utilizing sucrose density gradient centrifugation and protamine precipitation assay. J Urol 117:309-312, 1977.

34. Verhoeven G, Heyns W, DeMoor P: Ammonium sulfate precipitation as a tool for the study of androgen receptor proteins in rat prostate and mouse kidney. Steroids 26:149-168, 1975.

35. Blondeau JP, Corpechot C, le Goascogne C, Baulieu E-E, Robel P: Androgen receptors in the rat ventral prostate and their hormonal control. Vit Hormon 33:319-344, 1975.

36. Danzo BJ, Taylor AC, Schmidt WN: Binding of the photoaffinity ligand 17β-hydroxy-4,6-androstadien-3-one to rat androgen binding protein: Comparison with binding of 17β-hydroxy-5α-androstan-3-one Endocrinology 107:1169-1175, 1980.

37. Peck EJ Jr, Clark JH: Effect of ionic strength on charcoal adsorption assays of receptor estradiol complexes. Endocrinology 101:1034-1043, 1977.

38. Traish AM Muller RE, Wotiz HH: Binding of estrogen receptor to uterine nuclei. J Biol Chem 252:6823-6830, 1977.

39. Mauk LA, Day RN, Notides AC: Molybdate interaction with the estrogen receptor: Effects on estradiol binding and receptor activation. Biochemistry 21:1788-1793, 1982.

40. Dahmar MK, Quasney MW, Bissen ST, Pratt WB: Molybdate permits resolution of untransformed glucocorticoid receptors from the transformed state. J Biol Chem 256:9401-9405, 1981.

41. Tsai H, Steinberger A: Effect of sodium molybdate on the binding of androgen receptor complexes to germ cell and sertoli cell chromatin. J Steroid Biochem 17:131-136, 1982.

42. Traish AM, Wotiz HH: Unpublished observations.

43. Rennie P, Bruchovsky N: Studies on the relationship between androgen receptor and the transport of androgen in rat prostate. J Biol Chem 248:3288-3297, 1973.

44. Muller RE, Traish AM, Wotiz HH: Estrogen receptor activation precedes transformation. J Biol Chem 258:9227-9236, 1983.

45. Kumar SA, Beach T, Dickerman HW: Effects of chaotropic anions on the rate of dissociation of estradiol-receptor protein complexes of mouse uterine cytosol. Biochem Biophys Res Commun 84:631-638, 1978.

46. Hechter O, Mechaber D, Swick A, Campfield LA, Eychenne B, Baulieu E-E, Robel P: Optimal radio ligand exchange conditions for measurement of occupied androgen receptor sites in rat ventral prostate. Arch Biochem 224:49-68, 1983.

47. Williams D, Gorski J: Equilibrium binding of estradiol by uterine cell suspensions and whole uteri in vitro. Biochemistry 13:5537-5542, 1974.

48. Walters MR, Hunziker W, Clark JH: Hydroxylapatite prevents nuclear receptor loss during the exchange assay of progesterone receptors. J Steroid Biochem 13:1129-1132, 1980.

49. Krieg M, Szalay R, Voigt KD: Binding and metabolism of testosterone and 5α-dihydrotestosterone in bulbocavernosus ani (BCLA) of male rats. J Steroid Biochem 5:453-459, 1974.

50. Krieg M, Bartsch W, Janssen W, Voigt KD: A comparative study of binding, metabolism

48

and endogenous levels of androgens in normal, hyperplastic and carcinomatous human prostate. J Steroid Biochem 11:615-624, 1979.

51. Dahlberg E, Snochowski M, Gustafsson JA: Removal of hydrophobic compounds from biological fluids by a simple method. Anal Biochem 106:380-388, 1980.

52. King RJB, Mainwaring WIP: In: Steroid Cell Interactions. London: University Park Press, pp 25-101, 1974.

53. Wilson EW, Lea DA, French FS: Androgen-binding proteins of the male reproductive tract. In: Receptors and Hormone Action, O'Malley B, Birnbaumer L (eds). Vol. II, pp 491-531, 1978.

54. Bonne C, Raynaud JP: Methyltrienolone, a specific ligand for cellular androgen receptors. Steroids 26:227-232, 1975.

55. Pousette A, Snochowski M, Bression D, Hogberg B, Gustafsson JA: Partial characterization of [3H]-methyltrienolone binding in rat prostate cytosol. Biochem Acta 582:358-367, 1979.

56. Asselin J, Labrie F, Gourdeau Y, Bonne C, Raynaud JP: Binding of [3H]-methyltrienolone (R1881) in rat prostate and human benign prostatic hypertrophy (BPH). Steroids 28:449-459, 1976.

57. Zava DT, Landrum B, Horwitz KB, McGuire WL: Androgen receptor assay with [3H]-methyltrienolone (R1881) in the presence of progesterone receptors. Endocrinology 104:1007-1012, 1979.

58. Ho-Kim MA, Tremblay RR, Dube JY: Binding of methyltrienolone to glucocorticoid receptors in rat muscle cytosol. Endocrinology 109:1418-1423, 1981.

59. Rossini GP, Liao S: Intercellular inactivation, reactivation and dynamic status of prostate androgen receptors. Biochem J 208:383-392, 1983.

60. Heyns W, Peeters B, Mous J, Rombauts W, DeMoor P: Purification and characterization of prostatic binding protein and its subunits. Eur J Biochem 89:181-186, 1978.

61. Chen E, Schilling S, Hippakka RN, Huang I, Liao S: Prostate α-protein. J Biol Chem 257:116-121, 1982.

62. Lea OA, Petrusz P, French F: Prostatein: A major secretory protein of the rat ventral prostate. J Biol Chem 254:6196-6202, 1979.

63. Wotiz HH, Muller RE, Traish AM: A human prostatic steroid binding protein. Sixth International Congress on Hormonal Steroids. Jerusalem, Israel, September, 1982.

64. Traish AM, Muller RE, Burns ME, Wotiz HH: Steroid binding proteins in the rat and human prostate. In: The Prostatic Cell: Structure and Function. New York: Alan R Liss, Inc, Part A, pp 417-434, 1981.

65. Gaubert CM, Tremblay RR, Dube JY: Effect of sodium molybdate on cytosolic androgen receptors in rat prostate. J Steroid Biochem 13:931-937, 1980.

66. Noma K, Nakao K, Sato B, Nishizawa Y, Matsumoto K, Yamamura Y: Effect of molybdate on activation and stabilization of steroid receptors. Endocrinology 107:1205-1211, 1980.

67. Wright WW, Chan KC, Bardin W: Characterization of the stabilizing effect of sodium molybdate on the androgen receptor present in mouse kidney. Endocrinology 108:2210-2216, 1981.

68. McBlain WA, Toft DO, Shyamala G: Transformation of mammary cytoplasmic glucocorticoid receptors under cell free conditions. Biochemistry 20:6790-6798, 1981.

69. Blondeau JP, Baulieu E-E, Robel P: Androgen dependent regulation of androgen receptor in the rat ventral prostate. Endocrinology 110:1926-1932, 1982.

70. Coty W: Reversible dissociation of steroid hormone receptor complexes by mercurial reagent. J Biol Chem 255:8035-8037, 1980.

71. Banerji A, Kalimi M: Development of an [3H]-glucocorticoid exchange assay in rat liver cytosol. Steroids 32:409-421, 1981.

72. Massaro ER, Simpson RV, DeLuca H: Quantitation of endogenously occupied and unoccupied binding sites for 1,25-dihydroxy vitamin D_3 in rat intestine. Proc Natl Acad Sci USA 80:2549-2553, 1983.
73. Rennie P, Bruchovsky N: In vitro and in vivo studies on the functional significance of androgen receptors in rat prostate. J Biol Chem 247:1546-1554, 1972.
74. Clark JH, Paszko Z, Peck EJ Jr: Nuclear retention of the receptor estrogen complex: relation to the agonistic and antagonistic properties of estriol. Endocrinology 100:91-96, 1977.
75. Kim UH, Van Oosbree TR, Mueller GC: Influence of tetracaine on the structure and function of estrogen receptors. Endocrinology 111:260-268, 1982.
76. Muller RE, Mrabet N, Traish AM, Wotiz HH: The role of arginyl residues in estrogen receptor activation and transformation. J Biol Chem 258:11582-11589, 1983.
77. Okulicz WE, Robidoux WF, Leavitt WW: Measurement of nuclear estrogen receptor at low temperature. Validation of a new exchange assay using pyridoxal phosphate. Endocrine Society Meetings, Abstract #1035, 1983.

3. Chemotherapy in Prostatic Cancer

JOSEPH R. DRAGO *

1. BACKGROUND

Prostatic cancer is the third leading cause of cancer deaths in the United States, accounting for approximately 20 000 deaths per year [1].

Unfortunately, knowledge concerning the efficiency of cytotoxic agents used in the treatment of prostate cancer is limited. There are several reasons for this, but two are particularly prominent. The criteria for evaluation of responses to chemotherapy for prostatic cancer are sketchy, due to the fact that response parameters cannot be agreed upon [2, 3]. Also, very few of the available antitumor drugs have been sufficiently tested on prostate cancer patients.

In compiling data on the efficacy of recently researched drugs, the National Prostatic Cancer Project criteria for objective response of prostatic carcinoma to chemotherapy will be followed unless otherwise noted. The criteria are stated as follows [3, 4]:

A. *Complete remission*
1. Absence of clinically detectable soft tissue mass
2. Return of elevated acid phosphatase level to normal
3. Recalcification of all osteolytic lesions
4. Absence of evidence of progressive blastic lesions
5. Complete reduction in liver size and normalization of all pretreatment liver function abnormalities, if hepatomegaly is a significant indicator
6. Absence of new areas of neoplasia
7. Absence of significant weight loss

---

* Dr Drago is a member of the Specialized Cancer Research Center at The Milton S. Hershey Medical Center.

T. L. Ratliff and W. J. Catalona (eds), Urologic Oncology. ISBN 0-89838-628-4.
© *1984. Martinus Nijhoff Publishers, Boston. Printed in the Netherlands.*

B. *Partial objective response*
   1. 50% reduction in measurable or palpable soft tissue mass
   2. Return of elevated acid phosphatase level to normal
   3. Recalcification of some osteolytic lesions
   4. Reduction in liver size and at least 30% improvement of all pre-treatment liver function abnormalities, if hepatomegaly is a significant indicator
   5. Lack of increase in any other lesion and absence of new areas of neoplasia
   6. Absence of significant weight loss

C. *Objectively stable*
   1. Insufficient regression of the primary indicator lesion to meet criteria of previous categories
   2. Less than 25% increase in any measurable lesion
   3. Absence of significant weight loss (greater than 10%) and symptom or performance status deterioration

D. *Progression*
   1. Significant weight loss and symptom or performance status deterioration
   2. Appearance of new areas of malignant disease
   3. Increase in any previously measurable lesion (bone excluded) by more than 50% in two perpendicular diameters
   4. Increase in acid or alkaline phosphatase value alone is not considered an indication of progression; these measurements should be used in conjunction with other criteria.

Cyclophosphamide is the overall standard therapy in the treatment of prostatic cancer proven to be hormone resistant. There is no definitive proof, at this time, that this drug is superior to any other agents. Further investigation is necessary to properly evaluate the efficacy of this drug and others used in combination such as 5-Fu, doxorubicin, vincristine, methotrexate and cis-platinum.

The following is a general overview of the mode of action of some of the more commonly used chemotherapeutic agents.

Cyclophosphamide is an alkylating agent with chlorethylamine as the active alkyl group. It resulted from experiments with nitrogen mustard during World War II, when it was found that these were of therapeutic value. The major cause of its cytotoxicity may be the cross-linking of DNA by alkylation of the 7-nitrogen of guanine on adjacent strands. The alkylating agents cause profound chromosomal changes [5–7].

Doxorubicin or adriamycin and daunorubicin are glycoside antibiotics. These anthracycline agents bind DNA by intercalation between base pairs on adjacent strands. This results in uncoiling of the DNA helix and inhibition of DNA-directed RNA and DNA polymerases. The effects are maximal during the DNA synthesis phase of the cell cycle. These agents consist of chromophore and sugar (daunosamine moieties) [5, 6, 8–10]. The chromophore is the location of antitumor activity. Binding of daunosamine to myocardial fibers is the probable reason for the cardiac toxicity of these agents [6]. Their reversible side effects are bone marrow depression, stomatitis, and pronounced alopecia, and the major dose-limiting effect is myocardiopathy. This may lead to refractory congestive heart failure, especially at a cumulative dose of greater than 550 mg/m^2 [10]. Daunorubicin is mainly used for treatment of acute leukemia, but doxorubicin has varied antineoplastic activity.

Fluorouracil is a pyrimidine antagonist anti-metabolite. It is structurally similar to pyrimidine utilized by cells for metabolism and growth. Its intracellular conversion to nucleotide form causes incorporation of fluorouracil into RNA, which alters de novo RNA synthesis and function [3, 5, 6, 11]. Its major anti-neoplastic effect is due to inhibition of DNA synthesis after binding to thymidylate synthetase. The major toxicities of fluorouracil are bone marrow depression and mucositis; and its catabolism site is the liver.

Vincristine and vinblastine arrest mitosis by binding the microtubular protein of the mitotic spindle [5, 6]. The difference between the two agents is the methyl group in vinblastine and the formyl group in vincristine. They are both cleared from the blood by the liver and doses must be reduced if obstructive jaundice is present. The dose-limiting effects for vincristine are slowly reversible mixed sensory motor peripheral neuropathy, severe constipation, and adynamic ileus. Vincristine's major dose-limiting effect is bone marrow suppression.

Methotrexate is an anti-metabolite specific for the DNA synthesis phase of the cell cycle. It is most effective against malignancies with a high fraction of dividing cells. Methotrexate is a folic acid antagonist which binds to the enzyme dihydrofolate reductase and prevents conversion of folic acid to its active form of tetrahydrofolate [12]. It blocks DNA synthesis and has a lesser effect on RNA/protein synthesis. It causes a disproportionate growth with nucleocytoplasmic dissociation responsible for megaloblastic changes in bone marrow and cellular atypia. Its major dose-limiting toxic effects are bone marrow suppression and mucositis of the oral cavity and gastrointestinal tract. The principal route of excretion is through the urine. In the presence of impaired kidney function the plasma half-life may be prolonged; therefore, systemic toxicity may be increased [13]. Large doses may cause precipitation of methotrexate crystals in tubules with resulting renal toxicity. The use of folinic acid (formyl-tetrahydrofolic acid) may prevent toxic effects on bone marrow and mucous membranes and bypass the methotrexate-induced metabolic block [14].

Cis-platinum has biochemical properties with similarities to those of alkylating agents and acts by producing intrastrand and interstrand cross-links and interfering with DNA synthesis. For the most part, it is cell cycle non-specific. It concentrates mainly in the liver, kidneys, and large and small intestines. It is a heavy metal complex, and thus its major side effects are not surprising and include nephrotoxicity and ototoxicity. Hematologic side effects such as myelosuppression and leukopenia also can occur, as well as gastrointestinal side effects common to other chemotherapeutic agents.

Estramustine phosphate is a conjugate of steroid estradiol-17-beta and nitrogen mustard, an alkylating agent [15]. It has been used in Europe for several years. It has been hypothesized that estramustine phosphate would carry the cytotoxic agent directly to the steroid-dependent tumor cells, thereby decreasing its effect on other cells and lessening its side effects. Its exact mechanism of action has yet to be completely explained. In animals it has been shown to interfere with the uptake of estriol but not of testosterone and dihydrotestosterone. In other experimentation, estramustine has been shown to inhibit thymidine corporation in the rat ventral prostate more than estradiol does. It can be safely administered in the intravenous or the oral route. Occasionally, from local intravenous administration, thrombophlebitis may result. In general, estramustine is a well-tolerated drug; however, vomiting and other gastrointestinal side effects do occur as well as a low incidence of local thrombophlebitis at the site of i.v. administration. The main advantage in the use of estramustine has been that it has the potential theoretical advantage of combining the direct hormonal effect of estrogen as well as that of the chemotherapy of nitrogen mustard, and alkylating agent.

BCNU is one of the nitrosoureas that is highly soluble in alcohol and fully soluble in water. Its mode of action is that of an alkylating agent and alkylates DNA and RNA. It has also been shown to inhibit several enzymes by crabamoylation of amino acids and proteins. After intravenous administration, the drug is rapidly degradated. It is thought that its anti-neoplastic and toxic activities may be due to metabolites. Approximately 70% of the total dose is excreted in the urine in 96 hr. Its studies have been limited to a few series of patients with prostatic carcinoma. Major toxicities are those of the hemopoietic system, gastrointestinal and hepatic.

2. CLINICAL TRIALS

The Southeastern Cancer Study Group evaluated *5-Fu* alone and in combination with *cyclophosphamide* and *doxorubicin* (adriamycin) [16]. They found, by using the National Prostatic Cancer Project response criteria, that there is no significant difference between the survival curves of patients receiving combination chemotherapy or 5-Fu alone. In their study, 71 patients were selected using either prostatic acid phosphatase values (locally and at Minneapolis) [17] and/or National Prostatic Cancer Project criteria for objective stability. Thirty-two of these patients completed a six-week course of 5-Fu at a dosage of 600 mg/m^2. Thirty-nine completed a six-week course of combination chemotherapy with cyclophosphamide (500 mg/m^2), doxorubicin (50 mg/m^2), and 5-Fu (500 mg/m^2). In the patients receiving 5-Fu alone, an objective response (50% decrease in prostatic acid phosphatase) of 12% was seen and an objectively stable situation was induced in 50%. In the combination group, 60% were objectively stable and 32% experienced an objective response. The responding patients survived for a greater interval than either the non-responders ($p = 0.06$) or the progressors alone ($p = 0.03$). Prostatic acid phosphatase was used as an indicator. Toxicity was noted primarily in the combination chemotherapy patients, with most of the patients experiencing vomiting after each dose. The conclusion of this group of researchers is that there is no significant benefit to previously hormonally treated stage D prostatic cancer patients in combining cyclophosphamide and doxocuribin with 5-Fu (Table 1 and Table 2).

Also of note were studies done by the National Prostatic Cancer Project and the Eastern Cooperative Oncology Group. In the National Prostatic Cancer Project study, *cyclophosphamide, 5-Fu* and *imidazole carboxamide* were the agents utilized. Objective responses were obtained in 7%, 12% and

Table 1. Cyclophosphamide, 5-Fu, adriamycin.

Study (Reference)	No. of evaluable patients	Objective response		Subjective response	
		No.	%	No.	%
16	29	20	69	–	–
20	8	6	75	1	12.5
18	12	6	50	–	–
59	17	13	76	–	–
Total	66	45	68	1	12.5

Dose: initially – adriamycin 50 mg/m^2
　　　　　　cyclophosphamide 500 mg/m^2
　　　　　　5-Fu 500 mg/m^2
Dose: subsequently – adriamycin 60 mg/m^2
　　　　　　cyclophosphamide 600 mg/m^2
　　　　　　5-Fu 600 mg/m^2
Doses given at 3-week intervals.
If patients received > 3000 rads, initial dose was halved.

Table 2. 5-Fu.

Study (Reference)	Dose	No.of evaluable patients	Objective response		Subjective response (Pain relief)	
			No.	%	No.	%
16	600 mg/m^2 i.v. q week	29	14	48	–	–
7		33	12	36	21	64
26		66	19	29	–	–
27^a		14	14	100	–	–
30		16	7	44	–	–
Total		158	66	42	21	64

[a] Dose (Ref. 27): 15 mg/kg daily (constant infusion), then 2500 mg 5-Fu q 2 weeks through infusion catheters.

4% of the patients, respectively [18]. The Eastern Cooperative Oncology Group compared doxorubicin and 5-Fu and induced objective responses in 24% (mean survival of 31 weeks) in the doxorubicin patients and 8% (mean survival of 23 weeks) in the 5-Fu patients.

As is commonly the case in any study of metastatic adenocarcinoma of the prostate, a lack of clearly defined response criteria which correlates patient survival is a major problem. Usual response assessments cannot be made due to the fact that blastic skeletal metastases are frequently the only measurable parameters. In the following study done by Chlebowski and associates, cyclophosphamide alone was compared to the combination of cyclophosphamide, adriamycin (doxorubicin) and 5-Fu [18]. Twenty-seven patients with stage D metastatic prostate cancer resistant to hormone manipulation were entered into the trial. The National Prostatic Cancer Project criteria for objective response were used. Objective response was induced in 53% of the 15 patients in the cyclophosphamide group (800–1200 mg/m^2 i.v. q 3 weeks). The mean survival in this group was 45-plus weeks and the resonders lived significantly longer than the non-responders. Of the 12 patients in the combination group (cyclophosphamide 150–200 mg/m^2 p.o. days 3–6, 5-Fu 400–500 mg/m^2 i.v. days 1 and 8, and adriamycin 30–50 mg/m^2 i.v. day 1), 50% experienced an objective response. The mean survival was similar to the cyclophosphamide alone group and the responders did not live significantly longer than the non-responders. Twenty-four of the original 27 patients died by the publication of the study. The patients responding to cyclophosphamide lived significantly longer than the patients responding to the combination chemotherapy. In general, toxicity effects were mild in both groups, with nausea and vomiting seen in 60% of the cyclophosphamide patients and 57% of the patients treated with the combination. The combination group did not suffer any greater hematological toxicity than the cyclophosphamide alone group.

This study did not demonstrate significant advantage to a cyclophosphamide, 5-Fu, adriamycin regimen as compared to cyclophosphamide alone (Table 1).

External beam radiation and interstitial irradiation [^{125}I] in addition to *chemotherapy* with cyclophosphamide and doxorubicin were utilized in the experimental procedures at Boston University School of Medicine [22]. Thirty patients with clinically localized adenocarcinoma of the prostate underwent simultaneous staging pelvic lymphadenectomy and interstitial irradiation ([^{125}I] implants). Sixteen of these patients were upstaged to D, due to pelvic lymph node involvement (53.3%). Nine of these sixteen patients had disease progression (bone and soft tissue metastasis) and 12.2 months was the average time to progression. Three of these stage D patients have died, with an average time of 19.6 months to death. Cyclophosphamide (500 mg/m^2) and doxorubicin (50 mg/m^2), every three weeks for six months, were given to nine of the 16 upstaged patients and three of these had disease progression. Six of the seven upstaged patients not on chemotherapy developed metastasis. Of the original 30 patients, 18 received additional external beam irradiation for local tumor control (between 2000 and 4000 rad). There were 16 long-term complications in the 30 patients and 75% of these were those who received external beam irradiation. One of the 14 patients who had negative lymphadenectomies had disease progression (at 17 months), but there were no deaths. Several studies are ongoing to evaluate the use of adjunct chemotherapy in stage D prostatic cancer, especially in a less than well-differentiated tumor.

3. SINGLE AGENT TREATMENT

Cyclophosphamide has been used as a single agent in several clinical trials, with objective responses ranging from 25% to 53%, with a mean response of 37% of 185 evaluable patients. Subjective responses of pain relief and increases in ambulation have occurred from 17% to 54% [7, 18, 23, 24, 57] (Table 3).

Several clinical studies have evaluated the effects of cyclophosphamide with those of various other ablative therapies on patients with progressive prostatic carcinoma. The first of the randomized trials, conducted by the National Prostatic Cancer Project, compared cyclophosphamide or 5-fluorouracil with a variety of 'standard' non-chemotherapeutic treatments. The latter included cryosurgery, radiotherapy, and several treatments other than chemotherapy. Of the initial 110 evaluable endocrine-resistant prostatic

Table 3. Cyclophosphamide.

Study (Reference)	Dose	No. of evaluable patients	Objective response		Subjective response	
			No.	%	No.	%
7	1 gm/m^2 i.v. q 3 weeks	41	17	41	20/37	54
23	1 gm/m^2 i.v. q 3 weeks	35	9	26	8	23
24	1 gm/m^2 i.v. q 3 weeks	43	16	37	9	21
25	750 mg/m^2 i.v. q 3 weeks	17	9	53	3	18
18	800–1200 mg/m^2 i.v. q 3 weeks	15	8	53	–	–
57		35	9	26	6	17
Total		186	68	37	46/167	28

cancer patients, 41 received 1 gm/mm^3 cyclophosphamide i.v. every three weeks, 33 received 600 mg/m^2 5-Fu i.v. every week, and 36 received the standard treatment. Cyclophosphamide was significantly better than the standard treatment ($p<0.05$) in objective responses, which concluded stabilized disease and complete or partial regression. Survival rates were 46% for patients taking cyclophosphamide, 36% for 5-Fu treated patients, and 19% for the standard treatment. Both cyclophosphamide and 5-Fu showed significantly higher survival rates, primary tumor mass reduction, and increased pain relief compared with standard therapy ($p<0.05$). Toxicity was minimal for both agents administered, being confined to nausea, vomiting, and temporary leukopenia.

Adriamycin (doxorubicin HCl) has produced objective response rates of 22–50% in varying clinical series, with a mean response of 30% of 81

Table 4. Adriamycin (doxorubicin HCl).

Study (Reference)	Dose	No. of evaluable patients	Objective response		Subjective response	
			No.	%	No.	%
19		19	5	26		
26		9	2	22		
30	40–60 mg/kg i.v. q 3 weeks	12	6	50	30	
41		15	5	30		
62		26	6	23		
Total		81	24	30		

representative evaluable patients. Subjective responses parallel those seen with cyclophosphamide [19, 26, 30, 41, 62] (Table 4).

Estramustine phosphate has shown wide ranges of objective response rates from a low of 19% to a high of 81%. The mean response rate was 51% of 381 evaluable patients. This agent has shown great promise in multiple series. Subjective response rates have varied again, from a low of 10% to 53% for a mean of 34% of evaluable patients [15, 31, 33, 35, 37, 44, 45, 54-57] (Table 5).

Table 5. Estramustine phosphate.

Study (Reference)	Dose	No. of evaluable patietns	Objective response		Subjective response	
			No.	%	No.	%
31		51	35	69	5	10
33	600 mg/m² daily in 3 divided oral doses	27	7	60	5	21
36		54	26	48	–	–
37		30	12	40	16	53
44		17	16	94	8	47
45		44	8	19	15	36
46		20	8	27	10/30	33
54	5-15 mg/kg/day	48	39	81	–	–
55		44	28	64	–	–
57		46	14	30	14	30
Total		381	193	51	73/213	34

Prednimustine has been used in a significant number of patients, with objective responses ranging from 13% to 60% in 118 patients evaluated. Subjective responses have been reported by Dr Murphy of the National Prostatic Cancer Project [65], who found 32% of 62 patients experienced a marked decrease in pain [64, 65, 67] (Table 6). *Hydroxyurea* has been evaluated in some 58 patients, with objective response rates varying from 15%

Table 6. Prednimustine.

Study (Reference)	Dose	No. of evaluable patients	Objective response		Subjective response	
			No.	%	No.	%
64	25 mg/m² daily	23	3	13	–	–
65		62	8	13	20	32
67		10	6	60	–	–
Total		118	17	14	20	32

to 50%. Subjective responses were similar and ranged from 21% to 77%, with the mean being 50% of 58 patients evaluated [24, 63] (Table 11).

Cis-diamminedichloroplatinum produced objective response rates varying from 19% to 42% of the most recent 78 patients evaluated, and subjective response rates were approximately 40%. This agent shows promise as one of the most active single agents to be evaluated since the initiation of cyclophosphamide clinical trials [49, 56, 58] (Table 7). Cis-platinum's main promise, however, may be in its use as a combination agent combined with cyclophosphamide and adriamycin.

Table 7. Cis-platinum (cis-diamminedichloroplatinum).

Study (Reference)	Dose	No. of evaluable patients	Objective response		Subjective response	
			No.	%	N0.	%
49	1 mg/kg weekly for 6 weeks	45	19	42	18	40
56		12	4	33	8	32
58		21	4	19	–	–
Total		78	27	35	26/57	46

Table 8. Vincristine.

Study (Reference)	Dose	No. of evaluable patients	Objective response		Subjective response	
			No.	%	No.	%
26		22	2	9	–	–
33	1 mg/m^2 i.v. q 2 weeks	34	5	21	4	12
Total		56	7	13	4	12

Vincristine has been evaluated in smaller series, with objective response rates approximating 20%. It has appeared from these studies that reduction of pain has not been as dramatic as most of the other single agents [26, 33] (Table 8).

Objective have also been observed with the use of *methyl-CCNU* and approximated 23% of 57 recent patients evaluated [24, 26] (Table 9).

DTIC produced objective responses varying from 0% to 27% in 61 patients. In approximately one fourth of the patients studied there was a marked decrease in pain and increase in ambulation [23] (Table 10).

Carter and Wasserman reported the use of *nitrogen mustard* in a series of 31 patients, with an objective response rate of 39% [36]. In addition, several other small clinical series have evaluated *hexamethylmelamine* and

Table 9. Methyl-CCNU.

Study (Reference)	Dose	No. of evaluable patients	Objective response		Subjective response	
			No.	%	No.	%
24	175 mg/m^2 q 3 weeks	27	11	40	6/27	22
26		19	2	11	–	–
Total		57	13	23	6	22

Table 10. DTIC (imidazole carboxamide).

Study (Reference)	Dose	No. of evaluable patients	Objective response		Subjective response	
			No.	%	No.	%
26		6	0		–	–
23	200 mg/m^2 i.v. days 1–5 q 3 weeks	55	15	27	13	24
Total		61	15	26	13	24

Table 11.

Study (Reference)	No. of evaluable patients	Objective response		Subjective response	
		No.	%	No.	%
		BCNU			
26	15	2	14	–	–
		Nitrogen mustard			
26	31	12	39	–	–
		Melphalan			
51	15	1	7	1	7
		Hexamethylmelamine			
26	6	2	33	–	–
		Hydroxyurea			
24[a]	28	4	15	6/28	21
63	30	15	50	23/30	77

[a] Dose (Ref. 24): 3 gm/m^2 orally q 6 weeks.

BCNU. These latter agents have been used in small numbers of patients and do show some promise; however, numbers do not permit generalization regarding their objective and subjective response rates [26, 52] (Table 11).

Several clinical studies have been done to evaluate the efficacy of *5-Fu* used alone in the treatment of hormone-resistant stage D prostatic adenocarcinoma. In recent years 158 patients have been involved in these studies. A total of 66 had objective responses (including objective stability) or 42%. There have been 21 subjective responses (64%) which were judged on the basis of pain relief since this parameter was utilized in a majority of reports. Only one study listed subjective responses. The representative dose was 600 mg/m^2 i.v. every week [7, 16, 26, 27, 30] (Table 2).

Chloroethyl-cyclohexy-nitrosourea (CCNU) has produced objective responses in 30% [6] of 20 evaluable patients. There have been a total of three (or 15%) subjective responses. The dose used was 130 mg/m^2 orally every six weeks [57] (Table 12).

Table 12.

Study (Reference)	Dose	No. of evaluable patients	Objective response		Subjective response	
			No.	%	No.	%
Chloroethyl-cyclohexy-nitrosourea (CCNU)						
11	130 mg/m^2 orally every 6 weeks	20	6	30	3	15
Procarbazine						
23	100 mg/m^2 orally for 3 weeks of each 6-week treatment period	39	14	37	7	18
57		38	5	13	2	5

Procarbazine was reported by Schmidt et al. [57] to produce objective responses in 13% (or 5) of the 38 patients evaluated. A 5% subjective response rate was also seen in these patients. The patients received 100 mg/m^2 oral procarbazine for three weeks of each six-week treatment period (Table 12).

4. COMBINATION AGENTS

4.1 *5-Fu and cyclophosphamide*

In a total of 46 patients utilized in the evaluation of 5-Fu and cyclophosphamide in combination, four had objective responses (8.5%) and 12 had

Table 13. 5-Fu, cyclophosphamide.

Study (Reference)	No. of evaluable patients	Objective response		Subjective response	
		No.	%	No.	%
21 [a]	13	2	15.4	7	53.8
32	15	0	0	5	33
19	18	2	11	–	–
Total	46	4	8.7	12	42.8

[a] Dose (Ref. 21): i.v. 4 mg/kg cyclophosphamide for 5 days every 4 weeks + 8 mg/kg 5-Fu daily for 5 days every 4 weeks, starting on day 3.

subjective responses (42.8%). The objective responses in each individual study [19, 21, 32] ranged from zero to 15.4%. The doses utilized were approximately 4 mg/kg i.v. five days every four weeks for cyclophosphamide and 8 mg/kg 5-Fu daily for five days every four weeks (Table 13).

4.2 Adriamycin and cyclophosphamide

Objective responses utilizing adriamycin and cyclophosphamide ranged from 23.8% to 66.6%, with a mean of 42%. A total of 52 patients were evaluated. Of these, two studies listed subjective responses with a mean of 46.5%. The doses ranged from 100–500 mg/m^2 for cyclophosphamide and 30–50 mg/m^2 for adriamycin [21, 22, 38] (Table 14).

Table 14. Adriamycin, cyclophosphamide.

Study (Reference)	No. of evaluable patients	Objective response		Subjective response	
		No.	%	No.	%
21 [a]	21	5	23.8	8	38
22 [b]	9	6	66.6	–	–
38 [c]	22	11	50	12	54.5
Total	52	22	42	20	46.5

[a] Dose (Ref. 21): 40 mg/m^2 adriamycin every 3 weeks + 200 mg/m^2 cyclophosphamide daily for 4 days every 3 weeks, starting on day 3.
[b] Dose (Ref. 22): 500 mg/m^2 cyclophosphamide + 50 mg/m^2 adriamycin every 3 weeks for 6 months.
[c] Dose (Ref. 38): 30 mg/m^2 i.v. days 1 and 8 adriamycin, cyclophosphamide – 100 mg/m^2 p.o. days 1–14 of each 28-day cycle.
Adriamycin discontinued after total dose of 550 mg/m^2; cyclophosphamide alone at 1000 mg/m^2 i.v. every 3 weeks.

4.3 *Cis-platin and adriamycin*

Cis-platin used in combination with adriamycin has produced an objective response rate of 43% or nine patients out of 21 evaluated. The subjective response rate was 9.5%. The approximate dose utilized was 50–60 mg/m^2 i.v. every 3–4 weeks [61] (Table 15).

4.4 *Cyclophosphamide, methotrexate and 5-Fu*

In a recent study, cyclophosphamide, methotrexate and 5-Fu were used in combination and produced an objective response of 35% or seven patients out of 20. The subjective response was 35%. The drug doses used were 75 mg/m^2 p.o. days 1–14 cyclophosphamide, 45 mg/m^2 i.v. days 1 and 8 methotrexate, and 500 mg/m^2 cyclophosphamide, 45 mg/m^2 i.v. days 1 and 8 methotrexate, and 500 mg/m^2 i.v. days 1 and 8 5-Fu [11] (Table 15).

Additional randomized trials conducted by Muss et al. compared the effects of cyclophosphamide and the combination of cyclophosphamide, methotrexate and 5-Fu in advanced cases of prostatic cancer. Of 32 evaluable patients, all had progressive prostatic carcinoma and 97% had received hormonal therapy prior to the initiation of chemotherapy. Seventeen patients received cyclophosphamide and 15 patients received the combination chemotherapy. The doses of the combination chemotherapy were modified on the basis of drug toxicity. Response criteria were those used by the

Table 15.

Study (Reference)	No. of evaluable patients	Objective response		Subjective response	
		No.	%	No.	%
Cis-platin, adriamycin					
61	21	9	43	2	9.5
13 patients – 50–60 mg/m^2 i.v. every 3–4 weeks					
6 patients – <50 mg/m^2					
2 patients – 'modified regimens'					
Cyclophosphamide, methotrexate, 5-Fu					
11	20	7	35	7	35
Dose: cyclophosphamide 75 mg/m^2 p.o. days 1–14 + methotrexate 45 mg/m^2 i.v. days 1 and 8 + 5-Fu 500 mg/m^2 i.v. days 1 and 8 (each cycle repeated every 28 days)					
Cyclophosphamide, adriamycin, methotrexate					
60	12	9	75	10	83
Three-week courses: cyclophosphamide 600 mg/m^2 i.v., adriamycin 40 mg/m^2 day 1, methotrexate 15 mg/m^2 p.o. days 9, 13, 16, 20					
When adriamycin 500 mg/m^2 was reached, higher dose cyclophosphamide and methotrexate was used					

National Prostatic Cancer Project with the exception of the definition of stabilized disease as greater than three months with no change in bone or other lesions and no progression of symptoms. Subjective response rates for cyclophosphamide were 18%, and for the combination group 27%. Toxicity was moderate; there was no significant difference in toxicity between treatment groups. Objective response rates were not significantly different: cyclophosphamide 53% versus combination chemotherapy 54%; duration of stable response was 4.5 months for each group. Median survival for cyclophosphamide was longer than that of the combination, being 10.1 months and 8.8 months, respectively (Table 15).

4.5 Cyclophosphamide, adriamycin and methotrexate

Another combination of chemotherapeutic agents researched lately is cyclophosphamide, adriamycin and methotrexate. Of the 12 patients evaluated, 75% (9 patients) had objective responses and 83% (10 patients) had subjective responses. The drug doses used were: cyclophosphamide 600 mg/m^2 i.v., adriamycin 40 mg/m^2 day 1, methotrexate 15 mg/m^2 p.o. days 9, 13, 16 and 20 [60] (Table 15).

4.6 Cyclophosphamide, 5-Fu and adriamycin

Several studies have been done on cyclophosphamide, 5-Fu and adriamycin. The objective response rates ranged from 50% to 76%, with a mean of 68% (45 patients out of a total of 66). Only one study [20] listed subjective responses with a rate of 12.5%. Representative doses were adriamycin 50 mg/m^2, cyclophosphamide 500 mg/m^2, and 5-Fu 500 mg/m^2 [16, 18, 20, 59] (Table 1).

4.7 Procarbazine, imidazole carboxamide and cyclophosphamide

Schmidt and others compared the response of stage D prostatic cancer patients to procarbazine, imidazole carboxamide and cyclophosphamide [23]. The 129 evaluable patients had received hormonal therapy and had become resistant to this mode prior to the institution of chemotherapy. Patients were randomized, and 39 received cyclophosphamide (1 mg/m^2 i.v. q 3 weeks), 68 received DTIC (200 mg/m^2 i.v. days 1–5, 21-day rest, and then repeat the cycle), and 58 patients had procarbazine (100 mg/m^2 orally q day times 3 weeks, 3 weeks rest, and repeat cycle). Subjective response of pain relief and weight gain was approximately 20% for each group. More DTIC patients (45%) and cyclophosphamide patients (46%) had improved performance status compared to procarbazine (23%), with a significant difference between DTIC and procarbazine ($p < 0.05$). Procarbazine was found to be excessively toxic, and randomization of patients to this drug was discontinued halfway through the study.

Objective response of partial regression with stabilized disease in this group was: cyclophosphamide 26%, DTIC 27%, and procarbazine 14%. There was no significant reduction of primary mass size. At 30 weeks into the study, survival rates were: DTIC 62%, procarbazine 48%, and cyclophosphamide 37%. Crossover from DTIC to cyclophosphamide was associated with the highest survival rate. Although there was no significant difference in response rates, DTIC and cyclophosphamide did seem to have an advantage over the excessively toxic drug procarbazine. DTIC and cyclophosphamide are considered to be active agents in treatment of advanced prostatic carcinoma.

4.8 Hydroxyurea, methyl-chloroethyl-cyclohexy-nitrosourea (CCNU) and cyclophosphamide

Additional studies by Loening et al. compared hydroxyurea, methyl-chloroethyl-cyclohexy-nitrosourea and cyclophosphamide in patients with advanced prostatic carcinoma. Ninety-eight patients were evaluable and had previously received hormonal therapy and become resistant. There was a subjective improvement in performance status in approximately 20% of patients in each group; however, patients receiving hydroxyurea and methyl-CCNU experienced excessive toxicity; cyclophosphamide patients tolerated their dose well. Objective responses, characterized by stabilized disease or complete or partial regression, were observed in 35% of patients treated with cyclophosphamide, 30% of patients treated with methyl-CCNU, and only 15% of patients treated with hydroxyurea. Median survival rates were: 41 weeks for the cyclophosphamide group, 19 weeks for hydroxyurea, and 22 weeks for methyl-CCNU. Although these results were not significant by chi-square or the Fisher's exact test, there was an appreciable clinical subjective difference between the treatments. Patients treated with cyclophosphamide had a higher survival rate than those in the other groups ($p<0.01$) and methyl-CCNU ($p<0.05$).

4.9 DES, 5-Fu and cyclophosphamide

DES, 5-Fu and cyclophosphamide were reported by Mukamel et al. to produce a 100% objective response rate when used in combination. The subjective response value was 64% or 16 patients out of 25 evaluated. The DES dosage was 3 mg daily, plus weekly i.v. injections of 5-Fu (10 mg/kg) and cyclophosphamide (10 mg/kg) [39] (Table 16).

4.10 Estramustine phosphate, cyclophosphamide, 5-Fu and cis-platin

Twenty-five evaluable patients received 50 mg/m^2 cis-platin, 500 mg/m^2 5-Fu, and 500 mg/m^2 cyclophosphamide, all i.v. every three weeks. In addition, 600 mg/m^2 estramustine phosphate was administered orally in three

Table 16. DES, 5-Fu, cyclophosphamide.

Study (Reference)	No. of evaluable patients	Objective response		Subjective response	
		No.	%	No.	%
39	25	25	100	16	64

Dose: DES 3 mg daily + weekly i.v. injection of 5-Fu (10 mg/kg) and cyclophosphamide (10 mg/kg)

doses daily. Of these 25 patients, 10 had no prior treatment. There was a 100% objective response rate in this group and 100% subjective response. Fifteen of the 25 patients were hormonally unresponsive at the time of chemotherapy. The objective response rate in this group was 46% while the subjective response was 60% [50] (Table 17).

Table 17. Estramustine phosphate, cyclophosphamide, 5-Fu, cis-platin.

Study (Reference)	No. of evaluable patients	Objective response		Subjective response	
		No.	%	No.	%
50	25 A. no prior treatment (10)	10	100	10	100
	B. hormonally unresponsive (15)	7	46	9	60

Dose: cis-platin 40 mg/m^2 + 5-Fu 500 mg/m^2 + cyclophosphamide 500 mg/m^2, all i.v. every 3 weeks; estramustine phosphate 600 mg/m^2 orally in 3 doses daily

4.11 *5-Fu, methotrexate, vincristine, melphalan and prednisone*

Kane et al. studied the efficacy of 5-Fu, methotrexate, vincristine, melphalan and prednisone on hormonally unresponsive prostatic adenocarcinoma. Twenty-five patients were evaluated and the objective response rate was 72% (18 patients). The subjective response rate was 96% (24 patients). The doses used were: 5-Fu 500 mg/week orally, methotrexate 25 mg/week orally, vincristine 1 mg/week i.v. for the first four weeks and repeated every four months, melphalan 2 mg/day orally, and prednisone 40 mg/day for the first two weeks, then tapered during two months to a daily dosage of 5–10 mg [40] (Table 18).

4.12 *Bleomycin, 5-Fu, methotrexate, vincristine and prednisone*

Eight patients were involved in a study to evaluate bleomycin, 5-Fu, methotrexate, vincristine and prednisone on hormonally unresponsive pros-

Table 18.

Study (Reference)	No. of evaluable patients	Objective response		Subjective response	
		No.	%	No.	%

5-Fu, methotrexate, vincristine, melphalan, prednisone

| 40 | 25 | 18 | 72 | 24 | 96 |

Dose: 5-Fu 500 mg per week orally
methotrexate 25 mg per week orally
vincristine 1 mg per week i.v. for first 4 weeks and repeated every four months
melphalan 2 mg per day orally
prednisone 40 mg per day for first 2 weeks, then tapered during 2 months to daily dosage of 5–10 mg

Bleomycin, 5-Fu, methotrexate, vincristine, prednisone

| 43 | 8 | 1 | 12.5 | – | – |

Dose: vincristine days 1 and 8 of each course 1 mg i.v.
bleomycin followed vincristine by 1 hr 15 mg, discontinued after total dose of 210 mg
methotrexate 20 mg/m^2 p.o. days 2, 9, 16 of each course
prednisone 40 mg daily for 7 days, then tapered by 5 mg/week to 10 mg daily maintenance dose
5-Fu 500 mg/week orally

tatic adenocarcinoma. Objective response rate of 12.5% was obtained and no subjective responses were listed. The doses were as follows:

vincristine: days 1 and 8 of each course at 1 mg i.v.
bleomycin: followed vincristine by one hour at 15 mg, and was discontinued after a total dose of 210 mg
methotrexate: 20 mg/m^2 p.o. on days 2, 9 and 16 of each course
prednisone: 40 mg daily for seven days, then tapered by 5 mg/week to 10 mg daily maintenance dose
5-Fu: 500 mg/week orally [43] (Table 18).

During the last 10 to 15 years several studies have been initiated by various oncologic groups in a prospective fashion. The National Prostatic Cancer Project initially took the lead in this and has been instrumental in developing programs and protocols for the treatment of patients with prostatic carcinoma. As can be seen in several of the tables above, many patients experienced subjective responses and had objective improvement. Responses had included relief of pain, relief of hydronephrosis, improvement in their general condition, and stabilization or improvement in various biochemical parameters associated with metastatic prostatic carcinoma. 5-fluorouracil, cyclophosphamide and adriamycin have all been shown to be useful single agent therapies in 20% to 40–50% of patients treated. Mainly, patients have had partial responses and stabilization of disease. Combination chemotherapeutic agents including Emcyt (estramustine), a combination of estrogen and nitrogen mustard, and the combination of cyclophosphamide, 5-fluorouracil and adriamycin have also led to a high number of objective responders as well as a large number of patients who remain as subjective responders. Toxicities in these patients with metastatic prostatic carcinoma treated with various chemotherapeutic agents have been observed and various biochemical hematologic parameters must be monitored so as to avoid unnecessary toxicities. In all of the studies utilizing chemotherapy, these patients have had metastatic prostatic carcinoma unresponsive to hormonal manipulation, either orchiectomy or estrogen administration. Currently, several protocols are evaluating the use of early hormonal manipulation with chemotherapy, either single agent therapy or combination treatment in patients with stage D carcinoma. Perhaps this treatment rationale will yield longer survivorships of patients with newly diagnosed stage D carcinoma of the prostate and may lead to a higher percentage of patients with partial responses and, hopefully, some patients with complete responses. At present, patients who have failed hormonal therapy should be considered candidates for combination or single agent chemotherapy with the rationale that, at least, chemotherapeutic agents have served as a major modality for the reduction in pain and the decreased need for massive doses of analgesics, and second, that in a varying percentage of patients partial responses are seen. A large percentage of patients do remain stable in terms of disease progression for longer periods of time than the patients who are untreated, and an occasional long-term responder will be seen.

Promising new chemotherapeutic agents and new combinations must be evaluated in a prospective manner and strict criteria applied to the evaluation of such treatments so that an accurate comparison can be made between new treatments and protocols that have been previously utilized.

5. ANTI-ANDROGENS

The two most commonly used anti-androgens have been cyproterone acetate and flutamide (Sch 13521). Anti-adrogens have the effect of blocking the action of androgens at the target level by interfering with the intracellular events relating to androgenic action. These agents have been shown to be capable of blocking both exogenously administered androgen and endogenously secreted androgens [69–71]. No specific benefit has been observed with the use of cyproterone acetate in patients who have been previously treated with hormones or orchiectomy and have become unresponsive [72, 73]. Flutamide, similarly, has been evaluated by several investigators and also has been shown to have no more effect than standard hormonal treatment in the management of unresponsive stage D carcinoma of the prostate patients [71, 74, 75]. Its mechanism of action is that it interferes with the cellular uptake of testosterone and probably inhibits binding of 5-dihydrotestosterone via a cytosol receptor protein. It does have certain advantages over traditional hormonal therapies in that there is less fluid retention and a decreased incidence of thromboembolic effects [71, 74].

6. AMINOGLUTETHIMIDE

In stage D prostatic carcinoma patients with progression after primary hormonal therapy, a variety of medical treatments including chemotherapy, anti-androgens, and enzyme inhibitors as well as secondary major surgical ablative procedures such as hypophysectomy and adrenalectomy have been used with more or less equal success [75]. One can see from the previous description of the chemotherapeutic agents that the success rate varies from zero to as high as 61%. Median response rate for chemotherapy in patients who have become unresponsive after initial hormonal manipulation approximates 20–30%. Absolute comparisons of responses of various therapies is complicated by the wide variability in each patient's manifestations of their metastatic disease as well as their variability in response criteria used by different investigators. We have developed a 'medical adrenalectomy' using aminoglutethimide, an inhibitor of adrenal steroid biosynthesis and physiologic replacement of hydrocortisone [76–78]. The use of aminoglutethimide has been successful in treatment of metastatic breast carcinoma and has been previously reported in a smaller number of patients treated for stage D prostatic carcinoma [77–79]. Data on the most recent update of patients treated with aminoglutethimide include 39 patients, of which one is complete responder for more than 290 weeks, six patients are in the category of partial objective response, and 12 patients are objectively stable. This represents 48% of the patients who would be considered positive responders when utilizing the National Prostatic Cancer Project criteria. The range of the patients who have been partial objective responders is from 30 to 180 weeks, and the range of those patients who are objectively stable is 20–52 weeks, with a mean duration of response of 29 weeks. Forty-six percent of the patients, or 18, have progressed while on therapy. One patient has been lost to follow-up and one has been lost due to drug intolerance. All patients had been previously castrate, 92% had been tried on estrogen therapy, 10% had received previous chemotherapy, and 62% of the patients had received palliative radiation therapy. The main areas of metastatic involvement in this group of patients were: bone in 100%, liver and lung in 4%, extensive pelvic prostatic cancer in 8 % resulting in ureteral obstruction, and in one patient vena caval obstruction. The side effects of this drug regime have been well tolerated and have included nausea in roughly 30 %, a rash in one patient, and lethargy in approximately 40 % of the patients. Lethargy is one of the more pronounced side effects that can be ameliorated with decreasing the drug dosage and building tolerance up. However, our one drug intolerance patient did not show the expected response and continued to be lethargic even on small doses of aminoglutethimide, and therefore was discontinued. The response rate of the use of aminoglutethimide has compared favorably to patients treated with standard chemotherapy. A significant decrease in serum testosterone and dihydrotestosterone concentrations has been observed after aminoglutethimide therapy. Current evaluations do include the combination of aminoglutethimide and chemotherapy to see if improvements upon these results can be appreciated.

7. THE USE OF ANIMAL MODEL SYSTEMS FOR PROSTATIC ADENOCARCINOMA

As has been mentioned already in this chapter, chemotherapeutic trials have only come into vogue in the last 10–15 years. Several agents that are clinically active against other malignancies have not been studied extensively either as single agents or in combination treatment programs in patients with prostatic adenocarcinoma. The use of animal model systems may be beneficial not only in defining more clearly the relationship of the tumor – host response but also as a testing station for various chemotherapeutic programs [80–84]. Unfortunately, the ideal animal for the study of prostatic carcinoma does not exist today. However, there are several model systems that have aided in our understanding of receptors, tumor biology, and perhaps in predicting clinical response to various chemotherapeutic programs. The most commonly used models include the Noble rat, the Dunning-Copenhagen rat, the germ-free Wister rat prostatic model, and the AXC rat adenocarcinoma model. These model systems have both androgen-sensitive and androgen-insensitive tumor types and do allow for the evaluation of treatment programs involving both hormonal and chemotherapeutic treatments as well as the use of combination hormonal and chemotherapeutic treatments in the same tumor line. Hypothetically, perhaps through the use of these model systems the urologic community can gain some insight into various combinations including hormonal manipulation and chemotherapy treatments utilized together rather than sequentially. Future work in these areas is obviously necessary to prove or disprove their merit. This unit has extensively studied the Noble rat adenocarcinoma model system's response to chemotherapeutic and hormonal treatments and has found that the response rates generally parallel those seen clinically when treating patients with adenocarcinoma of the prostate [85].

8. FUTURE CLINICAL TRIALS

Partial tumor regression has been reported in patients treated with the various chemotherapeutic agents, either singly or in combination as mentioned above. Remissions of significant duration have been reported; however, they are not common. Recent evidence suggests that solid tumors are not responsive to chemotherapy because many of the malignant cells are either not cycling (Go) or cycled at a very small rate. Various protocols are currently being evaluated to determine whether or not the combination of hormonal manipulation and chemotherapy at an early stage of the disease might prove beneficial at a time at which the tumor burden is not large. Recently, Murphy et al. have reported the results of a randomized prospective trial (Protocol 500) conducted by the NPCP from July 1976 to September 1980. Criterion for entrance of patients was newly diagnosed, progressing metastatic stage D prostatic carcinoma with bony or demonstrable soft tissue metastasis that has not received any prior antitumor or prior hormonal therapy. The treatment arms of this protocol included diethylstilbestrol (DES) 1 mg orally three times a day or orchiectomy, DES, plus cyclophosphamide 1 mg/m^2 i.v. every three weeks or estramustine phosphate (Estracyt, EMCYT) 600 mg/m^2 orally in three divided doses plus cyclophosphamide (same dose schedule as arm above). Median survival times for all groups were 92, 91 and 94 weeks. The progression-free interval for responders in this protocol showed no difference between initial treatments, although nearly one half of patients are still in remission; hence, additional follow-up is necessary. Objective response rates for each treatment arm revealed no statistically significant differences. This protocol has begun to evaluate the use of combination therapy, hormones and chemotherapy in attempts at attacking the heterogeneous population of cells in prostate cancer patients' androgen-sensitive and androgen-insensitive cells. The advantage in survival for treatments containing anti-neoplastic agents in this protocol over hormonal therapy alone is nearly significant in terms of overall survival, but not yet statistically significant. Longer follow-up may prove this approach to be very useful in the early treatment of patients with stage D cancer of the prostate [86]. Additional protocols are being evaluated to see if it is possible to move the (Go) cells into a more active state of replication by means of stimulation with an androgen. Currently, our unit is evaluating the use of non-aromatizable androgens, fluoxymesterone, an oral androgen that can act without conversion to estrogen yet can suppress luteinizing hormone-releasing hormone (LH-RH). Cells so stimulated are then exposed to combinations of potent active chemotherapeutic agents. Currently, we are using 5-fluorouracil, adriamycin and cyclophosphamide in this study. These two protocols have too few patients to comment upon or perhaps can add to our results with future clinical trials in adequate numbers from which to draw conclusions.

REFERENCES

1. Williams SD, Einhorn LH: Prostate cancer: The current approach to diagnosis and treatment. Chicago: Bristol Laboratories, 1980.
2. Coffey DS et al.: Prostate tumor biology and cell kinetics – theory. Urology (Suppl) 17(3):40-53, 1981.
3. Gibbons RP: Cooperative clinical trial of single and combined agents protocols: Adjuvant protocols. Urology (Suppl) 17(4):48-52, 1981.
4. Schmidt JD, Gibbons RP, Johnson DE et al.: Chemotherapy of advanced prostatic cancer: Evaluation of response parameters. Urology 7:602-610, 1976.
5. Kiely JM: Clinical pharmacology: 12. Antineoplastic agents. Mayo Clin Proc 56:384-392, 1981.
6. Goodman LS, Gilman A: The Pharmacological Basis of Therapeutics, 5th ed. New York: MacMillan Publishing Co, 1975.
7. Scott WW, Johnson DE, Schmidt JE et al.: Chemotherapy of advanced prostatic carcinoma with cyclophosphamide or 5-Fu: Results of first national randomized study. J Urol 114:909-911, 1975.
8. Blum RH, Carter SK: Adriamycin: A new anticancer drug with significant clinical activity. Ann Intern Med 80:249-259, 1974.
9. Adamson RH: Daunomycin (NSC-82151) and Adriamycin (NSC-123127). An hypothesis concerning antitumor activity and cardiotoxicity (Letter to the editor). Cancer Chemother Rep 58:293-294, 1974.
10. Rinehart JJ, Lewis RP, Bakerzak SP: Adriamycin cardiotoxicity in man. Ann Intern Med 81:475-478, 1974.
11. Herr HW: Cyclophosphamide, methotrexate, and 5-Fu. Combination chemotherapy vs. chloroethylcyclohexynitrosourea in the treatment of metastatic prostate cancer. J Urol 127:462-465, 1982.
12. Bleyer WA: Methotrexate: Clinical pharmacology, current status, and therapeutic guidelines. Cancer Treat Rev 4:87-101, 1977.
13. Bleyer WA: The clinical pharmacology of methotrexate. New applications of an old drug. Cancer 41:36-51, 1978.
14. Skarin AT, Zuckerman KS, Pittman SW, Rosenthal DS, Moloney W, Frei E, III, Canelos GP: High dose methotrexate with folinic acid in the treatment of advanced non-Hodgkin lymphoma including CNS involvement. Blood 50:1039-1047, 1977.
15. Slack NH, Brady MF, Murphy GP: Observations of prolonged use of oral Emcyt in prostatic cancer patients. Urology 20(5):515-523, 1982.
16. Smalley RV, Bartolucci AA et al.: A phase II evaluation of a 3-drug combination of cyclophosphamide, doxorubicin and 5-fluorouracil and of 5-fluorouracil in patients with advanced bladder carcinoma or stage D prostatic carcinoma. J Urol 125:191-195, 1981.
17. Scott WW, Gibbons RP, Johnson DE, Prout GR, Schmidt JD, Saroff J, Murphy GP: The continued evaluation of the effects of chemotherapy in patients with advanced carcinoma of the prostate. J Urol 116:211-213, 1976.

74

18. Chlebowski RT, Hestorff R, Sardoff L, Weiner J, Bateman JR: Cyclophosphamide (NSC-26271) vs. the combination of adriamycin (NSC-123127), 5-fluorouracil (NSC-19893), and cyclophosphamide in the treatment of metastatic prostate Ca. Cancer 42:2546-2552, 1978.
19. Eagan RT, Hahn RG, Myers PP: Adriamycin vs. 5-Fu and cyclophosphamide in the treatment of metastatic prostate cancer. Cancer Treat Rep 60:115-117, 1976.
20. Collier D, Soloway MS: Doxorubicin hydrochloride, cyclophosphamide, and 5-Fu combination in advanced prostate and transitional cell carcinoma. Urology 8:459-464, 1976.
21. Merrin C, Etra W, Wajsman Z, Baumgartner G, Murphy G: Chemotherapy of advanced carcinoma of the prostate with 5-fluorouracil, cyclophosphamide and adriamycin. J Urol 115:86-88, 1976.
22. White R, Babaian RK, Feldman M, Krane RJ, Olsson CA: Adjunctive therapy with interstitial irradiation for prostate cancer. Urology 19(4):395-398, 1982.
23. Schmidt JD, Scott WW, Gibbons RP, Johnson DE, Prout GR Jr, Loening SA, Soloway MS, Chu TM, Gaeta JF, Slack NH, Saroff J, Murphy GP: Comparison of procarbazine, imidazole-carboxamide and cyclophosphamide in relapsing patients with advanced carcinoma of the prostate. J Urol 121:185-189, 1979.
24. Loening SA, Scott WW, DeKernion J, Gibbons RP, Johnson DE, Pontes JE, Prout GR, Schmidt JD, Soloway MS, Chu TM, Gaeta JR, Slack NH, Murphy GP: A comparison of hydroxyurea, methyl-chloroethyl-cyclohexy-nitrosourea and cyclophosphamode in patients with advanced carcinoma of the prostate. J Urol 125:812-816, 1981.
25. Muss HB, Howard V, Richards F, White DR, Jackson DV, Cooper MR, Stuart JJ, Resnick MI, Brodkin R, Spurr CL: Cyclophosphamide versus cyclophosphamide, methotrexate, and 5-fluorouracil in advanced prostatic cancer: A randomized trial. Cancer 47:1949-1953, 1981.
26. Carter SK, Wasserman TH: The chemotherapy or urologic cancer. Cancer 36:729-747, 1975.
27. Neuin JE, Hoffman AA: Use of arterial infusion of 5-Fu either alone or in combination with supervoltage radiation as a treatment for carcinoma of the prostate and bladder. Am J Surg 130:544-549, 1975.
28. Neuin JE, Melnick I, Baggerly JT Jr, Hoffman A, Landes RR, Easly C: The continuous arterial infusion of 5-fluorouracil as a therapeutic adjunct in the treatment of advanced carcinoma of the bladder and prostate: A preliminary report. Cancer 31:138-144, 1973.
29. Scott WW, Gibbons RP, Johnson DE, Prout GR, Schmidt JD, Chu TM, Gaeta JF, Joiner J, Saroff J, Murphy GP: Comparison of 5-fluorouracil (NSC-19893) and cyclophosphamide (NSC-26271) in patients with advanced carcinoma of the prostate. Cancer Chemother Rep 59:195-201, 1975.
30. DeWys WD, Bauer M, Colsky J, Cooper RA, Creech R, Carbone PP: Comparative trial of adriamycin and 5-Fu in advanced prostatic cancer – progress report. Cancer Treat Rep 61:325-328, 1977.
31. Benson RC, Ward JB, Gill GM: Treatment of stage D hormone-resistant carcinoma of the prostate with estramustine phosphate. J Urol 121:452-454, 1979.
32. Kuss R, Khoury S, Richard F, Fourcade R, Frantz P, Capelle JP: Estrogen-resistant prostate cancer with osseous metastasis: Pallative chemotherapy by 5-fluorouracil and cyclophosphamide. Nouv Presse Med 7:24-78, 1978.
33. Soloway MS, DeKernion JB, Gibbons RP, Johnson DE, Loening SA, Pontes JE, Proute GR, Schmidt JD, Scott WW, Chu TM, Gaeta JF, Slack NH, Murphy GP: Comparison of estramustine phosphate and vincristine alone or in combination for patients with advanced, hormone refractory, previously irradiated carcinoma of the prostate. J Urol 125:664-667, 1981.

34. Schmidt J: Chemotherapy of hormone-resistant stage D prostatic cancer. J Urol 123:797-805, 1980.

35. Murphy GP, Saroff J, Joiner JR, Prout GR, Gibbons RP, Schmidt JD, Johnson DE, Scott WW: Chemotherapy of advanced prostatic cancer by the National Prostatic Cancer Group. Semin Oncol 3(2):103-106, 1976.

36. Slack NH, Wajsman Z, Mittelman A, Bruno S, Murphy GP: Relationship of prior hormonal therapy to subsequent estramustine phosphate treatment in advanced prostatic cancer. Urology 14:549-554, 1979.

37. Kuss R, Khoury S, Richard F, Fourcade F, Frantz P, Capelle JP: Estramustine phosphate in the treatment of advanced prostatic cancer. Br J Urol 52:29-33, 1980.

38. Ihde DC, Bunn PA, Cohen MH, Dunnock NR, Eddy JL, Minna JD: Effective treatment of hormonally unresponsive metastatic carcinoma of the prostate with adriamycin and cyclophosphamide. Cancer 45:1300-1310, 1980.

39. Mukamel E, Nissenkorn I, Servadio C: Early combined hormonal and chemotherapy for metastatic carcinoma of prostate. Urology 16(3):257-260, 1980.

40. Kane RD, Stocks LH, Paulson DF: Multiple drug chemotherapy regimen for patients with hormonally unresponsive carcinoma of the prostate: A preliminary report. J Urol 117:467-471, 1977.

41. O'Bryan RM, Baker LH, Gottlieb JE, Balcerzak SP, Grumet GN, Salmon SC, Moon TE, Hoogstraten B: Dose response evaluation of adriamycin in human neoplasia. Cancer 39:1940-1948, 1977.

42. DeWys WD: Comparison of adriamycin (NSC-123127) and 5-fluorouracil (NSC-019893) in advanced prostatic cancer. Cancer Chemother Rep 59:215-217, 1975.

43. Paulson DF, Walker RA, Berry WR, Cox EB, Hinshaw W: Vincristine, belomycin, methotrexate, 5-Fu and prednisone in metastatic, hormonally unresponsive prostatic adenocarcinoma. Urology 17(5):443-445, 1981.

44. Fossa SD, Miller A: Treatment of advanced carcinoma of the prostate with estramustine phosphate. J Urol 115:406-408, 1976.

45. Mittleman A, Shukla SK, Murphy GP: Extended therapy of stage D carcinoma of the prostate with oral estramustine phosphate. J Urol 115:409-412, 1976.

46. Chisholm GD, O'Donoghue PN, Kennedy CL: The treatment of oestrogen-escaped carcinoma of the prostate with estramustine phosphate. Br J Urol 49:717-720, 1977.

47. Von Hoff DD, Rozencweig M, Slavik M, Muggia FM: Estramustine phosphate: A specific therapeutic agent? J Urol 177:464-466, 1977.

48. Merrin C: Treatment of advanced carcinoma of the prostate (stage D) with infusion of cis-diamminedichloroplatinum (II NSC-119875): A pilot study. J Urol 119:522-524, 1978.

49. Merrin CE, Beckley S: The treatment of estrogen-resistant stage D carcinoma of the prostate with cis-diamminedichloroplatinum. Urology 13:267-272, 1979.

50. Beckley S, Wajsman Z, Maeso E, Pontes E, Murphy G: Estramustine phosphate with multiple cytotoxic agents in treatment of advanced prostatic cancer. Urology 18(6):592-595, 1981.

51. Houghton AL, Robinson MR, Smith PH: Melphalan in advanced prostatic cancer: A pilot study. Cancer Treat Rep 61:923-925, 1977.

52. Torti FM, Carter SK: The chemotherapy of prostatic adenocarcinoma. Ann Intern Med 92:681-689, 1980.

53. Spector RE: Chemotherapy of prostatic cancer. J Iowa Med Soc 6:168-172, 1978.

54. Veronesi A, Zattoni F, Frustaci S, Gallagioni E, Tirelli U, Trovo G, Tumolo S, Merlo A, Artuso G, Cosciani-Cunico S, Grigoletto E: Estramustine phosphate (Estracyt®) treatment of T_3-T_4 prostatic cancer. Prostate 3:159-164, 1982.

55. Citrin DL, Cohen AI, Harberg J, Schlise S, Hougen C, Benson R: Systemic treatment of advanced prostatic cancer: Development of a new system for defining responses. J Urol 125:224-227, 1981.
56. Yagoda A, Watson RC, Natale RB, Burzell W, Sogani P, Grabstald H, Whitmore WF: A critical analysis of response criteria in patients with prostatic cancer treated with cis-diamminedichloride platinum II. Cancer 44:1553-1562, 1979.
57. Schmidt JD, Scott WW, Gibbons R, Johnson DE, Prout GR, Loening S, Soloway M, DeKernion J, Pontes JE, Slack NH, Murphy GP: Chemotherapy programs of the National Prostatic Cancer Project (NPCP). Cancer 45:1937-1946, 1980.
58. Rossof AH, Talley RW, Stephens R et al.: Phase II evaluation of cis-dichlorodiammineplatinum (II) in advanced malignancies of the genitourinary and gynecologic organs: A Southwest Oncology Group Study. Cancer Treat Rep 63:1557-1564, 1979.
59. Soloway MS, Tidwell M: Cytoxan, adriamycin and 5-fluorouracil combination chemotherapy in advanced cancer of the prostate. Proc Am Assoc Cancer Res 18:2-9, 1977.
60. Strauss MJ, Parmelee J, Olsson C, DeVere R, White R: Cytoxan, adriamycin, methotrexate (CAM) therapy of stage D prostate cancer. Proc Am Soc Clin Oncol 19:314-318, 1978.
61. Perloff M, Ohnuma T, Holland JF et al.: Adriamycin (ADM) and diamminedichloroplatinum (DDP) in advanced prostatic carcinoma (PC). Proc Am Soc Clin Oncol 18:333-337, 1977.
62. DeWys WD, Bogg CG: Comparison of adiramycin (ADRIA) and 5-fluorouracil (5-Fu) in advanced prostatic cancer. Proc Am Soc Clin Oncol 19:331-332, 1977.
63. Lerner HJ, Malloy TR: Hydroxyurea in stage D carcinoma of prostate. Urology 10:35-38, 1977.
64. Catane R, Kaufman JH, Magajewicz S, Mittleman A, Murphy GP: Prednimustine therapy for advanced prostatic carcinoma. Br J Urol 50:29-32, 1978.
65. Murphy GP, Gibbons RP, Johnson DE, Prout GR, Schmidt JD, Soloway MS, Loening SA, Chu TM, Gaeta JF, Saroff J, Wajsman Z, Slack N, Scott WW: The use of estramustine and prednimustine versis prednimustine alone in advanced metastatic prostatic cancer patients who have received prior irradiation. J Urol 121:763-766, 1977.
66. Tejada F, Eisenberger MA, Broder LA, Cohen MH, Simon R: 5-Fluorouracil versus CCNU in the treatment of metastatic prostatic cancer. Cancer Treat Rep 61:1589-1590, 1977.
67. Slack NH et al.: Prednimustine for prostate cancer therapy. Compr Ther 5(9):54-57, 1979.
68. Lerner H, Malloy T, Cromie W et al.: Hydroxyurea in stage D carcinoma of the prostate: A pilot study. J Urol 114:425-429, 1975.
69. Fang S, Liao S: Antagonistic action of anti-androgens on the formation of a specific dihydrotestosterone-receptor protein complex in rat ventral prostate. Mol Pharmacol 5:428-432, 1969.
70. Walsh PC, Korenman SG: Mechanism of androgenic action: Effect of specific intracellular inhibitors. J Urol 105:850-854, 1971.
71. Neri R, Florance K, Koziol P et al.: A biological profile of a non-steroidal antiandrogen SCH 13521 (4'-nitro-3'-trifluoromethylisobutyranilide). Endocrinology 93:427-428, 1972.
72. Smith RB, Walsh PC, Goodwin WE: Cyproterone acetate in the treatment of advanced carcinoma of the prostate. J Urol 110:106-111, 1973.
73. Geller J, Vazakas G, Fruchtman B et al.: The effect of cyproterone acetate on advanced carcinoma of the prostate. Surg Gynecol Obstet 127:748-753, 1968.
74. Stoliar B, Albert DJ: SCH 13521 in the treatment of advanced carcinoma of the prostate. Urology 111:803-807, 1974.
75. Resnick MI, Grayhack JT: Treatment of stage IV carcinoma of the prostate. Urol Clin North Am 2:141-160, 1975.

76. Santen RJ, Worgul TJ, Samojlik E, Interrante A, Boucher AE, Lipton A, Harvey HA, White DS, Smart E, Cox C, Wells SA: A randomized trial comparing surgical adrenalectomy with aminoglutethimide plus hydrocortisone in women with advanced breast cancer. N Engl J Med 305:545-549, 1981.

77. Santen RJ, Worgul TJ, Harvey H, Lipton A, Smart E, Boucher A, White D, Wells S: Aminoglutethimide as treatment of postmenopausal women with advanced breast carcinoma: Correlation of clinical and hormonal responses. Ann Intern Med (in press).

78. Sanford EJ, Drago JR, Rohner TJ Jr, Santen R, Lipton A: Aminoglutethimide medical adrenalectomy for advanced prostatic carcinoma. J Urol 115:170-174, 1976.

79. Worgul TJ, Santen RJ, Samojlik E, Veldhuis JD, Lipton A, Harvey HA, Drago JR, Rohner TJ: The clinical and biochemical effect of aminoglutethimide in the treatment of advanced prostatic carcinoma. J Urol (in press).

80. Noble RL: Tumors and hormones. In: Hormones, Pincus G (ed). New York: Academic Press, Vol 5, pp 559-579, 1964.

81. Pollard N, Luckert PH: Transplantable metastasizing prostate adenocarcinomas in rats. J Natl Cancer Inst 54:643-649, 1975.

82. Smolev KJ, Heston W, Scott WW et al.: Characterization of the Dunning R3327H prostatic adenocarcinoma: An appropriate animal model for prostatic cancer. Cancer Treat Rep 61:273-287, 1977.

83. Drago JR, Ikeda RM, Maurer RE, Goldman LB, Tesluk H: The Nb rat: Prostatic adenocarcinoma model. Invest Urol 16(5):353-359, 1979.

84. Shain SA, Boesel RW, Axelrod LA: Aging in the rat prostate. Reduction in detectable ventral prostate androgen receptor content. Arch Biochem Biophys 167:247-263, 1975.

85. Drago JR, Goldman LB, Gershwin ME: Chemotherapeutic and hormonal considerations of the Nb rat prostatic adenocarcinoma model. In: Models for Prostatic Cancer. New York: Alan R Liss, Inc, pp 325-363, 1980.

86. Murphy GP et al.: Treatment of newly diagnosed metastatic prostate cancer patients with chemotherapy agents in combination with hormones, versus hormones alone. Cancer 51:86-94, 1983.

Editorial Comment

JACK S. ELDER

1. INTRODUCTION

Dr Drago has presented a thorough summary of the reported clinical trials investigating the treatment of hormone-resistant prostatic cancer with single or combination drug cytotoxic chemotherapy. The results indicate that several drugs exhibit minor activity and a few drug combinations may be promising. A combination which was not mentioned is doxorubicin, mitomycin-C, and 5-Fu (DMF) which was evaluated recently at M.D. Anderson Hospital [1]. Of their 15 initial patients, nine (60%) showed a partial response and two additional patients were considered stable. Six of the nine responding patients had non-osseous metastases, and only three of the nine patients with osseous metastases alone had a partial regression.

The current results of chemotherapy in prostatic cancer cannot be compared to the results obtained with chemotherapy in certain other solid tumors such as testicular cancer or Hodgkin's disease. There have only been a handful of reported complete or nearly complete responses by hormone-resistant tumors to chemotherapy, and at present most of these patients can only look forward to a mean period of 6–12 months of improvement in quality of life or palliation with chemotherapy. I would like to review the reasons for these results plus other potential applications of chemotherapy in prostatic cancer.

2. CURRENT STATUS OF CHEMOTHERAPY IN PROSTATIC CANCER

Prostatic cancer is an aggressive disease that primarily affects older men. It constitutes the third leading cause of cancer death in men between 55 and 74 years of age and is second in men over 75 years [2]. Patients in these age groups are also susceptible to a variety of common medical conditions which may limit the amount of cancer therapy they may tolerate or which often result in patient demise prior to the malignancy. In fact, heart disease, cerebrovascular disease, pneumonia, chronic obstructive lung disease, and cirrhosis are more common causes of death than prostatic cancer in patients over 55 years [2].

In a recent survey by the American College of Surgeons' Commission on Cancer, 40%–54% of patients with prostatic cancer had stage C or D tumors [3], and in an older study by the VA Cooperative Group, greater than 80% had stage C or D disease [4], generally incurable with current therapy. Efforts at control of these extensive tumors have been directed at palliation, e.g., relief of obstructive symptoms from a bulky tumor by radiation therapy [5] or total prostatectomy [6] or relief of painful bony metastases by hormonal therapy [7]. These treatments often are successful in resolving the symptomatic problem temporarily but infrequently achieve regression or cure, which is the goal in more localized tumors in men less than 70 years without complicated medical problems.

These palliative treatments allow many patients with stage C and D tumors to live *with* their tumors for months to several years while remaining free of severe tumor-related symptoms or suffering from side effects of treatment. However, ultimately the hormone-resistant cells proliferate and result in painful metastases, anorexia, malaise, anemia, and other symptoms of systemic disease. It is at this terminal stage that chemotherapy has been utilized. At this late stage, which has been termed *stage E* [8], chemotherapy has shown some benefit in terms of subjective response with stabilization or occasionally partial regression of metastatic disease [9], but these results cannot be compared to the success obtained with chemotherapy in such solid tumors as testicular cancer and Hodgkin's lymphoma. There are several reasons for this:

1. First, cytotoxic chemotherapy in prostatic cancer is still in early stages of evaluation. In 1973, Yagoda reviewed the chemotherapy literature in prostatic cancer and found reports of a total of only 88 patients, with objective responses seen only with a few drugs, including nitrogen mustard, cyclophosphamide, and 5-fluorouracil [10]. In 1973, a cooperative study involving six major institutions, the National Prostatic Cancer Project (NPCP), was initiated to define the role of chemotherapy in endocrine-resistant prostatic cancer. This group has increased in size to 15 institutions and has completed ten prospective studies, most of which involve single drug agents given on an outpatient basis. They have carefully reviewed their data and established criteria for complete, partial, and stable response [9]. In these patients, the first evaluation for response is performed at 12 weeks. As Drago has reviewed, numerous agents have shown responses in up to 40% to 50% of patients, but these responses infrequently are prolonged. The successful management of other types of bulky tumors usually involves cycles of multiple cytotoxic agents, however, and trials of combination therapy in prostate cancer are just beginning. It is likely that experimental work in the Dunning tumor [11] and Nb rat adenocarcinoma model [12], both in studying tumor kinetics and adjuvant therapy, will be helpful in clarifying optimal uses of chemotherapy.

2. Insofar as *most patients* currently receiving chemotherapy are hormonal therapy failures, actually they have *failed another form of chemotherapy,* (i.e., hormones), and thus would be expected to have a dismal prognosis, as would patients with metastatic testicular cancer who have already failed a course of chemotherapy.

3. Many of the patients are elderly and have complicating medical problems which may limit the amount of adjuvant therapy they can receive safely. In addition, many patients with bulky tumors develop ureteral obstruction which results in deterioration of renal function. In the administration of cis-platinum, methotrexate, streptozotocin, and cyclophosphamide when patients have diminished renal function, therapy must be reduced or stopped.

4. In order to allow outpatient treatment and to minimize systemic toxic side effects few patients receive high doses of chemotherapy. The philosophy of minimizing risk to patients during these experimental trials has been justifiably maintained. In the treatment of other solid tumors, however, chemotherapy dosages generally have been higher (Table 1).

5. Many patients have received 4 000–6 000 rads of pelvic irradiation for control of their primary tumors. This limits the amount of myelosuppressive chemotherapy a patient may receive. The NPCP has utilized only a few such agents in these patients (cis-platinum in Protocol 1200 and cyclophosphamide in Protocol 1000). Interestingly, in two recent concurrent NPCP studies evaluating cis-platinum in irradiated (>2 000 rads to pelvis) (Protocol 1200) and non-irradiated patients (Protocol 1100), 39% of non-irradiated and only 19% of the irradiated group developed leukopenia, and 4% of non-irradiated and 10% of irradiated patients developed thrombocytopenia [13, 14]. Both groups received identical dosages except that the non-irradiated group received four treatments in the first 24 days of therapy and the irradiated group

Table 1. Comparison of dosages of chemotherapeutic agents used in prostatic cancer with dosages used in other solid tumors.

Agent	CA of prostate[a]	Other solid tumors
Cyclophosphamide	1 g/m^2 i.v. q 3 wk	400 mg/m^2 i.v. daily × 5 days[b]
5-Fu	600 mg/m^2 i.v. q wk or 700 mg/m^2 i.v. q 3 wk	15–20 mg/kg q wk[c] (max. dose 1 gram)
Methotrexate	60 mg/m^2 i.v. q wk or q 2 wk	50–250 mg/kg with leucovorin rescue[d]
Cis-platinum	60 mg/m^2 4 × 1st mo then q 1 mo	20 mg/m^2 daily × 5 days Repeat 5 day cycle q 3 wk (VBP Protocol for testis CA)[e]

[a] NPCP dosages.
[b] *Cancer: Principles and Practices of Oncology.* JP Lippincott Co, p 159, 1982.
[c] Cancer 39:34–40, 1977.
[d] N Engl J Med 197:630–634, 1977.
[e] Ann Intern Med 87:293–298, 1977.

received only two treatments during that time. The cis-platinum was subsequently administered on a monthly basis. In addition, there has been no difference in hematologic toxicity secondary to cyclophosphamide in Protocols 900 and 1000 (non-irradiated and irradiated patients) *. These data suggest that patients with prior pelvic irradiation may tolerate therapeutic dosages of myelosuppressive agents safely.

The reported early results in the treatment of hormone-resistant prostatic cancer are encouraging, but on the basis of tumor kinetic studies probably will not improve significantly, even with the use of multiple agents [15]. These data point out the need for developing methods for earlier diagnosis and better treatment of localized disease.

3. TUMOR KINETICS AND PROSTATIC CANCER

Studies of tumor cell kinetics have provided an important understanding of tumor growth and treatment [16]. One important principle is that one viable cancer cell which is capable of continued growth in time may kill the host [17]. In addition, in general, a single drug treatment kills a constant percentage of the tumor cell population, regardless of the total cell number at initiation of therapy [18]. For example, a tumor that is 1 cm^3 in size contains 10^9 (1 billion) cells. A particular treatment that kills 99.99% of the tumor would still leave 100 000 viable tumor cells which would, in time, overcome the host [19].

Charbit reported that the overall mean doubling time for human cancers is 58 days, although this figure varies with tumor grade and type [20]. When one cancer cell divides 25 times, the tumor volume becomes barely detectable at 33.5 million cells or 0.03 cc, the size of a matchhead [19]. By 30 cell divisions, the tumor volume increases to 1 cc. With ten additional divisions, the tumor mass is greater than 1 liter in volume, weighing 1 kg, which often is sizable enough to kill the host. Thus, with a mean tumor doubling time of 58 days, a tumor cell will

* Unpublished data from the NPCP.

develop into the size of a matchhead in 4 years, and with unrestricted growth would develop to a lethal size of 1 liter in just 2.4 further years [19]. However, the doubling time for prostatic cancer is unknown. In addition, tumors may outgrow their vascularity with resulting central tumor necrosis, or may move out of their growth phase, which would tend to slow the growth fraction and lengthen the tumor doubling time.

The Dunning R-3327 transplantable rat prostatic adenocarcinoma tumor model has been utilized in analyzing tumor growth curves [11. 21]. As the tumor enlarges in size, its observed doubling time or growth rate decreases and appears to result from lack of proper vascularity, cell death from overcrowding, and the presence of toxins or growth inhibitory factors [19]. Prostatic cancers generally appear to have relatively slow growth rates, and probably less than 5% of the cells are in DNA synthesis at a given time [19]. Since most drugs used in chemotherapy block DNA synthesis, it is to be expected that most used as single agents have little effect against prostatic cancer. Simarly, other human solid tumors such as colon cancer and lung cancer (excluding small cell carcinoma) have doubling times of approximately 60 days and tend to be resistant to anticancer drugs; in contrast, lymphomas and testicular cancers, with doubling times of 30 days or less, and childhood cancers frequently do respond to chemotherapy [22, 23]. The Dunning model has been used to evaluate possible combinations of surgery, chemotherapy, and immunotherapy to arrest tumor growth [11]. Other in vivo and in vitro experimental tumor models suggest that, after chemotherapy, although the kinetic properties of tumor cells do not change, biologic changes may occur within the surviving cells which make them resistant to further treatment by the same cytotoxic agent. For example, in leukemias which have become resistant to methotrexate, depleted intracellular drug transport and increased levels of dihydrofolate reductase have been found [15]. Elliot and Ling have shown that a change in the structure of the tumor cell membrane following exposure to a single anticancer drug can render tumor cells impermeable to a variety of such drugs [24]. In general, larger tumors are more resistant to chemotherapy, possibly because of an increased absolute number of resistant phenotypes. One mathematical model has shown that the probability of cure from chemotherapy drops sharply as the tumor grows, from a 95% probability to a 5% probability of cure with an increase in tumor cell number of only 1.8 logs [15]. This would argue for utilizing chemotherapy at an earlier stage of the disease.

The Dunning prostatic adenocarcinoma has been useful in characterizing tumor heterogeneity, in which there are both androgen-sensitive and androgen-insensitive cell populations and cells which may or may not be capable of metastasizing. This model also appears to apply to human prostatic cancer. Approximately 80% of the Dunning R-3327-H tumor is composed of androgen-sensitive cells [21, 25]. Starting with a population of five tumor cells, four of which are androgen-sensitive, after ten cell divisions, one would expect 5×2^{10} or 5120 tumor cells, of which 2^{10} or 1024 are androgen-insensitive. If bilateral orchiectomy is performed at that point, resulting in destruction of 80% of the tumor (i.e., the androgen-sensitive cells), then 1024 cells would remain. However, after just three more tumor doublings, the hormone-insensitive tumor cells would proliferate to 8192, or 160% greater than the overall size of the tumor at the time of castration. This illustrates what appears to occur clinically in human metastatic prostatic cancer, in that at some point following hormonal treatment the tumor recurs, resulting in a tumor which is quite resistant to further hormonal manipulation such as adrenalectomy or hypophysectomy. Thus, it would appear that orchiectomy in a patient with a tumor with 99% androgen-sensitive cells is going to result in a longer and more significant remission than a tumor with only 50% androgen-sensitive cells. Therefore, it would be useful to be able to distinguish which patients have tumors which are highly androgen-sensitive.

The prognosis for men with newly diagnosed metastatic prostatic cancer is quite variable: with hormonal therapy 10% survive less than 6 months and 10% survive greater than 10 years, with mean survival approximately 3 years [26]. In a retrospective study, there was no apparent tumor or patient characteristic which helped to predict which patients would enjoy prolonged survival [27]. However, recent studies have demonstrated nuclear androgen receptor levels in needle biopsy specimens appear to predict which patients will have prolonged responses, with higher androgen receptor levels associated with prolonged responses [28]. Another predictor of response may be relative nuclear roundness, which thus far has been able to show retrospectively manner which tumors in patients with localized prostatic cancer had the greatest metastatic potential [29, 30]. Essentially all patients have a subjective response to orchiectomy [28], but only 41% exhibit a partial or complete regression (utilizing NPCP criteria) [31]. If one could predict which patients would have a long-term remission of their tumors, then the remainder could be given cytotoxic chemotherapy at an earlier stage, thus utilizing a combined (hormonal plus chemotherapy) approach primarily to yield improved long-term survival [28]. In addition, from many of the cooperative studies it is known that certain characteristics in patients with stage D disease are associated with poor prognosis, namely anemia, radiation therapy, poorly differentiated tumor, positive bone marrow biopsy, extensive skeletal metastases, metastases to the femurs, and ureteral dilatation [8, 32]. These patients probably should receive early cytotoxic therapy also. Another reason to consider using chemotherapy at the time of initiation of hormonal therapy is that early hormonal therapy alone may have an adverse effect by allowing the androgen-independent tumor cell population to increase its growth rate by eliminating the adverse effects of tumor cell mass on growth rate [33].

4. WHEN SHOULD CHEMOTHERAPY BE USED IN PROSTATIC CANCER?

At present, the primary indication for chemotherapy is in hormone-resistant metastatic tumors (i.e., 'stage E') in which several single agents in various drug combinations have shown antitumor activity. In this group of patients, chemotherapy offers slightly prolonged survival, particularly in 'responders', and an improved quality of life [34]. The only alternative is palliative therapy, such as hypophysectomy, bromocriptine, radiation therapy directed at metastatic lesions, half or total body irradiation, or administration of corticosteroids. Ideally, patients receiving chemotherapy are entered into an established clinical trial of the NPCP, SWOG, ECOG, NCI-VA Group, or a single institution study.

For the reasons brought forth in the previous discussion, it seems apparent that the process of finding an effective combination of agents against hormone-insensitive tumors will take years. In the meantime, there are agents which have significant antitumor activity which may have application in earlier stages of the disease. It will be important for urologic oncologists to carefully consider using chemotherapy in earlier stages. Often in stage C and D1 tumors in which surgery and radiation only offer palliation and occasional cure, chemotherapy is not considered because of possible toxicity, 'lack of an effective agent', and because it may take 5–10 years to show significant benefit from the chemotherapy. Although the routine use of chemotherapy presently can only be recommended for patients with hormone-resistant tumors, its utilization in earlier stages should be evaluated in careful clinical trials with strictly defined response criteria and without injudicious use of hormones. Specifically, its efficacy as an adjuvant treatment should be assessed in patients with stage A2, C, and newly diagnosed metastatic disease (including D1) who otherwise would have an expected survival of 3–5 years or more.

4.1 Newly diagnosed metastatic prostatic cancer

In the past few years, several clinical trials utilizing chemotherapy in newly diagnosed metastatic disease have been reported (Table 2) [35]. Thus far, it has been difficult to separate the hormonal effect from the effect of chemotherapy, and only three studies have utilized a control arm (i.e. DES or orchiectomy alone). These studies are still in early stages of analysis.

Table 2. Chemotherapy in newly diagnosed stage D carcinoma of the prostate.

Author	Patients	Treatment	Results	Comments
Fossa [36]	2	Estracyt	2/2 – pain relief, decreased tumor size	1 patient died at 12 months 1 patient alive at 1.5 months
Nilsson [37]	38	Estracyt	36 – 'favorable' response 16 – PR of metastases	5 stage C tumors; median survival 2 years
Merrin [38]	34	Orch + DES + cis-platinum	PR 65% Stable 32%	Objective response lasted 3–29 months Mean objective response 9.3 months Survival not reported Short follow-up
Beckley [39]	10	Orch + Estracyt + cytoxan + 5-Fu	PR 70% Stable 30%	Response 12–64 weeks; average response 42 weeks; survival not reported % failing treatment not reported
Smith [40]	107 97	Estracyt Stilbestrol	21% progression 12% progression	Admittedly early data
Benson [41]	75 79	Estracyt DES	24% progression at 1st eval 33% progression at 1st eval	Mean duration to progression: DES 515 days Estracyt 868 days
Murphy [31]	96 104	DES + cytoxan Estracyt + cytoxan	CR 8%, PR 20%, stable 55% CR 8%, PR 17%, stable 57%	Duration of response: mean 79 wks Duration of response: means 83 wks
	101	DES/Orch	CR 12%, PR 29%, stable 40%	Duration of response: mean 92 wks
Servadio [42]	24	Orch + DES + 5-Fu + cytoxan	21/24 – acid phos returned to normal 19/24 – stabilization or regression of metastases	5 failed hormonal therapy Follow-up 42–72 mo; 63% 'cumulative' survival at 5 yrs and 51% at 6 yrs

PR = partial regression
CR = complete regression

4.2 *Stage D1 tumors*

At present, it is unclear whether radiation therapy is of benefit either in terms of prolonging the time to tumor progression or prolonging survival [43, 44]. In addition, radical prostatectomy in these patients has not been shown to increase survival [45]. deVere White and associates have reported a series of patients receiving interstitial [121]I with D1 disease in which only three of nine patients receiving adjuvant cyclophosphamide plus doxorubicin for 6 months developed distant metastases while six of seven not receiving chemotherapy showed disease progression [46]. Although the series is small, it demonstrates the potential benefits of chemotherapy in D1 disease. The NPCP currently has a protocol evaluating adjuvant estramustine phosphate and cyclophosphamide, in patients with B2, C, or D1 tumors undergoing radiation therapy.

4.3 *Radiorecurrent tumors*

Patients who have had radiation therapy to the prostate and/or hormonal therapy who develop obstructive symptoms, hematuria, or hydronephrosis secondary to ureteral obstruction may be candidates for hypogastric artery infusion of cis-platinum [47] or 5-Fu [48]. Scardino reported complete disappearance of local tumor in 2 of 15 patients with monthly infusions of cis-platinum. This type of treatment might be useful in the presence of recurrent or persistent local disease following external beam radiotherapy, interstitial ^{125}I, or [198]Au plus external radiation. Approximately one half of patients undergong ^{125}I therapy have biopsy-proven tumor 1 year or more after treatment [49], and following [198]Au plus external radiotherapy, biopsy-proven tumor is associated with decreased survival [50]. Giving adjuvant chemotherapy in this setting might result in significant local tumor destruction and delay or prevent later onset of metastatic disease.

4.4 *Radical prostatectomy with seminal vesicle invasion*

The optimal management of men with clinical stage B disease with expected survival of 10–15 years is radical prostatectomy [51]. In approximately 5% of clinical stage B1 tumors and in one half of clinical B2 tumors, seminal vesicle invasion is present [52, 53]. The outlook for these patients is poor, with only a 10% 15-year survival rate, compared to 50% 15-year tumor-free survival in patients with pathologic B tumors undergoing radical prostatectomy [53]. Postoperative radiation therapy has been utilized in those patients with pathologic C tumors [54]. Alternatively, this group might benefit from a short course of chemotherapy by hypogastric artery infusion or systemic chemotherapy postoperatively with less morbidity than radiation therapy. In colon cancer, umbilical vein perfusion of 5-Fu for 7 days postcolectomy has resulted in a significantly diminished incidence of liver metastases and tumor-related deaths [55]. In addition, in localized breast cancer, Nissen-Meyer reported the use of postoperative cyclophosphamide immediately after mastectomy and demonstrated a lower tumor recurrence rate and death rate from metastatic disease [56]. Finally, there is experimental evidence supporting adjuvant chemotherapy following surgery for prostatic cancer [57]. Thus, *some* patients with locally extensive prostatic cancer may benefit from postoperative local or systemic chemotherapy and clinical trials are encouraged.

In conclusion, chemotherapy in prostatic cancer is still in its early stages of evaluation and a 'magic bullet' which would provide prolonged objective remission in large numbers of men awaits discovery. In the meantime, some of the agents which have demonstrated antitumor activity in 'stage E' tumors may have benefit in earlier stages of the disease and should be evaluated.

REFERENCES

1. Logothetis CJ, von Eschenbach AC, Samuels ML, Trindade A, Johnson DE: Doxorubicin, mitomycin, and 5-Fu (DMF) in the treatment of hormone-resistant stage D prostate cancer: A preliminary report. Cancer Treat Rep 66:57-63, 1982.

2. Silverberg E: Cancer statistics. CA 32:15-31, 1982.
3. Murphy GP: Prostate cancer today. Urology 17 (March Suppl):1-3, 1981.
4. Veterans Administration Cooperative Urological Research Group: Treatment and survival of patients with cancer of the prostate. Surg Gynecol Obstet 124:1011-1017, 1967.
5. Gibbons RP, Mason JT, Correa RJ, Cumming KB, Taylor WJ, Hafermann MD, Richardson RG: Carcinoma of the prostate: Local control with external beam radiation therapy. J Urol 121:310-312, 1979.
6. Tomlinson RL, Currie DP, Boyce WH: Radical prostatectomy: Palliation for stage C carcinoma of the prostate. J Urol 117:85-87, 1977.
7. Huggins C, Stevens RE, Hodges CV: Studies on prostatic cancer. II. The effects of castration on advanced carcinoma of the prostate gland. Arch Surg 43:209-223, 1941.
8. Menon M, Catalona WJ: Interpreting response to treatment and advanced prostatic cancer. Rev Endocrine-Related Cancer 10:11-17, 1981.
9. Schmidt JD: Chemotherapy of hormone-resistant stage D prostatic cancer. J Urol 123:797-805, 1980.
10. Yagoda A: Non-hormonal cytotoxic agents in the treatment of prostatic adenocarcinoma. Cancer 32:1131-1140, 1973.
11. Weissman RM, Coffey DS, Scott WW: Cell kinetic studies of prostatic cancer: Adjuvant therapy in animal models. Oncology 34:133-137, 1977.
12. Drago JR, Ikeda RM, Maurer RE, Goldman LB, Tesluk H: The Nb rat prostatic adenocarcinoma model. Invest Urol 16:353-359, 1979.
13. Soloway MS, Beckley S, Brady MF, Chu TM, deKernion JB, Dhabuwala C, Gaeta JF, Gibbons RP, Loening SA, McKiel CF, McLeod DG, Pontes JE, Prout GR, Scardino PT, Schlegel JU, Schmidt JD, Scott WW, Slack NH, Murphy GP: A comparison of estramustine phosphate versus cis-platinum alone versus estramustine phosphate plus cis-platinum in patients with advanced hormone refractory prostate cancer who had had extensive irradiation to the pelvis or lumbosacral area. J Urol 129:56-61, 1983.
14. Loening SA, Beckley S, Brady MF, Chu TM, deKernion JB, Dhabuwala C, Gaeta JF, Gibbons RP, McKiel CF, McLeod DG, Pontes JE, Prout GR, Scardino PT, Schlegel JU, Schmidt JD, Scott WW, Slack NH, Soloway MS, Murphy JP: Comparison of estramustine phosphate (Emcyt), methotrexate, and cis-platinum in patients with advanced, hormone-refractory prostate cancer. J Urol 129:1001-1006, 1983.
15. Goldie JH: New thoughts on resistance to chemotherapy. Hosp Pract 18(May):165-177, 1983.
16. Drewinko B, Humphrey RM (eds): Growth Kinetics and Biochemical Regulation of Normal and Malignant Cells. Baltimore: Williams and Wilkins Company, 1977.
17. Skipper HE: Thoughts on cancer chemotherapy and combination modelity therapy. JAMA 230:1033-1035, 1975.
18. Skipper HE, Schabel FM Jr, Mellett LB, Montgomery JA, Wilkoff LJ, Lloyd HH, Brockman RW: Implications of biochemical, cytokinetic, pharmacologic, and toxicologic relationships in the design of optimal therapeutic schedules. Cancer Chemother Rep 54:431-450, 1970.
19. Coffey DS, Isaacs JT: Prostate tumor biology and cell kinetics – theory. Urology 17(March suppl):40-53, 1981.
20. Charbit A, Malaise E, Tubiana M: Relation between the pathological nature and the growth rate of human tumors. Eur J Cancer 7:307-315, 1971.
21. Smolev J, Heston W, Scott W, Coffey D: Characterization of the Dunning R-3327-H prostatic adenocarcinoma: An appropriate animal model for prostatic cancer. Cancer Treat Rep 61:273-287, 1977.
22. Tannock IF: Biology of tumor growth. Hosp Pract 18(April):81-93, 1983.

86

23. Tubiana M, Malaise EP: Growth rate and cell kinetics in human tumors. In: Scientific Formulations of Oncology, Symington T, Carter RL (eds). Chicago: Yearbook Medical Publishers, pp 126-136, 1976.
24. Elliott EM, Ling V: Selection and characterization of Chinese hamster ovary cell mutants resistant to melphalan (L-phenylalanine mustard). Cancer Res 41:393-400, 1981.
25. Smolev JK, Coffey DS, Scott WW: Experimental models for the study of prostatic adeno-carcinoma. J Urol 118:217-220, 1977.
26. Jordan WP Jr, Blackard CE, Byar DP: Reconsideration of orchiectomy in the treatment of advanced prostatic carcinoma. South Med J 70:1411-1413, 1977.
27. Reiner WG, Scott WW, Eggleston JC, Walsh PC: Long-term survival after hormonal therapy for stage D prostatic cancer. J Urol 122:183-184, 1979.
28. Trachtenberg J, Walsh PC: Correlation of prostatic nuclear androgen receptor content with duration of response and survival following hormonal therapy in advanced prostatic cancer. J Urol 127:466-471, 1982.
29. Diamond DA, Berry SJ, Jewett HJ, Eggleston JC, Coffey DS: A new method to assess metastatic potential of human prostatic cancer: Relative nuclear roundness. J Urol 128:729-734, 1982.
30. Diamond DA, Berry SJ, Umbricht C, Jewett HJ, Coffey DS: Computerized image analysis of nuclear shape as a prognostic factor for prostatic cancer. Prostate 3:321-332, 1982.
31. Murphy GP, Beckley S, Chu TM, deKernion JB, Gaeta JF, Gibbons RP, Loening SA, McKiel CF, McLeod DG, Pierce JM, Pontes JE, Prout GR, Scardino PT, Schlegel JU, Schmidt JD, Scott WW, Slack NH, Soloway MS: Treatment of newly diagnosed metastatic prostate cancer patients with chemotherapy agents in combination with hormones versus hormones alone. Cancer 51:1264-1272, 1983.
32. Torti FM, Carter SK: The chemotherapy of prostatic adenocarcinoma. Ann Intern Med 92:681-689, 1980.
33. Grayhack JT, Kozlowski JN: Endocrine therapy in the management of advanced prostatic cancer: The case for early initiation of treatment. Urol Clin North Am 7:639-643, 1980.
34. Slack NH, Mittelman A, Brady MF, Murphy GP, Investigators in the National Prostatic Cancer Project: The importance of the stable category for chemotherapy-treated patients with advanced and relapsing prostate cancer. Cancer 46:2393-2402, 1980.
35. Elder JS, Catalona WJ: Management of newly diagnosed metastatic carcinoma of the prostate. Urol Clin North Am (in press).
36. Fossa SD, Miller A: Treatment of advanced carcinoma of the prostate with estramustine phosphate. J Urol 115:406-408, 1976.
37. Nilsson T, Jonsson G: Primary treatment of prostatic carcinoma with estramustine phosphate: a preliminary report. J Urol 115:168-169, 1976.
38. Merrin CE: Treatment of previously untreated (by hormonal manipulation) stage D adenocarcinoma of prostate with combined orchiectomy, estrogen, and cis-diamminedichloroplatinum. Urology 15:123-126, 1980.
39. Beckley S, Wajsman Z, Maeso E et al.: Estramustine phosphate with multiple cytotoxic agents in treatment of advanced prostatic cancer. Urology 18:592-595, 1981.
40. Smith PH: Endocrine and cytotoxic therapy. Rec Res Cancer Res 78:154-172, 1981.
41. Benson RC Jr, Gill GM, Cummings KB: A randomized double-blind cross-over trial of diethylstilbestrol (DES) and estramustine phosphate (Emcyt) for stage D prostate carcinoma. Am Urol Assoc (Abstract). Kansas City, Missouri, p 152, 1982.
42. Servadio C, Mukamel E, Lurie H, Nissenkorn I: Early combined hormonal and chemotherapy for metastatic prostatic carcinoma. Urology 21:493-495, 1983.
43. Kramer SA, Cline WA Jr, Farnham R, Carson CC, Cox EB, Hinshaw W, Paulson DC: Prognosis of patients with stage D1 prostatic adenocarcinoma. J Urol 125:817-819, 1981.

44. Paulson DF, Cline WA Jr, Coefoot RB Jr, Hinshaw W, Stephani S, Uro-Oncology Research Group: Extended field radiation therapy versus delayed hormonal therapy in node-positive prostatic adenocarcinoma. J Urol 127:935-937, 1982.

45. Zincke H, Fleming TR, Furlow WL, Myers RP, Utz BC: Radical retropubic prostatectomy and pelvic lymphadenectomy for high-stage cancer of the prostate. Cancer 47:1901-1910, 1981.

46. deVere White R, Babaian RK, Feldman M, Krane RJ, Olsson CA: Adjunctive therapy with interstitial irradiation for prostate cancer. Urology 19:395-398, 1982.

47. Scardino PT, Lehane DE: Intermittent arterial infusion chemotherapy for advanced, hormonally risistant, radiorecurrent carcinoma of the prostate. Amurol Assoc (Abstract #222). Kansas City, p 113, 1982.

48. Nevin JE, Hoffman AA: Use of arterial infusion of 5-fluorouracil either alone or in combination with supervoltage radiation as a treatment for carcinoma of the prostate and bladder. Am J Surg 130:544-549, 1975.

49. Lytton B, Collins JT, Weiss RM, Schiff M Jr, McGuire EJ, Livolsi V: Results of biopsy after early stage prostatic cancer treatment by implantation of ^{125}I seeds. J Urol 121:306-309, 1979.

50. Wheeler TM, Scardino PT: Detailed pathologic review of prostate biopsy following irradiation for carcinoma of the prostate. Am Urol Assoc Annu Meeting (Abstract #298). Las Vegas, p 166, 1983.

51. Elder JS, Gibbons RP: Surgery for localized and disseminated cancer of the prostate. Clin Oncol 2:421-440, 1983.

52. Walsh PC, Jewett HJ: Radical surgery for prostatic cancer. Cancer 45:1906-1911, 1980.

53. Elder JS, Jewett HJ, Walsh PC: Radical perineal prostatectomy for clinical stage B2 carcinoma of the prostate. J Urol 127:704-706, 1982.

54. Taylor WJ, Richardson RG, Hafermann MD: Radiation therapy for localized prostate cancer. Cancer 43:1123-1127, 1979.

55. Taylor I, Rowling J, West C: Adjuvant cytotoxic liver perfusion for colorectal cancer. Br J Surg 66:833-837, 1979.

56. Nissen-Meyer R, Kjellgren K, Malmio K, Mansson B, Norin T: Surgical adjuvant chemotherapy: results with one short course with cyclophosphamide after mastectomy for breast cancer. Cancer 41:2088-2098, 1978.

57. Kadmon D, Heston WDW, Fair WR: Treatment of a metastatic prostate derived tumor with surgery and chemotherapy. J Urol 127:1238-1242, 1982.

4. In Vitro Assays for Directing Therapy of Genitourinary Cancers

JONATHAN FLEISCHMANN *, WARREN D. W. HESTON and WILLIAM R. FAIR

1. INTRODUCTION

There exist only speculative chemotherapy protocols for most genitourinary malignancies. With the exception of non-seminomatous testicular carcinoma, most patients with metastatic cancer will have an uncertain response to chemotherapy. While predictive in vitro chemosensitivity testing for various malignancies has lately been exploited at the commercial level, no one type of test has gained the confidence accorded disc sensitivity testing for infectious diseases.

Several methods of in vitro chemosensitivity testing of solid tumors, effusions, and bone marrow aspirations have evolved in the past 25 years. Almost all rely on initial mechanical or enzymatic degradation of the tumor before proceding with the actual test. These procedures discount the well-documented contention that most tumors are a heterogeneous composition of cellular subpopulations with different biologic potentials for growth or metastasis [1]. This is a critical issue when one considers the clinical applicability of these in vitro assays, especially those assays measuring tumor growth such as the 'clonogenic' stem cell assay. For example, Tsuruo and Fidler [2] demonstrated differences in chemosensitivities between a 'parental' tumor and its 'daughter' metastases. Heterogeneous responses of this type can be magnified in those tests which employ intact solid tumor slices to assess metabolic parameters or peripheral cellular outgrowth following drug exposure. Within this context emerges the companion controversy surrounding in vitro drug exposure protocols and attempts to apply test results to clinical situations [3]. Some of the factors which must be considered in formulating an in vitro chemosensitivity protocol include tumor cell growth rate, cycle-specificity of the drug, concentration of the drug over time

---

* National Kidney Foundation Fellow (1981–1983).

T. L. Ratliff and W. J. Catalona (eds), Urologic Oncology. ISBN 0-89838-628-4.

(CXT), and what drug concentrations would best correspond to actual plasma or in vivo tumor concentrations [4]. To date there has been no comprehensive answer to these issues.

Each type of in vitro test is designed to measure either cellular damage, cell kill, or lack of reproductive ability following drug exposure or radiation. Data has been collated using morphologic, metabolic or radiobiologic parameters. This chapter will examine the various methods and current status of in vitro chemosensitivity testing for human genitourinary malignancies with particular emphasis on the 'human tumor stem cell assay' as developed by Salmon and Hamburger [5].

2. MORPHOLOGIC ASSAYS

Morphologic evaluations of tumor appearance and growth following exposure to chemotherapeutic agents were among the first assays to be developed [6, 7]. Monolayer cultures as outgrowths of tissue slices [8] or dispersed cells [9] would be scored by cell counts or other criteria for cellular damage. Drug exposures varied but usually lasted at least 24 hours. Microscopic evaluation of the drug effects requires a skilled technician or pathologist, but some investigators have used trypan blue exclusion [10] or autoradiography [11] to better define viable cell populations. Despite initial enthusiasm, most investigators have now concluded that the in vitro morphologic tests correlated poorly with clinical course following assay-directed chemotherapy.

The poor predictive results may be explained by recognizing that assay systems based on monolayer cultures are encumbered by technical and logistical problems. First, monolayer culture allows for growth of both malignant and non-malignant cells. Fibroblasts may overgrow the tumor and not all tumors 'grow' in this system; slow growing renal cell carcinomas and testicular carcinomas have had among the worse records for proliferation or clinical correlations [7, 10, 12]. Secondly, drug effects are scored in subjective fashion, and the expert required for such tasks further adds to the cost of the assay. Finally, these subjective scorings are difficult to standardize as are the size and uniformity of tissue slices or dispersed cellular elements.

3. VISUAL INDICATOR TESTS

Whether cytostatic or cytotoxic, chemotherapeutic agents will alter or inhibit some phase of cellular metabolism. In 1954 Black and Speer [13] correlated a drug's inhibition of carbohydrate metabolism to subsequent clinical trials. Methylene blue dye was used as a substrate for cellular dehydrogenase; the lack of dye reduction (to a clear color) indicated decreased dehydrogenase activity. Their large series of primary tumors also included bladder, non-seminomatous testicular, and renal cell carcinomas, but no in vitro results correlated accurately with clinical responses. Modifications by DiPaolo [14] employed a disc sensitivity technique applied to monolayer cultures which would yield a blue 'zone of inhibition' corresponding to inhibition of dehydrogenase. An interesting study by Kondo [15] measured inhibition of succinate dehydrogenase and lysosomal acid phosphatase in colorometric assays performed on tumor cell suspensions and also tested patients' normal liver as a predictive gauge of toxicity. The in vitro/in vivo comparisons were encouraging but no specific data on genitourinary tumors were presented. One may criticize these assays for their inability to distinguish the metabolism of tumor from non-tumor cells, and that the tests do not account for those tumor cells which may have been damaged temporarily.

Dye exclusion or vital staining assays have been similarly used to ascertain the functional integrity of the cell following drug exposure. Trypan blue exclusion testing has been used extensively in parts of other in vitro assays as a viability 'check' [3, 5, 16-18] and in some studies has assumed a primary role in assessing drug effect. There is disagreement as to whether vital staining techniques are capable of accurately gauging cell injury or death. Roper and Drewinko [16] used a human lymphoma cell line maintained in liquid monolayer culture to compare colony formation in agar with tritiated thymidine uptake, labeling index (autoradiography), [51]chromium release, and exclusion dye testing by trypan blue and eosin Y following drug exposure. They found that 90% to 100% of tumor cells exposed to high or low drug concentrations were able to exclude dyes but colony formation decreased with increasing drug concentration. The other parameters tested also did not correlate well with colony formation. However, Durkin et al. [19] exposed primary lymphoma tumors to adriamycin or BCNU for 2 days in liquid medium then tested the tumor cells' ability to exclude trypan blue. They found significant clinical correlations in subsequent chemotherapy trials. Using an 'internal control' with duck erythrocytes Weisenthal et al. [20] corrected for 'pitfalls' associated with other trypan blue assays and concluded that fast green dye exclusion can correlate well with soft agar clonogenic assays of tissue culture cell lines. Our experience with primary genitourinary tumors indicates that trypan blue exclusion fails to predict ability to form colonies in the 'human tumor stem cell assay'. Buick et al. [21] examined transitional cell carcinoma cells obtained by bladder barbotage and found that cell viability 'by trypan blue exclusion was consistently greater than 85%', but subsequent colony growth varied widely.

4. ASSAYS USING RADIOACTIVE COMPOUNDS

Indirect methods to assess drug effects include measurement of cellular uptake, incorporation, or release of selected radioactive compounds. The ^{51}Chromium assay measures cell death by the release of ^{51}Chromium from membrane damaged cells. Tritiated thymidine, uridine and adenine have been used to assess nucleotide synthesis. ^{14}Carbon has been employed in measuring nucleotide synthesis, protein synthesis, and carbohydrate metabolism. The 'scintillation index' is a reflection of the incorporation of tritiated compounds into proliferating versus dormant cells as measured by a scintillation counter. The 'labeling index' is similar to the scintillation index but is obtained by analysis of autoradiographs (film exposed by beta particle emission).

These tests have been incorporated as part of cell slice, monolayer, cell suspension, or 'clonogenic' assay techniques [16, 22-24]. In common with other 'metabolic' assays, they have been criticized for an inability to distinguish permanent from transient damage, or in selecting temporarily non-cycling tumor cells from live non-tumor cells. For example, a decreased incorporation of tritiated thymidine may have been a result of a drug-related membrane transport defect without a companion defect in the cell's proliferative capacity [25]. Conversely, nucleotide salvage pathways may speciously account for increased cellular incorporation despite a crippled reproductive potential [26]. It is not surprising, then, that there are conflicting reports on the clinical usefulness of these assays [28, 32].

In 1966 Bickis et al. [22] collated 10 patients' in vitro/in vivo responses to chemotherapeutic agents using [^{14}C]-labeled amino acids and glucose. Tumor cell suspensions were incubated in the presence of the radiolabeled precursors and drug for 2 hours, followed by measurement of [^{14}C]-incorporation into protein, lipids and nucleotides. Two in vitro/in vivo correlations with renal cell carcinoma patients were inconclusive as were studies with other tumors. Tchao et al. [29] tested hormone effects on organ cultures of normal kidney and renal cell carcinoma and found good correlation between histological and [^{3}H]-scintillation index criteria, but in vivo correlations were also inconclusive. In contrast, the group for Sensitivity Testing of Tumors (KSST) [27] conducted in vitro/in vivo correlations on 155 patients, 72 of whom had metastatic ovarian carcinoma. They found the in vitro tests predicted most of the 'remissions' and almost all of the 'resistances' following cytoxan and adriamycin therapy for ovarian carcinoma.

In an experimental setting, recent enthusiasm for these assays has been generated from good correlations with the results of the in vitro soft agar clonogenic assay [23, 24] and a modified monolayer assay [30]. The relatively 'rapid' scintillation labeling index techniques have been proposed as a substitute means for accurately predicting the results of the 'slow' clonogenic assay. However, Shrivastav and Paulson [17] obtained mixed results when testing bladder tumors obtained from patients and tissue culture cell lines. They reported that drug-treated cells occasionally yielded higher nucleotide incorporation rates than controls. Tannock [31] noted that the labeling indices for large tumors tended to be less than that for smaller tumors; and in bladder tumors, increasing histologic grades tended to yield higher labeling indices. This paradox underscores the questionable value of radioisotope assays in light of the various clinical presentations of bladder cancer.

5. HORMONE RECEPTOR ASSAYS

Estrogen and progesterone receptor assays for breast cancer are routine procedures in most large medical centers. Almost all clinical correlations are based on the estrogen or progesterone receptor content of the cytosol as derived from various modifications of a dextran-coated charcoal assay. The predictive value of these assays are well known [33]. A much smaller body of data has been generated for clinical correlations of hormone receptor assays in genitourinary cancer.

Although renal cell carcinoma has, on occasion, responded to endocrine manipulation, the majority of patients will not respond [34]. Pearson et al. [35] attempted to correlate responses to provera with measurements of estrogen and progesterone receptors in renal cell carcinoma specimens. Their assay employed tritiated estradiol and progesterone in a 'dextran radioimmunoassay'. They noted that few tumors had measurable estrogen or progesterone receptors, and that normal kidney tissue, more likely than tumor, was receptor-positive. This was also a disappointing study because none of the 26 patients responded to hormonal therapy.

Receptor assays have had more promise when applied to prostatic carcinoma. Ekman et al. [36] used the dextran-coated charcoal assays to correlate prostatic cancer biopsy specimens' methyltrienolone (androgen) receptor content in the cytosol with hormonal therapy. Fifteen of 18 patients with receptor-positive cytosols responded to therapy. Of 5 patients with receptor-negative cytosols, only one responded to therapy. Trachtenberg and Walsh [37] refined this method to a 'microassay' technique and measured both cytosol and nuclear androgen receptor content in 23 prostatic cancer specimens. All biopsies were receptor-positive; significantly, the cytosol fraction data did not correlate with clinical data, but the nuclear androgen receptor content had excellent predictive value. This may prove a useful clinical tool if the assay procedures are simplified.

6. CLONOGENIC ASSAYS

The 'human tumor stem cell assay', 'clonogenic assay', or 'double-layer soft agar assay' are all synonyms for a method of in vitro chemosensitivity testing which evolved in the 1970s. Salmon et al. [5] began a movement within the scientific community toward this type of assay system which demonstrated good positive and even better negative in vitro/in vivo retrospective correlations for ovarian cancer patients. The initial enthusiasm for this assay prompted numerous protocols for clonogenic assay-directed chemotherapy in this country and in Europe. Advertisements by commercial laboratories offering the assay 'service' began appearing in medical journals. However, persistent technical difficulties found by other investigators and the fact that not all tumors will grow in soft agar forced a retrenchment of opinion and appreciation for the assay's limitations [38, 39]. Selby, Buick and Tannock [40] have summarized these problems in a recent review and state that use of the assay 'in routine selection of anticancer drugs is premature'. Our own experience with this assay for genitourinary tumors has led us to similar conclusions, and renal cell carcinoma is particularly unsuitable for the clonogenic assay system as described in the literature.

The double layer of soft agar offers an advantage over monolayer cultures because it allows growth of primary tumors and prevents fibroblast proliferation. The technique is as follows: tumor in any form is disaggregated by mechanical and/or enzymatic means to obtain a theoretical single cell suspension. After a cell count, aliquots of 1.5×10^6 epithelial cells are incubated for one hour in the presence of a chemotherapeutic agent(s). The original 1.5×10^6 cell aliquot is then divided equally into three fractions such that 5×10^5 cells are layered, in an agar suspension, over a 'feeder' underlayer in 35 mm petri dishes. An alternative to the one hour drug exposure is the 'continuous' drug incubation for the duration of the assay. Colony formation (30 to 50 cells) is assessed at various intervals over the following two or three week period. Presumably only those cells capable of dividing at least 5 times (stem cells) will form colonies. Colony formation from drug-treated cells is compared to controls and a relative percent chemosensitivity is derived. Similar to other in vitro assays, the concept is simple but each step is fraught with difficulties which have formed the basis for the current controversy. This will be examined in detail.

6.1 *Preparation of the single cell suspension*

Mechanical degradation of a solid tumor will not usually yield a homogeneous single cell suspension [41]. Cell clusters are often present and will interfere with accurate assessment of colony growth. Repeated passage of the cell suspension through a 25 gauge needle will disperse most cell clusters, but some tumors require enzymatic degradation for remaining clusters [42]. Enzymatic degradation of tumor, however, will increase cell membrane permeability [43]. We have noted that enzymatic degradation or enzymatic treatment of an already dispersed cell suspension results in a decrease in trypan blue exclusion. It is uncertain to what extent chemosensitivity testing would be altered from enzymatic treatment for want of data comparing enzymatic degradation with a better mechanical means of generating single cell suspensions.

Ideally, cell dispersion would result in only single cells obtained with a minimum of trauma, and these single cells would remain dispersed to form 'clusterless' plates such that no doubt existed as to which cells grew into colonies. This can be the case for tissue culture cell lines harvested from liquid medium as depicted in Figures 1 and 2, but primary tumors will not behave in this matter. Clusters are more of a problem with necrotic tumors or tumors with stromal elements such as prostate carcinomas. Even single cell suspensions generated enzymatically from these tumors tend to reaggreagate during the course of the assay.

After mechanical or enzymatic degradation, most clonogenic assay protocols require a centrifugation step to concentrate the single cell suspension before division into aliquots of 1.5×10^6 cells. We have observed that tumors with a high lipid and glycogen content, such as a clear cell renal carcinoma, will be composed of at least two types of epithelial cell popula-

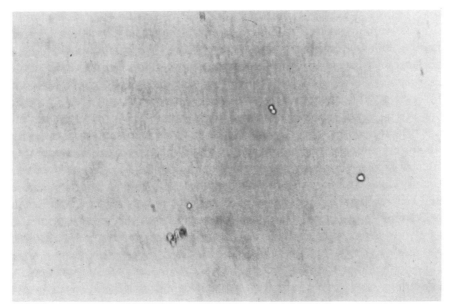

Figure 1. Photomicrographic of the Copenhagen rat R3327 MAT-Lu tumor in the upper agar layer on the day of plating.

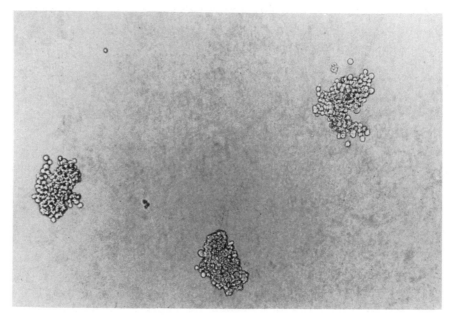

Figure 2. Photomicrograph of the same Copenhagen rat R3327 MAT-Lu tumor (as seen in Figure 1) seven days later.

tions – some of which float and the others pellet during centrifugation. Figures 3 through 5 exemplify this phenomenon for a mixed clear cell/granular cell renal carcinoma. Figure 3 depicts the 'homogeneous' cell suspension; Figure 2, following centrifugation at $200 \times g$ for 10 min – note the cell pellet and layer of film on the surface of the supernatant. Figure 3 is a photomicrograph of the lipids and epithelial cells taken from this supernatant film. It is obvious that these cells would be lost by discarding the supernatant. We have occasionally harvested these cells from the supernatant and plated them in soft agar. They did not form 'true' colonies, but some of the cell clusters increased to colony size as recognized by an automated colony counter. This observation regarding 'floater' epithelial cells may partially explain why Hamburger et al. [44] reported that some tumors, including renal cell carcinoma, had improved colony formation following enzymatic dispersion. As discussed previously, however, it is difficult to accurately assess the benefits of enzymatic versus mechanical methods of tumor degradation.

The epithelial cell 'floater' phenomenon of renal cell carcinomas explains our findings that predominantly clear cell carcinomas have lower growth rates than predominantly granular cell carcinomas (Table 1), and that duplicated cell aliquots (control and drug treated) will often yield disparate colony counts (Table 3). We had partially ameliorated this problem by minim-

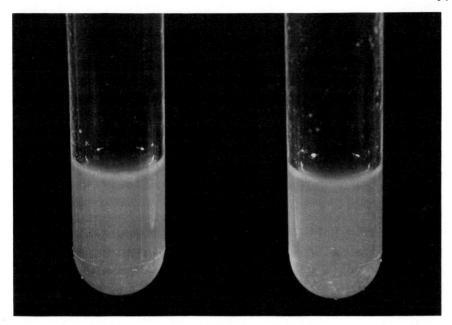

Figure 3. Freshly prepared 'single cell' suspension of a mixed granular/clear cell renal carcinoma.

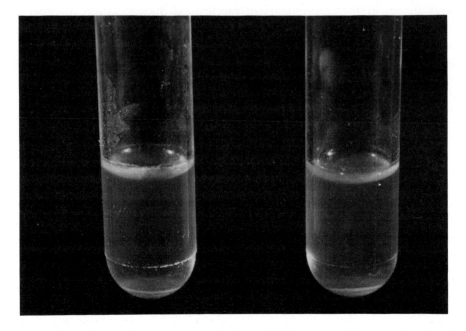

Figure 4. The 'single cell' suspension seen in Figure 3 following centrifugation. Note the cell pellet and the layer of film at the top of the supernatant.

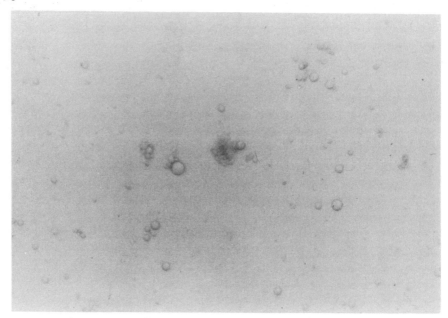

Figure 5. Photomicrograph of the supernatant film as seen in Figure 4. Note the lipid droplets and epithelial cells.

izing the medium requirements of mechanical disaggregation in order to avoid the initial centrifugation step. The one hour assay, however, includes a centrifugation and washing procedure to purge the drug from the cell suspension and causes variable amounts of cell loss. We have tried addition of a detergent, NP-40, to the cell/drug suspension to disintegrate the lipid–

Table 1. Histology of renal cell carcinoma.

		Predominately clear cell	Predominately granular cell	Mixed clear/ granular	Predominately spindle cell
Number of tumors	IC[a]	7/12	4/4	7/10	0/2
Forming colonies/total	MC[b]	0/3	2/3	1/2	1/2
Average cloning	IC[a]	0.036 range (0.008–0.13)	0.11 range (0.008–0.24)	0.054 range (0.01–0.1)	0
Efficiency (%) of tumors forming colonies	MC[b]	0	0.013 range (0.095–0.017)	0.023	0.01

[a] Investigator counted (7/81–6/82).
[b] Machine counted (7/82–).

Table 2. Methodologic comparisons.

Patient	47-year old white female			10-year old white female			72-year old white female			71-year old white male		
Method	A	B	C	A	B	C	A	B	C	A	B	C
Best cloning efficiency (%)	0.096	0.032	0.176	0.065	0.025	0.029	0.011	0.015	0.013	0.058	0.076	0.035
Drug-sensitivity (% of control)												
Adriamycin	73	0	37	6	18	88	53	63	3	75	91	78
BCNU	73	0	53	32		93	38	62	26	54	78	60
Bisantrene		65	62	59	65	47	69	53	64	39	87	32
Bleomycin			25	10		82	23	41	0	98	163	74
Cis-platinum	39		94	55	15	45	40	98	0	120	90	35
DTIC	55	65	16	57		108	74	76	18	117	66	88
5-Fu	98			12	19	67	20	40	0	73	92	114
Methyl-gag	38		61	58		77	44	39	77	71	31	47
Melphalan	40		38	16	102	52	43	84	53	85	62	53
Mito-C			45	20	121	59	28	48	0	69	60	49
Mitoxantrone			44	8	83	44	51	54	38	79	49	77
MTX		73	67	73	48	75	19	79	0	98	66	71
Velban			19	20	27	26	47	34	0	41	29	61
Vindescine	65	100	28	46		54	42	59	33	89	74	49
	NP-40 1×10^{-3}%			NP-40 1×10^{-3}%			NP-40 5×10^{-4}%			NP-40 7.5×10^{-4}%		

A = one hour.
B = one hour + NP-40.
C = continuous.

Table 3. Duplicated control aliquots.

Patient	Method	No. of colonies/plate (average)
47-year old white female	A	482, infected
	B	78, 21
	C	881, 578
70-year old white female	A	40, 323
	B	123, 66
	C	143, 74
72-year old white female	A	57, 21
	B	76, 44
	C	63, 28
71-year old white male	A	290, 191
	B	378, 342
	C	177, 172

A = one hour.
B = one hour + NP-40.
C = continuous.

cellular interactions and this resulted in improved cell recovery. Unfortunately, NP-40 is toxic and the less toxic concentrations (7.5×10^{-4}%) do not optimize cell recovery. Table 2 details the results of comparing the one hour assay (column A) to the one hour assay with NP-40 (column B) and the continuous assay (column C). Among other observations from this data, one notes the relative 'toxic' effect of NP-40 at 1×10^{-3}%, and the discordance of colony growth and chemosensitivities between the three methods.

To summarize: preparation of a single cell suspension is difficult and almost impossible for some primary tumors. Some epithelial cells may be lost, resulting in poor colony formation; for this reason alone renal cell carcinoma is particularly unsuitable for the 'standard' clonogenic assay protocol. Any 'chemosensitivities' may be a function of cell loss rather than drug-induced inhibition of colony formation.

6.2 *Drug incubations*

The methodology of the clonogenic assay provided no new insight as to what single in vitro drug dose would correspond to the clinical situation. As originally envisioned by Salmon et al. [5], a one hour drug incubation period in liquid medium was sufficient for cellular uptake of most chemotherapeutic agents. Excess drug would then be washed out of the liquid medium before resuspending the cells in the upper soft agar layer. Drug concentrations and CXT estimates were designed to bracket the achievable plasma concentrations in vivo [45]. The alternative 'continuous' drug incubation method provides drug exposure in the soft agar from the time of upper layer plating to the final colony counts. This method discounts the value of CXT calculations, but data presented by Salmon's research group indicates no substantial differences in colony counts from cells exposed for one hour or continuously to several chemotherapeutic agents [46]. The theoretical limitations of drug effects seen with cycle-specific drugs in a one hour assay or colony inhibition from low doses of a rapidly biodegraded agent in a continuous assay have not been resolved. Unlike bacterial sensitivity testing, no 'minimum inhibitory concentration' for any chemotherapeutic agent has been found.

We compared the two drug incubation schedules in testing primary renal cell carcinoma. Following the recommendations of Salmon's group [45], we used the 'single-point assay' drug concentrations for the one hour assay (column A) and the suggested 1/200 dilution of those concentrations for the continuous assay (column C) as represented in Table 2. As can be seen, the cloning efficiencies varied widely as did the drug sensitivities. We have already pointed out the pitfalls associated with the one hour assay, but we conclude from this and other data (not shown) that one method is not demonstrably better than the other. However, the continuous assay is easier to do and has less potential for technical difficulties. One would suppose that eliminating any centrifugation step would improve the internal consistency of the assay results, but our results indicate otherwise. Table 3 presents the raw data from duplicated controls and suggests that other problems with the assay (making of single cell suspensions or colony counting) overshadow the unique problems associated with renal cell carcinoma. Other genitourinary tumors behave similarly.

We have now modified our continuous assay drug concentrations to equal 1/4 that of the one hour assay in an effort to ferret out any potential sensitivities from the notoriously chemoresistant genitourinary tumors. When possible, we have used more than one concentration per drug as a further check on the internal consistency of the assay. As other investigators have noted, we have found that some low dose drug concentrations will occasionally inhibit colony formation better than the next higher dose. We have no explanation for this phenomenon but have observed it in our cell line cultures (Figures 1 and 2) as well as primary tumors.

6.3 Colony counting

The most controversial aspect of the clonogenic assay has been the counting of colonies. The clonogenic assay was developed experimentally with cultured cell lines which easily dispersed into homogeneous single cell suspensions and retained this quality during the plating procedure. Investigator-counted colony formation under these circumstances was accurate and reproducible. As discussed previously, however, a single cell suspension derived from a primary tumor is illusory, and despite all reasonable efforts, some cell clusters will be present in the upper layer at the time of plating. In many instances, especially with necrotic or fibrous tumors, the colony or near colony-sized cluster counting may number in the hundreds per plate. 'Plating' or 'cloning' efficiency is defined as a percent of the number of colonies formed per number of cells plated. Human primary tumors reportedly range 0.001 to 0.1%, with genitourinary tumors tending toward the lower end of the scale [18, 47]. Therefore, there is a very small margin for assessing colony formation beyond the clusters usually present at plating. We have found that the majority of genitourinary malignancies tested did not form at least 50 colonies (cloning efficiency 0.01%) per plate.

The obvious approach to this problem is to count the clusters at the time of plating and subtract this number from the final colony count to yield the 'actual' colony growth. Early publications [3, 5] regarding the stem cell assay did not address this issue nor present data on quantifying clusters at the time of plating by investigator or machine (Omnicon FAS-II Scanner) counts. Some tumors were reported to have 'grown' with as few as 5 colonies per plate [18] which partially accounts for the inflated figures stating that the vast majority of tumors were able to 'grow' in the soft agar. For example, Stanisic and Buick [48] reported 'growth' from bladder urothelial cells obtained by bladder barbotage in 9 of 9 patients with biopsy-proven carcinoma of the bladder and in 3 of 17 patients with normal urothelium and no previous evidence of malignancy.

Even with the subtraction method of colony assessment, investigator-counted data is suspect. Table 1 details our results over an 18 month period for renal cell carcinomas and illustrates the differences between investigator and machine counts. Direct comparisons of investigator and machine counts yielded similar findings.

Colony counting by the subtraction method, however, is not able to distinguish colonies which arise from single cells or from smaller-than-colony-sized clusters not scored at the time of plating. True colonies should reflect the reproductive potential of the 'stem cells' within the tumor since these are the cells thought to be responsible for the uncontrolled (cancerous) growth in vivo. In keeping with the stem cell model, Selby et al. [40] point out that small clusters of the so-called 'transitional cells', capable of only 2 or 3 cell divisions, may form 'colonies' which masquerade as stem cell-derived colonies. To add to the confusion, it is also possible for so-called 'end cells', incapable of reproduction, to have formed colony-sized clusters at the time of plating and then shrink or disappear over the course of the one to two week incubation period. Furthermore, Rosenblum et al. [50] have demonstrated the misleading appearance of tumor 'giant' cells which have not divided but increased in size so as to be recognized as a colony by an automated colony counter. Salmon's research group [49] has also reported that some amyloid producing myeloma 'colonies' are actually composed of myeloma cells and macrophages (not tumor) in a symbiotic relationship. In short, the subtraction method is not a straightforward solution to the problem of determining colony formation, but it is clear that investigator-counted data is unreliable compared to machine-counted data.

Alley, Uhl and Lieber [38] addressed these problems and attempted to solve them by incorporating a vital staining technique (INT dye) which allows the automated colony counter to ignore the unstained (dead?) cells or clusters and only count the stained (live) colonies. Their techniques appeared to improve the internal consistency of the assay for in vitro cell cultures and help distinguish the cluster debris from the viable colonies in primary tumor cultures. We have also tested this staining method and have found that the automated colony counter will distinguish stained from unstained clusters/colonies, but there are some cell cluster/colony formations in the 'gray' area which are only partially stained. This suggests, among other possibilities, that tiny 2 to 3 cell clusters present during plating could have been composed of a combination of 'stem' cells and 'transitional' cells or 'end' cells. Also, we have noted that cell clusters unstained by INT may still harbor live cells capable of metabolizing 5-fluorescinediacetate or rhodamine 123 [51]. Our data for duplicated controls or drug-treated cell aliquots from primary tumors has not improved with the INT staining technique, but further investigations are in order.

6.4 *Clinical correlations*

Very little data regarding genitourinary tumors is in the literature. There are anecdotal cases of patients with metastatic renal cell carcinoma having a 'partial' response following assay-directed chemotherapy, but these data are not substantive. One major reason for this lack of clinical data is that only a minority of tumors will form colonies in soft agar, and of those, few display any chemosensitivities. Considering the technical problems of the assay, especially with renal cell carcinoma, it is not surprising that few positive correlations exist.

In the only clinical report of in vitro/in vivo correlations for a genitourinary tumor, Stanisic et al. [52] in a later study collated data on 5 patients with transitional cell carcinoma of the bladder. They obtained cells by bladder barbotage and performed one hour assays. They defined 'sensitivity' to adriamycin, mitomycin C or thiotepa as a 50% or greater reduction in colony formation compared to control. Only 10 of 20 assays yielded colony growth. Trypan blue exclusion testing on cell suspensions before plating showed 10% to 90% 'viability' in both 'growth' and 'no-growth' cultures. Retrospective and prospective sensitivity correlations were reported as 'correct' in 7 of 9 instances, but on a case-by-case basis the assay results did not predict or influence the clinical course in 4 of 5 patients. It was also unclear which patients had 'growth' or 'no-growth' cultures during their respective clinical courses.

Other non-genitourinary carcinoma data does not encourage a role for the clonogenic assay as a reliable clinical tool [40], but efforts toward eliminating the technical problems may prove fruitful. The greatest obstacle to reliability for the clonogenic assay is the failure to atraumatically generate and maintain a single cell suspension from a solid tumor.

7. CONCLUSION

In vitro assays to direct chemotherapy or hormonal therapy are still in developmental stages. The need for these assays has stimulated investigations along several avenues, some of which have already demonstrated clinical potential such as the hormone receptor assay for prostatic carcinoma developed by Trachtenberg and Walsh [37]. The clonogenic assay has demonstrated its worth as a research tool in selected circumstances, but it will be difficult to overcome the burden of evidence detailing the methodologic shortcomings and lack of predictive successes in primary tumors. As with any other in vitro test, clinical data generated under stringently controlled in vitro and in vivo protocols will be required to establish the predictive value of the assay.

Although the 'stem cell' concept may yet be the best approach to addressing the problems of tumor heterogeneity and measurement of reproductive potential, only a minority of genitourinary tumors form colonies in vitro. One of the current research challenges is to identify growth factors that will accelerate stem cell proliferation and to make this assay a useful clinical tool for the majority of specimens submitted [47, 53]. This approach may also aid in the discovery of new chemotherapeutic agents, but the best retrospective data generated by the clonogenic assay has been in negative correlations [3, 5]. Perhaps the value of the clonogenic assay will be recognized for sparing patients ineffective or toxic chemotherapy.

ACKNOWLEDGEMENTS

We gratefully acknowledge the pathologic specimen reviews by Walter Bauer, M.D. of the Department of Surgical Pathology at Washington University and Barnes Hospital.

The Emerson Electric Company of St. Louis generously donated the funds for purchase of the Bausch and Lomb Omnicon FAS-II Scanner used for automated colony counting.

A special thanks to Ms Ann Zito for preparation of this manuscript.

REFERENCES

1. Dexter DL, Calabresi P: Intraneoplastic diversity. Biochem Biophys Acta 695:97-112, 1982.
2. Tsuruo T, Fidler IJ: Differences in drug sensitivity among tumor cells from parental tumors, selected variants, and spontaneous metastases. Cancer Res 41:3058-3064, 1981.
3. Von Hoff DD, Casper J, Bradley E, Sandbach J, Jones D, Makuch R: Association between human tumor colony-forming assay results and response of an individual patient's tumor to chemotherapy. Am J Med 70:1027-1032, 1981.
4. Alberts DS, Salmon SE, Chen HSG, Moon TE, Young L, Surwit EA: Pharmacologic studies of anticancer drugs with the human tumor stem cell assay. Cancer Chem Pharm 6:253-264, 1981.
5. Salmon SE, Hamburger AW, Soehnlen B, Durie BGM, Alberts DS, Moon TE: Quantification of differential sensitivity of human tumor stem cells to anticancer drugs. N Engl J Med 298(24):1321-1327, 1978.
6. Wright JC, Cobb JP, Gumport S, Golomb FM, Safadi D: Investigation of the relation between clinical and tissue culture response to chemotherapeutic agents on human cancer. N Engl J Med 257:1207-1211, 1957.
7. Wright JC, Cobb JP, Gumport SL, Safadi D, Walker DG, Golomb FM: Further investigation of the relation between the clinical and tissue culture response to chemotherapeutic agents on human cancer. Cancer 15:284-293, 1962.
8. Hurley JD, Yount LJ: Selection of anticancer drugs for palliation using tissue culture sensitivity studies. Am J Surg 109:39-42, 1965.
9. Dendy PP, Bozman G, Wheeler TK: In vitro screening test for human malignant tumors before chemotherapy. Lancet 2:68-72, 1970.
10. Lazarus H, Tegeler W, Mazzone HM, Leroy JG, Boone BA, Foley GE: Determination of sensitivity of individual biopsy specimens to potential inhibitory agents: evaluation of some explant culture methods as assay systems. Can Chem Rep 50(8):543-555, 1966.
11. Wheeler T, Dendy P, Dawson A: Assessment of an in vitro screening test of cytotoxic agents in the treatment of adrenal malignant disease. Oncology 30:362-376, 1974.
12. Berry RJ, Laing AH, Wells J: Fresh explant culture of human tumors in vitro and the assessment of sensitivity to cytotoxic chemotherapy. Br J Cancer 31:218-222, 1975.
13. Black MM, Speer FD: Further observations of the effects of cancer chemotherapeutic agents on the in vitro dehydrogenase activity of cancer tissue. J Natl Cancer Inst 14(5):1147-1158, 1954.
14. DiPaolo JA: Analysis of individual chemotherapy assay system. Natl Cancer Inst Monogr 34:240-245, 1971.
15. Kondo T: Prediction of response of tumor and host to cancer chemotherapy. Natl Cancer Inst Monogr 34:251-256, 1971.
16. Roper PR, Drewinko B: Comparison of in vitro methods to determine drug-induced cell lethality. Cancer Res 36:2182.2188, 1976.
17. Shrivastav S, Paulson DF: In vitro chemotherapy testing of transitional cell carcinoma. Invest Urol 17(5):395-400, 1980.

18. Sarosdy MF, Lamm DL, Radwin HM, Von Hoff DD: Clonogenic assay and in vitro chemosensitivity testing of human urologic malignancies. Cancer 50:1332-1338, 1982.
19. Durkin WJ, Ghanta VK, Balch CM, Davis DW, Hiramoto RN: A methodological approach to the prediction of anticancer drug effect in humans. Cancer Res 39:402-407, 1979.
20. Weisenthal LM, Dill PL, Kurmick NB, Lippman ME: Comparison of dye exclusion assays with a clonogenic assay in the determination of drug-induced cytotoxicity. Cancer Res 43:258-264, 1983.
21. Buick RN, Stanisic TH, Salmon SE, Trent JM, Krasovich P: Development of an agarmethylcellulose clonogenic assay for cells in transitional cell carcinoma of the human bladder. Cancer Res 39:5051-5056, 1979.
22. Bickis IJ, Henderson IWD, Quastel JH: Biochemical studies of human tumors (II). Cancer 19:103-113, 1966.
23. Tanigawa N, Kern DH, Hikasa Y, Morion DL: Rapid assay for evaluating the chemosensitivity of human tumors in soft agar culture. Cancer Res 42:2159-2164, 1982.
24. Friedman HM, Glaubiger DL: Assessment of in vitro drug sensitivity of human tumor cells using [^{3}H]-thymidine incorporation in a modified human tumor stem cell assay. Cancer Res 42:4683-4689, 1982.
25. Bender RA, Bleyer WA, Drake JC, Ziegler JL: In vitro correlates of clinical responses to methotrexate in acute leukemia and Burkitt's lymphoma. Br J Cancer 34:484-492, 1976.
26. Von Hoff DD, Weisenthal L: In vitro methods to predict for patient response to chemotherapy. Adv Pharm Chem 17:133-156, 1980.
27. Group for Sensivity Testing of Tumors (KSST): In vitro short-term test to determine the resistance of human tumors to chemotherapy. Cancer 48:2127-2135, 1981.
28. Hart JS, George SL, Frei E, Bodney GP, Nickerson RC, Freirich EJ: Prognostic significance of pretreatment proliferative activity in adult leukemia. Cancer 39:1603-1617, 1977.
29. Tchao R, Easty GC, Ambrose EJ, Raven RW, Bloom HJG: Effect of chemotherapeutic agents and hormones on organ cultures of human tumors. Eur J Cancer 4:39-44, 1968.
30. Shrivastav S, Bonar RA, Stone KR, Paulson DF: An in vitro assay procedure to test chemotherapeutic drugs on cells from human solid tumors. Cancer Res 40:4438-4442, 1980.
31. Tannock I: Cell kinetics and chemotherapy: a critical review. Cancer Treat Rep 62(8):1117-1133, 1978.
32. Livingston RB, Titus GA, Heilbrun LK: In vitro effects on DNA synthesis as a predictor of biological effect from chemotherapy. Cancer Res 40:2209-2212, 1980.
33. De Sombre ER, Carbone PP, Jensen EU, McGuire WL, Wells SA, Wittliff JL, Lipsett MB: Steroid receptors in breast cancer. N Engl J Med 301:1011-1012, 1979.
34. Bloom HJG: Hormone-induced and spontaneous regression of metastatic renal cancer. Cancer 32:1066-1071, 1973.
35. Pearson J, Friedman MA, Hoffman PG: Hormone receptors in renal cell carcinoma. Cancer Chem Pharm 6:151-154, 1981.
36. Ekman P, Snochowski M, Zetterberg A, Hogberg B, Gustafsson JA: Steroid receptor content in human prostatic carcinoma and response to endocrine therapy. Cancer 44:1173-1181, 1979.
37. Trachtenberg J, Walsh PC: Correlation of prostatic nuclear androgen receptor content with duration of response and survival following hormonal therapy in advanced prostatic cancer. J Urol 127:466-471, 1982.
38. Alley MC, Uhl CB, Lieber MM: Improved detection of drug cytotoxycity in the soft agar colony formation assay through use of a metabolizable tetrazolium salt. Life Sci 31:3071-3078, 1983.
39. Editorial: Clonogenic assays for the chemotherapeutic sensitivity of human tumors. Lancet 3:780-781, 1982.

40. Selby P, Buick RN, Tannock I: A critical appraisal of the 'human tumor stem cell assay'. N Engl J Med 308:129-134, 1983.
41. Dow LW, Bhakta M, Wilimas J: Clonogenic assay for Wilm's tumor: improved technique for obtaining single cell suspensions and evidence for tumor cell specificity. Cancer Res 42:5262-5264, 1982.
42. Slocum HK, Pavelic ZP, Kanter PM, Nowak NJ, Rustum YM: The soft agar clonogenicity and characterizations of cells obtained from human solid tumors by mechanical and enzymatic means. Cancer Chem Pharm 6:219-225, 1981.
43. MacKintosh FR, Evans TL, Sikic BI: Methodologic problems in clonogenic assays of spontaneous human tumors. Cancer Chem Pharm 6:205-210, 1981.
44. Hamburger AW, White CP, Tencer K: Effect of enzymatic disaggregation on proliferation of human tumors in soft agar. AACR Abstracts 73:182, 1982.
45. Alberts DS, Salmon SE, Chen HSG, Moon TE, Young L, Surwit EA: Pharmacologic studies of anticancer drugs with the human tumor stem cell assay. Cancer Chem Pharm 6:253-264, 1981.
46. Ludwig R, Alberts DS, Miller TP, Salmon SE, Wood DA: The schedule dependency (SD) of anticancer drugs in the human tumor stem cell assay (HTSCA). AACR Abstracts 73:718, 1982.
47. Lieber MM, Kovach JS, Soft agar clonogic assay for primary renal carcinoma: in vitro chemotherapy drug sensitivity testing. Invest Urol 19:111-114, 1981.
48. Stanisic TH, Buick RN: An in vitro clonal assay for bladder cancer: clinical correlation with the status of the urotheliam in 33 patients. J Urol 124:30-33, 1980.
49. Durie BGM, Persky B, Soehnlen BJ, Grogan TM, Salmon SE: Amyloid production in human myeloma stem-cell culture, with morphologic evidence of amyloid secretion by associated macrophages. N Engl J Med 307:1689-1692, 1982.
50. Rosenblum ML, Dougherty DV, Reese C, Wilson CB: Potentials and possible pitfalls of human stem cell analysis. Cancer Chem Pharm 6:227-235, 1981.
51. Darznkiewicz Z, Traganos F, Staiano-coico L, Kapuscinski J, Melamud MR: Interactions of rhodamine 123 with living cells studied by flow cytometry. Cancer Res 42:799-806, 1982.
52. Stanisic TH, Owens R, Graham AR: Use of clonal assay in determination of urothelial drug sensitivity in carcinoma in situ of the bladder: clinical correlations in five patients. J Urol (in press).
53. Sherwin SA, Twardzik DR, Bohn WH, Cockley KD, Todaro GJ: High-molecular-weight transforming growth factor activity in the urine of patients with disseminated cancer. Cancer Res 43:403-407, 1983.

108

Editorial Comment

MICHAEL M. LIEBER

Most patients with metastatic transitional cell carcinoma, renal cell carcinoma, and hormonally unresponsive prostate cancer have not had objective tumor responses when treated by the cytotoxic chemotherapy regimes used up to the present. Therefore, it is a high priority to identify new active agents with which to treat patients with advanced genitourinary malignancies. It is also a high priority to develop laboratory tests which could individualize chemotherapy selection for a given patient. Indeed, a laboratory technique which would achieve such individualization of anticancer drug treatment would revolutionize the treatment of advanced genitourinary cancer. This profound clinical need is responsible for the intense research and commercial activity associated with in vitro assays with Drs. Fleischmann, Heston and Fair describe in their chapter.

The Urology Research Laboratory at the Mayo Clinic has had an active interest in in vitro chemotherapy sensitivity testing for GU tumors over the last 5 years. With the publication of Salmon's encouraging report in the summer of 1978 [1], our efforts to apply soft agar colony formation assays to genito-urinary tumors got started at the Mayo Clinic.

Our laboratory performs the soft agar colony formation/drug sensitivity testing assays for all solid tumors removed at our institution for which adequate tumor tissue remains after diagnostic pathology examination. To date we have studied over 5500 different human tumors by this technique and are currently assessing new tumors at the rate of 2000 per year. Our laboratory also has received a contract from the National Cancer Institute to use the soft agar colony formation assay in a screening mode to search for new chemical agents which might be active against primary human tumors of various histologic types. So my comments are based on a perspective gained from the experience cited above (as of March, 1984).

There are numerous technical problems in the performance of soft agar colony formation assays which Fleischmann and colleagues rightly emphasize. These problems were originally overlooked by the assay's proponents but have become more and more apparent as other laboratories around the world have tried to apply soft agar colony formation chemotherapy sensitivity testing to a variety of human tumor types. The main technical problems with the assay to date have been: 1) common inability to prepare healthy, proliferative single cell suspensions from the vast majority of human solid tumors and effusions; 2) the fact that colony formation observed in soft agar cultures of primary human tumors appears to derive from the enlargement of pre-existing seeded small cell aggregates rather than from the clonal growth of individual 'stem cells' [2]; 3) arbitrary drug concentration and time of drug exposure considerations compared to in vivo circumstances; and 4) difficulty in assessing drug 'killing' effects on cell colonies by visual or computerized image analysis methods [3].

Our laboratory has encountered the same sorts of technical problems in these assays described so clearly by Fleischmann and co-authors. There is no question that these technical problems need to be resolved before soft agar colony formation assays for drug sensitivity testing are marketed as clinically useful tests. Nevertheless, we remain guardedly optimistic that the technical problems can be reliably solved and that these assays can then come to clinical testing. At present we believe that: 1) tumor tissue must be taken from the patient to the laboratory as quickly as possible and immediately processed by a brief enzymatic exposure into single cells and small cell aggregates; 2) several steps of filtration must be performed to reduce the initial seeding of cell aggregates which could be mistaken for colonies; 3) drugs to be tested should be overlaid onto the soft agar cultures after seeding rather than pre-incubated with the tumor cells before seeding; 4) drugs should be tested at several concentrations to determine if a dose response curve is present; 5) all experiments should contain positive cytotoxic control compounds such as sodium azide, mercuric chloride or other universal toxins which must reliably eliminate colony formation in valid experiments; 6) plates should be counted the day after set-up to eliminate the inclusion of large cell aggregates in the assays; 7) vital staining techniques such as use of the vital stain INT [3] need to be used to differentiate between living and dead colonies after 5–10 days of cell incubation.

With such technical changes, our laboratory has been able to perform evaluable chemotherapy sensitivity experiments for human GU tumors in slightly more than 50% of tumors submitted to the laboratory in the past year [4]. Using 'conventional' techniques described several years ago, we rarely found even one drug active in vitro; with newer techniques we now find one or more drugs active in vitro in a majority of tests.

We are presently designing prospective phase II clinical trials in which the results from in vitro chemotherapy sensitivity testing will be used to select treatment for patients with advanced GU tumors. The urologic clinician should await the results from such trials before submitting his patients' tumors to this type of test at commercial laboratories which at present have not been using the most advanced technical refinements and which charge from $ 1000–$ 2000 per tumor test. We believe that clinicians should adopt an attitude of 'cautious skepticism' [5] to in vitro chemotherapy sensitivity assays as they are presently performed until there are clear data which demonstrate the utility of these tests in selecting therapy for patients with advanced GU tumors. Such data does not exist at the present time.

In vitro chemotherapy sensitivity testing for GU tumors is just in its infancy. The Salmon assay was marketed as a finished product with proven technical details and clinical utility. This simply is not the case! But tumor cells from all the difficult genitourinary tumors with which urologists must deal will proliferate for a short time in vitro in soft agar cultures. Further laboratory and clinical research is necessary to find out if this in vitro proliferation capacity can (or cannot) be used to select clinically useful chemotherapy. The answer to this question is not available at present.

REFERENCES

1. Salmon SE, Hamburger AW, Soehnlen B, Durie BGM, Alberts DS, Moon TE: Quantification of differential sensitivity of human tumor stem cells to anticancer drugs. N Engl J Med 298(24):1321–1327, 1978.
2. Agrez MV, Kovach JS, Lieber MM: Cell aggregates in the soft agar 'human tumour stem-cell assay'. Br J Cancer 46:880–887, 1982.
3. Alley MC, Uhl CB, Lieber MM: Improved detection of drug cytotoxicity in the soft agar colony formation assay through use of a metabolizable tetrazolium salt. Life Sci 31:3071–3078, 1982.
4. Lieber MM: Soft agar colony formation assay for in vitro chemotherapy sensitivity testing of human renal cell carcinomas: Mayo Clinic experience. J Urol (submitted).
5. Editorial: Clonogenic assays for the chemotherapeutic sensitivity of human tumors. Lancet 3:780–781, 1982.

5. Tumor Markers in Genitourinary Cancer

H. BARTON GROSSMAN

1. INTRODUCTION

Tumor markers have become increasingly important in the management of genitourinary malignant neoplasms. For the purpose of this discussion, I will use a broad definition of tumor markers that is based on their potential clinical use. With this perspective, a tumor marker may be defined as any biochemical, hormonal, or immunologic assay which provides information regarding the diagnosis and/or prognosis of a malignant neoplasm. In addition to the obvious potential clinical importance of tumor markers, they may also prove to be useful tools for basic scientists in the study of the pathophysiology of human malignancy. Tumor markers may be highly specific for a given neoplasm or may be quite non-specific. However, their clinical relevance, which does not always correlate with specificity, will determine whether they will be incorporated into the urologic oncologist's armamentarium or not. A number of factors will determine whether an individual tumor marker will be clinically accepted. Obvious relevant factors include the prevalence of the neoplasm; its actual or perceived impact on the population at risk; and the sensitivity and specificity of the tumor marker itself. Sensitivity refers to the accuracy of the tumor marker in detecting neoplasm when it is actually present. An insensitive test will produce false negative results, i.e., failure to detect neoplasm when it is actually present. Specificity on the other hand, concerns itself with the accuracy of the tumor marker in determining which patients are truely free of neoplasm. Failures of specificity are termed false positive results.

Although, it would be ideal to have a completely sensitive and specific test for all neoplasms or for that matter for any neoplasm, this is not the case. False negative and false positive results occur with all currently used tumor markers. Nevertheless, these markers do have clinical usefulness and have in many cases proved to be of great benefit to patients with a wide variety of tumors.

T. L. Ratliff and W. J. Catalona (eds), Urologic Oncology. ISBN 0-89838-628-4.
© 1984. Martinus Nijhoff Publishers, Boston. Printed in the Netherlands.

2. PROSTATE CANCER

2.1 *Acid phosphatase*

The extensive experience with acid phosphatase as a tumor marker for the evaluation of adenocarcinoma of the prostate testifies to both the clinical usefulness and pitfalls associated with the application of tumor markers (Table 1). Acid phosphatase has long been used as a clinical aid for the evaluation of prostatic carcinoma. Previously untreated patients with disseminated disease frequently have serum elevations of this enzyme. With a good response to hormonal or other forms of therapy, inidividuals with disseminated prostatic adenocarcinoma often exhibit a decrease in serum acid phsophatase which may return to normal values. Unfortunately, exceptions to this clinical scenario frequently exist. Patients who relapse after being treated frequently do not again manifest elevations of acid phosphatase. In addition, serum acid phosphatase may be elevated in a variety of other pathologic states besides metastatic carcinoma of the prostate [1].

With increasing knowledge about serum acid phosphatase, the usefulness of this marker has become progressively less clear. What is termed acid phosphatase by routine enzymatic assay is actually a group of isoenzymes that are produced by a variety of histologically different tissues [1]. Various modifications of the enzymatic assays have been evaluated to produce a test which was more specific for prostatic acid phosphatase. However, these enzymatic alterations have not been consistently better than the measurement of total serum acid phosphatase. More recently, immunologic assays with greater specificity and sensitivity for prostatic acid phosphatase have been developed. A variety of immunologic techniques for the measurement of prostatic acid phosphatase including counter-immunoelectrophoresis, radioimmunoassay, and solid-phase immunoassay have been described [2].

Table 1. Prostate cancer markers.

	Blood	Urine	Tissue	Prostatic fluid
Acid phosphatase	√		√	
Prostate specific antigen	?		√	
Monoclonal antibodies	?		?	
Hormone receptors			?	
Hormones	?	?		
Hydroxyproline		?		
Sialic acid	?			
Lactic dehydrogenase isoenzymes				?
Complement				?
Transferrin				?
Creatine kinase-BB	?		?	
Cholesterol		?		

However, complete specificity for prostatic acid phosphatase has not been achieved because low but measurable amounts of acid phosphatase can be detected in normal females [3]. Despite the theoretical advantages of immunoassays over enzymatic assays, clinical problems remain with their application. One new problem that resulted from their sensitivity was the occasional presence of elevated prostatic acid phosphatase in patients without metastatic spread [4]. Although the increase in sensitivity of the immunoassays were theoretically advantageous, this finding blurred the usefulness of this enzyme as a determinant of distant metastases [5]. Attempts to take advantage of the increased sensitivity of the immunoassays to detect prostate cancer at an earlier stage have also been unsuccessful [6]. Calculations using a theoretical sensitivity of 70% and a specificity of 94% have shown that the radioimmunoassay for prostatic acid phosphatase is not an effective clinical screening test for asymptomatic men [7].

The greater specificity of the immunoassays as compared to the enzymatic methods has been demonstrated to be useful in the measure of bone marrow acid phosphatase. Bone marrow acid phosphatase measurement has been sought as a potentially more sensitive method of determining early metastatic skeletal spread. Conventional enzymatic assays have not been reliable measures of bone marrow acid phosphatase because of the frequent occurrence of positive results in patients without disseminated prostatic cancer [8, 9]. The specificity of the immunoassay gives more accurate measurements of bone marrow acid phosphatase. However, the clinical relevance of this application still remains to be defined. It has been suggested that elevations of the bone marrow acid phosphatase by radioimmunoassay is an early demonstration of bone marrow metastasis which may occur prior to changes detected by bone scan [10]. One short-term study tends to support this hypothesis [11]. In a group of 118 patients, 94% were followed for a mean of 23 months. All patients had bone marrow acid phosphatase determined by radioimmunoassay. Patients with stage D1 disease who had elevated bone marrow acid phosphatase had a much higher chance of developing skeletal metastases during this short follow-up than patients who had normal values (36 and 3% respectively). Nevertheless, in several instances, false positive elevations were also seen. Other investigators, however, comparing serum acid phosphatase and bone marrow acid phosphatase measured by radioimmunoassay have noted little difference between these studies, either in amount of enzyme assayed or percent of patients with abnormal elevation [12]. Further clinical follow-up is required before this diagnostic procedure is accepted for routine clinical use.

On a microscopic scale, immunohistochemical localization of acid phosphatase has been useful for demonstrating the presence of prostatic cancer in metastatic tumors [13]. Caution, however, must be used in interpreting the results because metastatic breast carcinomas occasionally reacted weakly with this assay. The intensity of the staining by prostatic cancer is correlated with the degree of differentiation of the neoplasm [14]. Adenocarcinomas that are well differentiated usually demonstrate intense staining with minimal variability. As these neoplasms become poorly differentiated, the intensity becomes much weaker and the variability of staining increases. Therefore, the analysis of metastatic lesions, particularly when less differentiated tumors are being evaluated, remains a difficult problem.

Acid phosphatase represents a microcosm of the clinical applicability of almost all tumor markers. While it has demonstrated usefulness on both a serologic and histologic basis, there are enough exceptions producing both false positive and false negative results to make a clinical decision solely on an isolated value hazardous. Whether radioimmunoassay is superior to enzymatic assay remains a moot point [15]. The one widely accepted precaution of not drawing blood for serum acid phosphatase after performing a digital rectal examination of the prostate may, in fact, not be relevant. Routine rectal examination rarely causes an elevated serum acid phosphatase [16, 17]. However, more vigorous prostatic manipulation by massage, cystoscopic examination, or biopsy may cause elevations of this enzyme [17, 18]. Despite the limitations inherent in this test, it does give a useful correlation with the presence of metastatic disease and is valuable in monitoring the response to therapy when combined with other monitors of disease activity [19].

2.2 Prostate antigens

In 1979, Wang and associates described the purification of a human prostatic-specific antigen that was distinct from acid phosphatase [20]. The antigen is a glycoprotein with a molecular weight of approximately 34 000 [21]. Antibodies raised to this antigen have been demonstrated to be useful for identifying prostate cancer cells on histologic sections and for measuring the serum level of this antigen [22, 23]. Preliminary studies suggest that serum levels of this antigen may be useful in monitoring the clinical course of some patients and demonstrate that an elevated serum level is an ominous prognostic sign [24]. Monoclonal antibodies have recently been produced to this prostate antigen [25]. A sandwich radioimmunoassay using these antibodies was able to detect 5 ng of prostate antigen per milliliter in patients' serum. Nevertheless, only 25% of patients with metastatic disease had elevations of this antigen. The monoclonal antibody failed to react with membrane preparations of prostate suggesting that the prostate antigen being defined is primarily intracellular.

Several other prostate associated antigens have recently been defined by monoclonal antibodies produced through the hybridoma technique. Ware and associates have produced an antibody designated αPro3 which defines a 54 000 molecular weight antigen that is present on a wide variety of cells including prostatic carcinoma [26]. Quantitatively, the antigen appears to be more prevalent upon poorly differentiated prostatic cancer cells. Clark and associates produced an antibody which reacts with differentiated prostatic epithelial cells [27]. Mild degrees of reactivity were seen with extracts of other normal tissues. Starling and associates have characterized a mono-clonal antibody which is present on several human prostate and bladder carcinoma cell lines [28]. The antibody also reacts with a cell line transformed by cytomegalovirus.

The ultimate role of these prostatic antigens as tumor markers remains to be defined. The prostatic antigen defined by Wang and associates has already been shown to have some relevance histologically. Whether it will prove to be a useful serum marker as well remains to be seen. The usefulness of monoclonal antibody production to define a variety of antigens present on prostatic cancer cells is just recently being exploited. Significant problems include defining the specificity of the antibodies being produced and determining the usefulness of these antibodies in a clinical setting.

2.3 Hormone receptors and hormones

Hormone receptors have been studied primarily as a means of selecting which patients will respond to hormonal manipulation of their neoplasm. Levels of total androgen receptors in patients with benign prostatic hyperplasia were not found to be statistically different from patients with either treated or untreated prostatic cancer [29]. Analysis by R1881 binding of tumor cytosols has shown a better correlation with clinical response to hormonal treatment. Ekman found that 18 of 21 patients who were receptor positive had a good response to hormonal therapy (86%) [30]. On the other hand, only 3 of 8 (37%) receptor negative patients had similar favorable responses to therapy. The duration of response in these patients did not correlate with the content of cytosolic receptors. Trachtenberg and Walsh have studied the nuclear androgen receptor content as well as cytosolic and total cellular androgen receptor content in prostatic cancer cells [31]. Twenty-three men with metastatic prostatic cancer were evaluated with prostatic biopsy before treatment. All patients had measurable levels of androgen receptor in their biopsy specimens and all patients demonstrated a good response to hormonal therapy. Total response was measured by duration of the response and survival following hormonal manipulation. As would be expected, patient survival correlated with the duration of response. Total cellular and cytosolic androgen receptor content did not correlate with response. Higher nuclear androgen receptor levels correlated with greater duration of response and prolonged survival.

Plasma and urine hormone levels have been analyzed as possible markers for prostatic cancer. Hoisaeter measured follicle stimulating hormone, luteinizing hormone, prolactin, testosterone, estradiol, and sex hormone binding globulin in 100 consecutive patients with prostatic cancer [32]. None of the hormones measured could distinguish between different stages or grades of prostatic cancer. Rannikko and associates similarly studied plasma and urine levels of a number of hormones [33]. Urine hormone excretion of androgens, estrogens, and their metabolites were measured. Patients with T1 and T2 disease had significantly higher urinary levels of 17-ketosteroids, etiocholanolone, dehydroepiandrosterone, and 17-ketogenic steroids than patients with T3 and T4 tumors. Nevertheless, there was considerable overlap of these values. Plasma estradiol was significantly greater in patients with metastases than in patients with localized tumors. Patients without metastatic disease had higher ratios of plasma testosterone/plasma estradiol than patients with metastatic disease. Plasma testosterone/plasma estrone plus estradiol ratios were higher both in patients without metastases and in patients with well-differentiated tumors. The role of hormone measurement at this point is unclear. It appears that isolated hormone values appear to have little prognostic value. Marked daily variation in hormone levels certainly compounds this problem. Whether ratios of various hormones will prove more useful remains to be determined.

2.4 Non-specific markers

A number of substances have been analyzed which, although they are not specific for prostatic cancer, appear to offer the potential for clinical relevance. One of these is urinary hydroxyproline. This amino acid is present throughout the body in collagen, and its measurement may be used as an index of turnover of bony matrix. Because of the propensity for prostatic cancer to metastasize to bone, this amino acid may prove to be a useful marker. Total hydroxyproline excretion in the urine and urinary hydroxyproline/creatinine ratios have been reported to be elevated in patients with prostatic cancer who have active skeletal metastases [34, 35]. Serial spot urinary hydroxyproline/creatinine ratios have been demonstrated to correlate with bone scans as a measure of osseous metastasis [36]. Although individual exceptions were present, increasing, stable, or decreasing ratios were usually indicative of progression, stability, or regression on sequential bone scans respectively.

Similar to the findings with hydroxyproline, sialic acid (N-acetylneuraminic acid) is another non-specific substance which may have clinical relevance. This serum glycoprotein has been demonstrated to be elevated in a wide variety of malignant tumors as well as benign disease processes. Elevated serum levels have been recorded in patients with prostatic cancer and appear to correlate with clinical stage [37]. Although the data is not available for prostatic cancer, in other neoplasms serial measurements of sialic acid have been useful as a measure of total body tumor burden (vide infra).

Other studies using non-specific markers have been performed in attempts to discover prostatic neoplasia at an early stage. Lactic dehydrogenase (LDH) isoenzymes, complement components C3 and C4, and transferrin have been measured in the prostatic fluid of patients clinically determined to be at high risk for prostatic cancer [38]. High levels of LDH-5/LDH-1, C3, C4 and transferrin in the prostatic fluid correlated with a high incidence of neoplasia.

Serum levels of creatine kinase-BB have been reported to be elevated in some patients with prostate cancer. However, a prospective study evaluating acid phosphatase and creatine kinase-BB has shown neither of these enzymes to be useful as a screening test [39]. The number of patients with elevated levels of creatine kinase-BB was small. For patients with stages A, B, C, and D, the percent of patients with elevated levels were 7.7, 4.0, 15.4, and 21.1% respectively. Abnormal acid phosphatase values ranging from 6.2% of the patients with stage A to above 65% for stage D with either the enzymatic assay or radioimmunoassay were recorded. As noted in other reports, the percent of patients with abnormal elevation of acid phosphatase was similar regardless whether an enzymatic assay or radioimmunoassay was used.

A histologic evaluation of creatine kinase in benign prostatic hyperplasia and carcinoma of the prostate demonstrated that creatine kinase-BB accounted for 98% of the creatine kinase activity in both prostatic carcinoma and benign hyperplasia [40]. Carcinomas, however, contained less creatine kinase activity (units/g) than hyperplastic prostatic glands. Large variations were seen from different specimens regardless whether the neoplasia was benign or malignant. Because of this large variation, it was suggested that if this enzyme were to be useful at all, it would be most useful in longitudinal studies of individual patients.

Another screening tool for patients with suspected prostatic carcinoma has been the measurement of urinary cholesterol. Total cholesterol was elevated in 52% of patients with stages A and B carcinoma of the prostate and 63% of patients with stages C and D [41]. However, similarly elevated levels were seen in patients with benign prostatic hyperplasia with residual urine. Individuals with benign prostatic hyperplasia without urinary retention had normal levels of urinary cholesterol. Other possible causes for elevated urinary cholesterol include neoplasms of the testis, kidney, and urothelium (vide infra).

3. BLADDER CANCER

3.1 *Cellular antigens*

In 1968, a mixed cell agglutination reaction was described in which the distribution of blood group antigens could be determined on histologic sections of a variety of tissues [42] (Table 2). In this report, it was demonstrated that urothelium normally exhibited the blood group antigen appropriate for that individual. In addition, it was noted that transitional cell carcinomas of the bladder may or may not demonstrate the blood group antigen on the tumor cell surface. This was interpreted as a loss of differentiation by some neoplastic cells. In 1975, this phenomenon was further examined by another group of investigators, and it was determined that the absence of the appropriate blood group antigen on urothelial carcinomas correlated with a tendency to subsequently develop invasive cancer [43]. This finding was subsequently demonstrated with upper urinary tract neoplasms as well as bladder cancer [44]. More recently, the assay has been improved through the use of the immunoperoxidase technique [45]. The cause for antigen deletion remains unclear. It may result from a specific defect in biosynthesis and/or accelerated degradation of blood group antigen substances [46].

Numerous investigators have confirmed the usefulness of the red cell adherence assay. This was recently reviewed by Catalona [47]. In addition to differences in local invasion, the tendency for tumor recurrence in blood group antigen positive and negative neoplasms is strikingly different. Patients with blood group positive tumors have approximately a 46% recurrence rate while individuals with blood group negative tumors have a 90% recurrence rate. Although blood group antigen analysis of tumor cells has

Table 1. Prostate cancer markers.

	Blood	Urine	Tissue	Prostatic fluid
Acid phosphatase	√		√	
Prostate specific antigen	?		√	
Monoclonal antibodies	?		?	
Hormone receptors			?	
Hormones	?	?		
Hydroxyproline		?		
Sialic acid	?			
Lactic dehydrogenase isoenzymes				?
Complement				?
Transferrin				?
Creatine kinase-BB	?		?	
Cholesterol		?		

shown a strong correlation with the subsequent development of invasive disease, it is by no means perfect. Approximately 5% of patients whose tumors demonstrate the appropriate blood group antigen will subsequently develop invasive disease. On the other hand, up to one third of those individuals with blood group antigen negative neoplasms will not develop aggressive disease. At this point in the analysis, it appears that patients with blood group antigen negative neoplasms are at higher risk both for recurrence and subsequent development of invasive tumors. These patients certainly need to be followed very closely and possibly selected for adjuvant therapy of some sort. However, it appears premature at this time to arbitrarily take patients with superficial tumors that are antigen negative and submit them to aggressive extirpative therapy such as radical cystectomy. These conclusions are a result of the extensive study of A, B, and O(H) antigens on human bladder carcinomas. A similar evaluation of the T-antigen is currently being performed [48].

Grossman has reported a monoclonal antibody that reacts on direct serologic testing with only one human bladder cancer cell line [49]. When the same antibody was analyzed with a more sensitive absorption technique, it was found to define an antigen present on 2 of 6 human bladder cancer cell lines and a human cervical cancer cell line. It was not present on a wide variety of other normal and malignant cultured cells. Starling and associates have reported a monoclonal antibody which reacts with some prostate and bladder cancer cell lines as well as a cytomegalovirus transformed cell line [28]. This antibody also did not exhibit significant reactivity with a wide variety of other normal and malignant cell lines.

A polyclonal antibody has been produced against bladder tumor-associated antigens present in urine [50]. This antibody preparation is nonreactive in gel diffusion assays against urine specimens from normal individuals but reacts with 61% of patients with papillomas and carcinoma in situ and 95% of patients with overt bladder cancer. However, individuals with urinary tract infections also demonstrated 37% reactivity in gel diffusion assays. Patients with bladder neoplasia could be differentiated from normals and inviduals with urinary tract infection more clearly when complement fixation assays were used.

3.2 Non-specific markers

Urinary immunoglobulin A has been described to be elevated in patients with bladder cancer [51]. Although urinary levels of IgA are elevated in individuals with urinary tract infection, the levels are still significantly less than in individuals with overt bladder neoplasms. Whether this will be clinically useful in patients with incipient neoplasia remains to be determined.

Urinary polyamines have been measured in an effort to gain more useful prognostic information [52]. The level of putrescine in 24 hr urine specimens were determined in 54 patients with bladder cancer prior to therapy. Elevated levels of putrescine correlated both with stage and grade. In addition, individuals having elevated levels prior to therapy were more likely to develop clinical relapse at six months than those with normal preoperative levels. Of 21 patients with disease recurrence or progression, 20 had preoperatively elevated putrescine levels. On the other hand, of 8 patients remaining disease free, 6 had normal preoperative levels.

Urinary cholesterol has been evaluated as a possible screening tool for genitourinary carcinomas. As such, it has not been effective in an unselected population because of the low incidence of neoplasia and because benign diseases of the kidney and urinary retention are documented causes for abnormal results [53]. On the other hand, in selected populations with microscopic hematuria, elevations of urinary cholesterol were commonly seen with neoplasms of the bladder, prostate, and kidney [54]. The sensitivity of the assay for genitourinary carcinomas was 80% with a specificity of 90%. Patients with urinary catheters, urinary fistulae, or gross hematuria were not included in this study and limit the clinical population for which it is applicable.

Carcinoembryonic antigen (CEA) has been reported to be elevated in the urine and plasma of patients with bladder cancer. However, recent studies have shown that these measurements have little value clinically [55, 56]. A major problem with urinary CEA assays is the abnormal elevation seen in patients with urinary tract infections. Immunoperoxidase localization of CEA on histologic sections of normal and metaplastic urothelial lesions demonstrate that CEA is seen in squamous metaplasia but not in other normal and metaplastic lesions of the bladder [57]. Immunohistochemical evaluation of CEA on 150 transitional cell carcinomas has shown that high stage, high grade tumors are more likely to contain CEA [58]. The percent of grade 1, 2, and 3 neoplasms containing CEA are 24, 72, and 76% respectively. The results for stages Ta, T1, and T2-3 are 34, 59, and 80% respectively.

A variety of urinary proteins were studied by O'Brien and associates as possible tumor markers. Although elevated urinary proteins were seen in many patients, similar patterns of response were seen as well in patients with urinary tract infection [59]. Urinary fibrinogen degradation products have been reported to be elevated in 32% of patients with low stage superficial bladder tumors [60]. Urinary fibrinogen degradation products when coupled with cytology increased the accuracy of the positive results to 80% compared with 71% for cytology alone. Acute phase reactant proteins (acid glycoprotein, antichymotrypsin, and C-reactive protein) are elevated in approximately 60% of patients with advanced bladder cancer (T3 and T4 disease) [61]. It has not been determined whether these proteins will be of any significant use in the monitoring of the course of patients with advanced disease.

Hypercalcemia has been associated with isolated cases of uroepithelial neoplasms. This may be caused by parathormone production by the tumor [62]. Urothelial neoplasms may produce other hormones as well. Human chorionic gonadotropin-like substance has been documented to be produced by some urothelial neoplasms [63].

Serum rheumatoid factor has been measured in individuals with bladder neoplasms [64]. Elevated levels of rheumatoid factor were commonly seen. However, most of these reactions were with undiluted serum. High titer reactions were more uncommon. Individuals without rheumatoid factor in their serum tended to have a lower tumor recurrence rate than individuals with rheumatoid factor.

Lymphocyte adenosine deaminase is an enzyme that appears to play a role in normal lymphocyte function. Sufrin and associates demonstrated that elevations of this enzyme correlated with progressive disease in patients with bladder cancer [65]. Patients with high stage tumors had higher enzyme levels than patients with low stage tumors. Tumor grade did not correlate with lymphocyte adenosine deaminase levels.

Serum sialic acid (N-acetylneuraminic acid) has been shown to correlate with the clinical course of patients with advanced bladder cancer undergoing systemic chemotherapy [66]. This non-specific measure of tumor burden when measured in serial specimens correlates well with disease response. Although, high values do occur in patients with greater amounts of disease, isolated values may not accurately reflect clinical status.

3.3 Cytologic studies

In the late 1960s it was determined that aneuploid transitional cell carcinomas were more often associated with histologic invasion while near diploid neoplasms tended to be non-invasive [67]. Additional studies determined that abnormal chromosomes (markers) were a poor prognostic finding [68]. While only one of 18 papillary bladder tumors without markers recurred, 11 of 32 papillary neoplasms with markers recurred and became invasive. Another study of 40 patients with non-invasive tumors has confirmed these findings [69]. Twenty patients without markers had a 10% recurrence rate while patients with markers had a recurrence rate of 90%.

The use of flow cytometry has expedited the DNA analysis of exfoliated cells. This technique has demonstrated that aneuploid tumors tend to have higher grade and higher S-phase fractions [70]. Follow-up of patients with flow cytometry has demonstrated that patients with consistently diploid

DNA analysis did not have tumor progression [71]. Individuals with tetraploid DNA patterns developed progression in 10% of the cases while 51% of individuals with aneuploid, non-tetraploid cases developed progression. However, even patients with diploid patterns may be at risk because some patients with an initial diploid pattern may change to an aneuploid DNA pattern with time.

4. RENAL CANCER

4.1 *Hormones*

Renal carcinoma may be associated with a wide variety of paraneoplastic endocrinopathies. A number of hormone and hormone-like substances have been reported in isolated cases. These include substances that are identical with or function similar to parathormone, erythropoietin, renin, gonadotropin, placental lactogen, prolactin, enteroglucagon, insulin, adrenocorticotropic hormone, and prostaglandins [72]. Although in theory any of these substances could act as a tumor marker, their clinical relevance is limited because most of these endocrinopathies are rare. In selected patients, however, these substances may be useful to follow (Table 3).

Hypertension associated with elevated plasma renin values has been recorded in some patients with renal carcinoma. Nephrectomy has been documented to cure the hypertension and return renin values to normal. In addition, tissue renin has been documented to be elevated in tumor extracts from a nephrectomy specimen [73]. Sufrin and associates evaluated a group of 57 patients with renal adenocarcinoma for plasma renin, erythropoietin, and chorionic gonadotropin [74]. Elevated renin levels were found in 37% of patients and were associated with high stage tumors and a poor prognosis. In this study, the renin elevation was unrelated to blood pressure. Erythropoietin was elevated in 63% of patients and did not correlate with stage, prognosis, or hemoglobin. None of the patients had elevated chorionic gonadotropin levels.

Table 3. Renal cancer markers.

	Serum	Urine	Tissue
Hormones	?		
Hormone receptors			?
Fibrinogen	?		
Haptoglobin	?		
β_2-microglobulin	?		
Polyamines		?	
Cholesterol		?	

Ectopic parathormone production has been reported with renal adenocarcinoma associated with hypercalcemia. In a patient with this syndrome, nephrectomy resulted in return of calcium and immunologically measured parathormone to normal [75]. Furthermore, extract of the renal tumor contained material that was immunologically similar to human parathyroid hormone.

Steroid receptors have also been examined in renal carcinomas. Concolino and associates studied the cytosol of 23 renal carcinomas for estradiol and progesterone receptors [76]. Each receptor was found in 61% of the neoplasms. Both receptors were found in 39% and neither were found in 17%. Progestational therapy was carried out in 18 patients. Three of the four patients who were receptor negative did not respond to treatment. Thirteen of fourteen patients with either or both receptors were alive 8 to 36 months following the treatment. Di Fronzo and associates evaluated estrogen receptors in 31 renal carcinomas [77]. Using a charcoal absorption technique, no receptors were detectable in 19 samples, and, in the remainder, the values were very low. Progesterone and dihydrotestosterone receptors were studied in four cases and were negative. Chen and associates evaluated the presence of estradiol, androgen, and dexamethasone in 10 primary and 6 metastatic renal carcinomas [78]. Cytosols from all tumors were negative for estrogen receptors. Four samples had low levels of progesterone receptors. Nine had dihydrotestosterone receptors, and 11 had dexamethasone receptors. A competition assay demonstrated that progestin competed for dexamethasone receptors in the cytosol in 7 tissue samples that were so tested. It was hypothesized that the effect of progestational agents in some patients may be explained by the ability to block the activity of glucocorticoid receptors of these tumors.

4.2 Non-specific markers

Non-hormonal substances have been examined as well for possible use as tumor markers. Plasma fibrinogen levels of patients with high stage tumors are significantly higher than normal [79]. In addition, patients with progressive disease had higher fibrinogen levels than patients with stable disease who in turn had higher levels than control subjects. In a similar fashion, serum haptoglobin levels have been correlated with clinical stage [80]. Just as with fibrinogen, patients with low stage disease had significantly lower levels than patients with high stage disease. Eighty-seven percent of patients with stage I disease had normal preoperative haptoglobin levels while all 6 patients with stage IV disease had elevated values. A recent report by Babaian and Swanson measured haptoglobin in 116 patients with renal carcinoma [81]. Normal levels of haptoglobin were found in 87.2% (34/39) of patients who underwent nephrectomy and were clinically free of disease.

Abnormal elevations were present in 58% (45/77) of patients who had unresected tummors or metastatic disease. With increasing tumor burden, higher levels of serum haptoglobin were recorded. However, considerable overlap of values occurred. Serial measurements of serum haptoglobin correlated well with the clinical course and may prove useful for following patients with renal carcinoma.

Serum β_2-microglobulin has been examined in a small group of patients with renal cancer [82]. In three patients with renal carcinoma examined postoperatively who had normal renal function, elevated serum β_2-microglobulin was universally present. However, 8 other patients with renal carcinoma could not be evaluated because of elevated serum creatinine following nephrectomy. Because of the pronounced effect of decreased renal function on serum β_2-microglobulin level, it was concluded that this would severely limit the usefulness of this marker for urologic neoplasms. Similarly, urinary cholesterol has been reported as useful, but only in selected populations (vide supra).

Sanford and associates have measured the urinary polyamines putrescine, spermine, and spermidine in the urine of patients with renal cell carcinoma [83]. Elevated urinary polyamine levels were found in all stages of renal carcinoma (9/11, 82% elevated). One patient with elevated preoperative values underwent curative surgical therapy and had normal values postoperatively. In contrast to this, a patient with metastatic disease continued to have elevated values after undergoing nephrectomy.

5. ADRENAL CANCER

Functioning adrenal neoplasms produce a variety of hormones which may serve as useful markers (Table 4). Malignant tumors of the adrenal medulla include the neuroblastoma and pheochromocytoma. The former neoplasm

Table 4. Adrenal cancer markers.

	Serum	Urine
Vanilmandelic acid		√
Homovanilic acid		√
Metanephrine		√
Catecholamines	√	
17-Ketosteroids		√
17-Hydroxycorticoids		√
Hormones	√	√
17-Ketogenic steroids		√

occurs in infancy and childhood while the latter is more common in the adult population. Neuroblastomas are malignant counterparts of the benign ganglioneuroma. Pheochromocytomas are usually benign with the incidence of malignancy being approximately 10–20% [84, 85]. Both neuroblastomas and pheochromocytomas are diagnosed by the determination of catecholamines and their metabolites. Neuroblastomas have been diagnosed by urinary levels of vanilmandelic acid (VMA) and homovanilic acid (HVA). VMA as measured in the urine is a reliable measure of its production because of the rapid turnover of this substance [86]. Eighty percent of patients with neuroblastoma will excrete one or both of these substances [87]. In addition, the VMA/HVA ratio has been demonstrated to have some prognostic value. In patients with stage IV disease, high VMA/HVA ratios correlated with an improved prognosis [88]. It has been suggested that this supports the concept that tumors which are biochemically primitive, i.e., deficient in dopamine β-hydroxylase, are biologically more malignant.

The traditional method for diagnosing pheochromocytomas has also been the urinary measure of catecholamines and their metabolites. While VMA and HVA have been used, urinary metanephrine levels are much more reliable [89]. A 10-year experience using urinary metanephrine levels as a screening procedure for pheochromocytoma revealed that false positive studies occurred at a rate of 1.9% [90]. Many of these false positive results were drug related. All patients with histologically confirmed pheochromocytoma were tested on multiple occasions and had elevated urinary metanephrine levels. Multiple studies are important because some of these patients did have occasional normal metanephrine excretion. More recently, the use of plasma catecholamines has been assessed. Bravo and associates compared plasma catecholamines with the urinary catecholamine metabolites VMA and metanephrine [91]. Resting, supine plasma catecholamines were more useful than either or both urinary metabolites. Plasma catecholamines were reliable even in normotensive patients and thus can eliminate the need for potentially dangerous provocative testing. Nevertheless, when such testing was performed with glucagon, increases in plasma catecholamine levels correlated with increases in blood pressure. Provocative testing may be required when plasma catecholamine values are between 1000 and 2000 ng/l. This is important because 15% of hypertensive individuals without pheochromocytoma will have elevated plasma catecholamines with levels ranging up to 1500 ng/l [92].

Adrenal cortical carcinoma may produce any of the hormones normally secreted by the adrenal cortex. These hormones include corticosteroids, mineralocorticoids, androgens, and estrogens. These tumors are classified as functioning or non-functioning depending on whether or not a clinical syndrome caused by hormonal excess is present. Although non-functioning tumors do not have obvious hormonal excess, increased levels of hormonally inactive precursors may be present [93]. Patients with functional carcinomas commonly have increased levels of urinary 17-ketosteroids [94]. Abnormal elevations of 17-ketosteroids may also occur in some patients with clinically non-functioning tumors [95]. In addition to the 17-ketosteroids, other abnormalities may include elevations of urinary 17-hydroxycorticoids and urinary free cortisol. It has been suggested that 17-ketogenic steroids may be more useful than 17-hydroxycorticoids because the former test also includes pregnanetriol which is a metabolite of 17-hydroxyprogesterone [96]. A report of a child with a virilizing adrenal cortical carcinoma documented the usefulness of serum testosterone in monitoring the subsequent development of recurrent disease [97].

6. TESTICULAR CANCER

6.1 *AFP and HCG*

When urologists think of tumor markers, alpha-fetoprotein (AFP) and the beta subunit of human chorionic gonadrotropin (HCG) immediately come to mind (Table 5). The specificity, sensitivity, and clinical relevance of these markers has been outstanding. Nevertheless, false positive and negative studies do occur. The reasons for this have been well documented and are instructive.

Alpha-fetoprotein is a glycoprotein with a half-life of five days. It is elevated in up to 75% of patients with non-seminomatous germ cell carcinomas (NSGCC) but is not present in patients with seminomas [98]. In fact, patients with histologically pure seminoma and elevated AFP must be suspected of harboring an occult NSGCC. An exception to this rule, however, has been described in a patient with a pure seminoma with liver metastases whose elevated AFP was related to active liver regeneration [99]. Localiza-

Table 5. Testicular cancer markers.

	Serum	Urine	Tissue
Alpha-fetoprotein	√		√
Human chorionic gonadotropin	√	?	√
Pregnancy specific beta-1 glycoprotein	?		?
Lactic dehydrogenase	?		
Sialic acid	?		
β_2-microglobulin	?		
Placental alkaline phosphatase	?		?

tion of AFP by immunohistologic study of 21 patients revealed that AFP is present in and presumably is produced by mononuclear embryonal cells within embryonal carcinoma and endodermal sinus tumor [100]. In addition, AFP has been shown to be present in cylindric epithelia in two of seven immature teratomas [101].

Human chorionic gonadrotropin is a glycoprotein composed of two dissimilar subunits. The whole molecule has a half-life of approximately 24 hr [98]. The alpha subunit has a half-life of 20 min and is similar to the alpha subunit of luteinizing hormone, follicle-stimulating hormone, and thyrotropic hormone [102]. An interesting use of the alpha subunit of HCG was reported in an individual who had tumor localization by measurement of this substance. Selective catheterization and venous sampling of the right ascending lumbar vein was performed in a patient with disease in the right lateral pelvis. The short half-life of the alpha subunit permitted localization of disease to this area [100]. The beta subunit is unique for HCG and has a half-life of 60 min. Using an immunoperoxidase technique, HCG has been identified within syncytiotrophoblastic giant cells in association with embryonal carcinoma and occasionally endodermal sinus tumor and seminoma [100]. HCG has also been localized to the syncytiotrophoblastic cells in choriocarcinoma. Testicular tumors have been demonstrated to synthesize AFP and HCG in vitro [103].

AFP and the beta subunit of HCG have received wide clinical use in the management of patients with testicular germ cell neoplasms. Patients with seminoma frequently have normal levels of AFP and HCG. Elevated levels of AFP must be considered to represent an occult focus of NSGCC unless liver metastases are present. Approximately 10% of patients with seminoma will have elevated serum levels of HCG. However, high levels should raise the suspicion of an undetected focus of choriocarcinoma [104].

While the incidence of elevated AFP and HCG in seminomas is low, these markers are commonly elevated in non-seminomatous testicular tumors. The percent of patients with elevated markers increases with the stage of disease [105]. Elevation of markers is seen in approximately 20% of the patients with stage I disease prior to orchiectomy. Stage II and stage III patients will have approximately 60 and 90% abnormal increases in one or both markers respectively. The measurement of HCG and AFP has proved to be an accurate diagnostic test. In a group of 37 patients with retroperitoneal metastases, 73% had elevated markers while only 59% had abnormal clinical studies consisting of excretory urography (IVP) and lymphangiography [106]. When both clinical studies and tumor markers were combined, the accuracy was increased to 86%. Because of the high correlation of metastatic disease with elevated tumor markers, the measurement of AFP and HCG have become crucial in the staging of this disease. Markers have also been used extensively to follow patients' clinical courses, and frequently, recurrent disease will be associated with elevation of these tumor markers [98]. However, this is not always the case. Tumors may recur without abnormal AFP or HCG, and their measurement cannot be used as the sole method for follow-up. Serum levels of AFP and HCG frequently are normal even in the presence of residual tumor in patients undergoing chemotherapy [107].

There have been several sources for error noted with the measurement of HCG and AFP. Some of these are on a technical basis. This particularly involves the measurement of HCG where elevations may be seen due to cross-reactivity with luteinizing hormone when assays are used that are not completely specific for the beta subunit [108]. If this is suspected, suppression of luteinizing hormone may be carried out by the administration of testosterone. An alternative method is to have the studies repeated at a reference laboratory [109]. Measurement of AFP is not susceptible to these cross-reactivities and hence has been much more reliable [110].

False negative studies may occur because the tumor either does not produce AFP or HCG or does so in very low amounts. It would be expected, therefore, that individuals with small amounts of tumor would have fewer elevations of serum markers. In a study of 60 patients with retroperitoneal lymphatic metastases, the percent of patients with elevated AFP or HCG correlated directly with the amount of disease present [111]. When only one lymph node was positive, there was a 9% incidence of elevated markers. As lymphatic involvement increased the percent positive elevation increased up to 89%. Determination of simultaneous serum and tumor cytosol levels of HCG and AFP has demonstrated that elevated levels are more commonly seen in the tumor cytosol than in the serum [112]. A recent study also showed that urine levels of HCG measured by a carboxyl-terminal radioimmunoassay are more sensitive than serum levels using a double antibody radioimmunoassay [113].

Measurement of AFP and HCG half-lives may have some prognostic benefit as well. Although the initial half-life after onset of chemotherapy has not been helpful in determining prognosis [114], measurement of AFP half-life 21 to 42 days after onset of chemotherapy revealed prolongation of AFP half-life in patients who relapsed or had persistent disease compared with patients who became tumor free [115]. The role of half-life determination of tumor markers in testicular cancer remains to be defined. Variables that have a crucial impact on the calculation of marker half-life include the point where calculation begins, the frequency of specimen collection, and the point where calculation terminates [116]. When these factors are better defined in prognostic studies, the clinical relevance of these calculations can then be more accurately appraised.

6.2 Other markers

Pregnancy specific beta-1 glycoprotein (SP1) has been localized by immunoperoxidase studies to the syncytiotrophoblastic component of choriocarcinoma and in syncytiotrophoblastic giant cells associated with embryonal carcinoma with or without teratoma [117]. Although SP1 is most commonly elevated in concordance with HCG, exceptions have been documented both in serum levels and by immunoperoxidase assays of tumor specimens [118, 119]. Human placental lactogen (HPL) has also been evaluated as a serum marker for testicular neoplasms. Just as with SP1, there is a marked concordance of elevations of HCG and HPL. However, occasional discordance of serum levels do occur and two patients have been documented in which HPL was elevated when HCG was normal [120].

Serum lactic dehydrogenase (LDH) has been reported to be a valuable measure of gross tumor burden [121]. In patients with stages B and C disease, elevated total LDH that persisted during therapy was a poor prognostic sign and signified the presence of persistent disease and lack of response to treatment. Total LDH, however, did not always reliably predict the presence of disease or disease recurrence.

Just as with bladder cancer, serial measurements of serum sialic acid (N-acetylneuraminic acid) have proved useful in a patient with metastatic embryonal cell carcinoma [66]. In this individual, elevation of sialic acid was a more sensitive indicator of disease recurrence then either AFP or HCG (Figure 1).

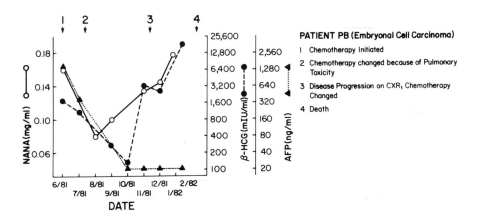

Figure 1. Serial serum levels of sialic acid (N-acetylneuraminic acid [NANA]), alpha-fetoprotein (AFP), and the beta subunit of human chorionic gonadotropin (β-HCG) in a patient with embryonal carcinoma of the testis. An increasing serum sialic acid was the first indicator of relapse. Reprinted with permission from Khanderia et al. [66].

Serum β_2-microglobulin has been evaluated in patients with testicular neoplasms [122]. Only 12.5% of the patients had elevated serum β_2-microglobulin and all these patients had advanced disease. Nevertheless, even with advanced disease, only 3 of 13 patients had elevated levels of β_2-microglobulin.

Immunoperoxidase localization of the placental (Regan) isoenzyme of alkaline phosphatase has demonstrated this substance to be present on approximately 90% of seminomas. It was not present on embryonal carcinomas or interstitial cell tumors [123]. Elevated serum levels of placental alkaline phosphatase have been found in 43% (9/21) of patients with initially diagnosed seminoma (pre-orchiectomy sera) and in 75% (9/12) of patients with metastatic seminoma [124]. Just as with AFP and HCG in NSGCC, serial measurements of placental alkaline phosphatase were useful in following patients with seminoma.

Serum calcitonin has been documented in a single case report to be a useful marker of disease in a patient with extragonadal seminoma [125]. In this individual with elevated serum calcitonin and initially elevated serum calcium, serial measurement of calcitonin proved valuable in following the course of his disease despite the fact that the serum calcium was normal.

7. CONCLUSION

The use of biologic tumor markers has enormous potential to aid the clinician in the management of malignant disease. On a microscopic basis, markers may not only offer clues to the site of origin of metastatic disease, but may yield significant prognostic information as well. Serum and urine markers are potentially useful both in staging disease and in follow-up as an aid in determining the effectiveness of therapeutic intervention and in detecting early recurrent disease. Although no currently available markers are completely specific and sensitive for any neoplasm, usefulness for the above purposes has been repeatedly demonstrated for a variety of substances. However, because of the inherent limitations in sensitivity and specificity, it is appropriate that the clinician be cautious before embracing any new putative markers. Examples of false negative and false positive assays abound, and interpretation of results even with widely used markers may at times be extremely difficult. As can be seen by a casual glance at Tables 1–5, markers which have strongly documented clinical usefulness as indicated by a checkmark are scarce. Nevertheless, with increased sophistication of use of markers and the development of monoclonal antibodies, it appears that tumor markers will gain an ever increasing clinical role in the future.

REFERENCES

1. Yam LT: Clinical significance of the human acid phosphatase. A review. Am J Med 56:604-616, 1974.
2. Chu TM, Wang MC, Lee CL, Killian CS, Valenzuela LA, Wajsman Z, Slack N, Murphy GP: Enzyme markers for prostate cancer. Cancer Detect and Prev 2:693-706, 1979.
3. Goldenberg SL, Silver HBK, Sullivan LD, Morse MJ, Archibald EL: A critical evaluation of specific radioimmunoassay for prostatic acid phosphatase. Cancer 50:1847-1851, 1982.
4. Lee CL, Chu TM, Wajsman LZ, Slack NH, Murphy GP: Value of new fluorescent immunoassay for human prostatic acid phosphatase in prostate cancer. Urology 15:338-341, 1980.
5. Bruce AW, Mahan DE, Sullivan LD, Goldenberg L: The significance of prostatic acid phosphatase in adenocarcinoma of the prostate. J Urol 125:357-360, 1981.
6. Quinones GR, Rohner TJ Jr, Drago JR, Demers LM: Will prostatic acid phosphatase determination by radioimmunoassay increase the diagnosis of early prostatic cancer? J Urol 125:361-364, 1981.
7. Watson RA, Tang DB: The predictive value of prostatic acid phosphatase as a screening test for prostatic cancer. N Engl J Med 303:497-499, 1980.
8. Pontes JE, Choe B, Rose N, Pierce JM Jr: Reliability of bone marrow acid phosphatase as a parameter of metastatic prostatic cancer. J Urol 122:178-179, 1979.
9. Romas NA, Veenema RJ, Hsu KC, Tomashefsky P, Lattimer JK, Tannenbaum M: Bone marrow acid phosphatase and prostatic cancer: An assessment by immunoassay and biochemical methods. J Urol 123:392-395, 1980.
10. Cooper JF, Foti A, Herschman H: Combined serum and bone marrow radioimmunoassay for prostatic acid phosphatase. J Urol 122:498-501, 1979.
11. Belville WD, Mahan DE, Sepulveda RA, Bruce AW, Miller CF: Bone marrow acid phosphatase by radioimmunoassay: Three years of experience. J Urol 125:809-811, 1981.
12. Vihko P, Kontturi M, Lukkarinen O, Vihko R: Radioimmunoassayable prostate-specific acid phosphatase in peripheral and bone marrow sera compared in diagnosis of prostatic cancer patients. J Urol 128:739-741, 1982.
13. Li CY, Lam KW, Yam LT: Immunohistochemical diagnosis of prostatic cancer with metastases. Cancer 46:706-712, 1980.
14. Bates RJ, Chapman CM, Prout GR Jr, Lin C-W: Immunohistochemical idenfication of prostatic acid phosphatase: correlation of tumor grade with acid phosphatase distribution. J Urol 127:574-580, 1982.
15. Sarosdy MF, Kledzik G, Lamm DL: Serum and bone marrow radioimmunoassay of acid phosphatase in prostatic cancer. Urology 19:33-36, 1982.
16. Khan AN, Lee GS, Jackett DMR, Newcombe RG, Pathy MS: The effect of routine digital examination of the prostate on serum acid phosphatase. Br J Urol 50:182-184, 1978.
17. Vihko P, Lukkarinen O, Contturi M, Vihko R: The effect of manipulation of the prostate gland on serum prostate-specific acid phosphatase measured by radioimmunoassay. Invest Urol 18:334-336, 1981.
18. Pearson JC, Dombrovskis S, Dreyer J, Williams RD: Radioimmunoassay of serum prostatic acid phosphatase after prostatic massage. Urology 21:37-41, 1983.
19. Johnson DE, Prout GR, Scott WW, Schmidt JD, Gibbons RP, Murphy GP: Clinical significance of serum acid phosphatase levels in advanced prostatic carcinoma. Urology 8:123-126, 1976.
20. Wang MC, Valenzuela LA, Murphy GP, Chu TM: Purification of a human prostate specific antigen. Invest Urol 17:159-163, 1979.
21. Papsidero LD, Kuriyama M, Wang MC, Horoscewicz J, Leon SS, Valenzuela L, Murphy

GP, Chu TM: Prostate Antigen: A marker for human prostate epithelial cells. J Natl Cancer Inst 66:37-42, 1981.

22. Nadji M, Tabei SZ, Castro A, Chu TM, Murphy GP, Wang MC, Morales AR: Prostatic-specific antigen: An immunohistologic marker for prostatic neoplasms. Cancer 48:1229-1232, 1981.

23. Wang MC, Papsidero LD, Kuriyama MM, Valenzuela LA, Murphy GP, Chu TM: Prostate antigen: A new potential marker for prostatic cancer. Prostate 2:89-96, 1981.

24. Kuriyama M, Wang MC, Lee C, Papsidero LD, Killian CS, Inaji H, Slack NH, Nishiura T, Murphy GP, Chu TM: Use of prostate-specific antigen in monitoring prostate cancer. Cancer Res 41:3874-3876.

25. Frankel AE, Rouse RV, Wang MC, Chu TM, Herzenberg LA: Monoclonal Antibodies to human prostate antigen. Cancer Res 42:3714-3718, 1982.

26. Ware JL, Paulson DF, Parks SF, Webb KS: Production of monoclonal antibody αPro3 recognizing a human prostatic carcinoma antigen. Cancer Res 42:1215-1222, 1982.

27. Clark SM, Merchant DK, Starling JJ: Monoclonal antibodies against a soluble cytoplasmic antigen in human prostatic epithelial cells. Prostate 3:203-214, 1982.

28. Starling JJ, Sieg SM, Beckett ML, Schellhammer PF, Ladaga LE, Wright GL Jr: Monoclonal antibodies to human prostate and bladder tumor-associated antigens. Cancer Res 42:3084-3089, 1982.

29. Ghanadian R, Auf G, Williams G: Relationship between prostatic cytoplasmic and nuclear androgen receptors in patients with carcinoma of the prostate. Eur Urol 7:39-40, 1981.

30. Ekman P: Steroid receptors in urological malignancies. Acta Obstet Gynecol Scand (Suppl) 101:87-92, 1981.

31. Trachtenberg J, Walsh PC: Correlation of prostatic nuclear androgen receptor content with duration of response and survival following hormonal therapy in advanced prostatic cancer. J Urol 127:466-471, 1982.

32. Hoisaeter PA, Haukaas S, Bakke A, Hoiem L, Segadal E, Thorsen T: Blood hormone levels related to stages and grades of prostatic cancer. Prostate 3:375-381, 1982.

33. Rannikko S, Kairento A-L, Karonen S-L, Adlercreutz H: Hormonal pattern in prostatic cancer. I. Correlation with local extent of tumour, presence of metastases and grade of differentiation. Acta Endocrinol 98:625-633, 1981.

34. Mooppan MMU, Wax SH, Kim H, Wang JC, Tobin MS: Urinary hydroxyproline excretion as a marker of osseous metastasis in carcinoma of the prostate. J Urol 123:694-696, 1980.

35. Rinsho K, Aoyagi K: Urinary hydroxyproline excretion as a marker of bone metastasis in prostatic cancer. Tohoku J Exp Med 137:461-462, 1982.

36. Hopkins SC, Nissenkorn I, Palmieri GMA, Ikard M, Moinuddin M, Soloway MS: Serial sport hydroxyproline/creatinine ratios in metastatic prostatic cancer. J Urol 129:319-323, 1983.

37. Moss AJ Jr, Bissada NK, Boyd CM, Hunter WC: Significance of protein-bound neuraminic acid levels in patients with prostatic and bladder carcinoma. Urology 13:182-184, 1979.

38. Grayhack JT, Wendel EF, Oliver L, Lee C: Analysis of specific proteins in prostatic fluid for detecting prostatic malignancy. J Urol 121:295-299, 1979.

39. Fair WR, Heston WD, Kadmon D, Crane DB, Catalona WJ, Ladenson JH, McDonald JM, Noll BW, Harvey G: Prostatic cancer, acid phosphatase, creatinine kinase-BB and race: A prospective study. J Urol 128:735-738, 1982.

40. Pretlow TG II, Whitehurst GB, Pretlow TP, Hunt RS, Jacobs JM, McKenzie DR, McDaniel HG, Hall LM, Bradley EL Jr: Decrease in creatinine kinase-BB in human prostatic carcinoma compared to benign prostatic hyperplasia. Cancer Res 42:4842-4848, 1982.

41. Juengst D, Pickel A, Elsaesser E, Marx FJ, Karl HJ: Urinary cholesterol excretion in men with benign prostatic hyperplasia and carcinoma of the prostate. Cancer 43:353-359, 1979.

42. Kovarik S, Davidsohn I, Stejskal R: ABO antigens in cancer. Detection with the mixed cell agglutination reaction. Arch Pathol 86:12-21, 1968.

43. Decenzo JM, Howard P, Irish CE: Antigenic deletion and prognosis of patients with stage a transitional cell bladder carcinoma. J Urol 114:874-878, 1975.

44. Hall L, Faddoul A, Saberi A, Edson M: The use of the red cell surface antigen to predict the malignant potential of transitional cell carcinoma of the ureter and renal pelvis. J Urol 127:23-25, 1982.

45. Wiley EL, Mendelsohn G, Droller MJ, Eggleston JC: Immunoperoxidase detection of carcinoembryonic antigen and blood group substances in papillary transitional cell carcinoma of the bladder. J Urol 128:276-280, 1982.

46. Limas C, Lange P: Altered reactivity for A, B, H antigens in transitional cell carcinomas of the urinary bladder. A study of the mechanisms involved. Cancer 46:1366-1373, 1980.

47. Catalona WJ: Practical utility of specific red cell adherence test in bladder cancer. Urology 18:113-117, 1981.

48. Javadpour N: Immunocytochemical localization of various markers in cancer cells and tumors. Diagnostic and therapeutic strategy in urologic cancers. Urology 21:1-7, 1983.

49. Grossman HB: Hybridoma antibodies reactive with human bladder carcinoma cell surface antigens. J Urol 130:610-614, 1983.

50. Gozzo JJ, Cronin WJ, O'Brien P, Monaco AP: Detection of tumor-associated antigens in urine from patients with bladder cancer. J Urol 124:804-807, 1980.

51. Betkerur V, Baumgartner G, Talluri K, Sharifi R, Nagubadi S, Guinan P: Urinary immunoglobulin A in the diagnosis of bladder cancer. J Surg Oncol 16:215-217, 1981.

52. Pastorini P, Milano G, Toubol J, Raymond G, Cambon P, Lalanne CM: The diagnostic and prognostic value of urinary polyamine measurement in bladder cancer. Urol Res 9:13-16, 1981.

53. Jungst D, Tauber R, Osterholzer M, Karl HJ: Is urinary cholesterol determination a possible screening test for urological carcinomas? Urol Res 9:1-3, 1981.

54. Jungst D, Osterholzer M, Tauber R, Karl HJ: Urinary cholesterol in cancer screening. Urology 20:495-498, 1982.

55. Murphy WM, Vandevoorde JP, Rao MK, Soloway MS: The clinical value of urinary carcinoembryonic antigen-like substances in urothelial cancer. J Urol 118:806-808, 1977.

56. Glashan RW, Higgins E, Neville AM: The clinical value of plasma and urinary carcinoembryonic antigen (CEA) assays in patients with hematuria and urothelial carcinoma. Eur Urol 6:344-346, 1980.

57. El-Sayed LH, Hassan EM, Amin AM, Ismail AA: Immunocytochemical studies of carcinoembryonic antigen (CEA) in bilharzial bladder. Neoplasma 29:233-235, 1982.

58. Jautzke G, Altenaehr E: Immunohistochemical demonstration of carcinoembryonic antigen (CEA) and its correlation with grading and staging on tissue sections of urinary bladder carcinomas. Cancer 50:2052-2056, 1982.

59. O'Brien P, Gozzo JJ, Monaco AP: Urinary proteins as biological markers: Bladder cancer diagnosis versus urinary tract infection. J Urol 124:802-803, 1980.

60. Wajsman Z, Williams PD, Greco J, Murphy GP: Further study of fibrinogen degradation products and bladder cancer detection. Urology 12:659-661, 1978.

61. Bastable JRG, Richards B, Haworth S, Cooper EH: Acute phase reactant proteins in the clinical management of carcinoma of the bladder. Br J Urol 51:283-289, 1979.

62. Mandell J, Magee MC, Fried FA: Hypercalcemia associated with uroepithelial neoplasms. J Urol 119:844-845, 1978.

134

63. Kitajima K, Satoh Y, Okada K, Kishimoto T: Human chorinic gonadotropin-like substance (hCG-LS)-producing urothelial carcinoma: Immunohistological location of hCG-LS. Jpn J Clin Oncol 12:49-56, 1982.
64. Gupta NP, Malaviya AN, Singh SM: Rheumatoid factor: Correlation with recurrence in transitional cell carcinoma of the bladder. J Urol 121:417-418, 1979.
65. Sufrin G, Tritsch GL, Mittleman A, Murphy GP: Adenosine deaminase activity in patients with carcinoma of the bladder. J Urol 119:343-346, 1978.
66. Khanderia U, Keller JH, Grossman HB: Serum sialic acid is a biologic marker for malignant disease. J Surg Oncol 23:163-166, 1983.
67. Lamb D: Correlation of chromosome counts with histological appearances and prognosis in transitional-cell carcinoma of bladder. Br Med J 1:273-277, 1967.
68. Sandberg AA: Chromosome markers and progression in bladder cancer. Cancer Res 37:2950-2956, 1977.
69. Summers JL, Falor WH, Ward R: A 10-year analysis of chromosomes in non-invasive papillary carcinoma of the bladder. J Urol 125:177-178, 1981.
70. Tribukait B, Gustafson H, Esposti P: Ploidy and proliferation in human bladder tumors as measured by flow-cytofluorometric DNA analysis and its relations to histopathology and cytology. Cancer 43:1742-1751, 1979.
71. Gustafson H, Tribukait B, Esposti PL: DNA profile and tumour progression in patients with superficial bladder tumours. Urol Res 10:13-18, 1982.
72. Altaffer LF III, Chenault OW Jr: Paraneoplastic endocrinopathies associated with renal tumors. J Urol 122:573-577, 1979.
73. Lebel M, Talbot J, Grose J, Morin J: Adenocarcinoma of the kidney and hypertension: report of two cases with special emphasis on renin. J Urol 118:923-927, 1977.
74. Sufrin G, Mirand EA, Moore RH, Chu TM, Murphy GP: Hormones in renal cancer. J Urol 117:433-438, 1977.
75. Buckle RM, McMillan M, Mallinson C: Ectopic secretion of parathyroid hormone by a renal adenocarcinoma in a patient with hypercalcaemia. Br Med J 4:724-726, 1970.
76. Concolino G, Marocchi A, Conti C, Tenaglia R, Di Silverio F, Bracci U: Human renal cell carcinoma as a hormone-dependent tumor. Cancer Res 38:4340-4344, 1978.
77. Di Fronzo G, Ronchi E, Bertuzzi A, Vezzoni P, Pizzocaro G: Estrogen receptors in renal carcinoma. Eur Urol 6:307-311, 1980.
78. Chen L, Weiss FR, Chaichik S, Keydar I: Steroid receptors in human renal carcinoma. Isr J Med Sci 16:756-760, 1980.
79. Sufrin G, Mink I, Fitzpatrick J, Moore R, Murphy GP: Coagulation factors in renal adenocarcinoma. J Urol 119:727-730, 1978.
80. Vickers M Jr: Serum haptoglobins: A preoperative detector of metastatic renal carcinoma. J Urol 112:310-312, 1974.
81. Babaian RJ, Swanson DA: Serum Haptoglobin: A nonspecific tumor marker for renal cell carcinoma. South Med J 75:1345-1348, 1982.
82. Bunning RAD, Haworth SL, Cooper EH: Serum beta-2-microglobulin levels in urological cancer. J Urol 121:624-625, 1979.
83. Sanford EJ, Drago JR, Rohner TJ, Kessler GF, Sheehan L, Lipton A: Preliminary evaluation of urinary polyamines in the diagnosis of genitourinary tract malignancy. J Urol 113:218-221, 1975.
84. Duckett JW, Koop CE: Neuroblastoma. Urol Clin North Am 4:285-295, 1977.
85. Gittes RF, Mahoney EM: Pheochromocytoma. Urol Clin North Am 4:239-252, 1977.
86. LaBrosse EH, Imashuku S, Fineberg SE: Distribution and turnover of 7-^{3}H-methoxy-4-hydroxymandelic acid in a patient with ganglioneuroma. J Clin Endocrinol Metab 35:753-761, 1972.

87. Evans AE: Staging and treatment of neuroblastoma. Cancer 45:1799-1802, 1980.
88. Laug WE, Siegel SE. Shaw KNF, Landing B, Baptista J, Gutenstein M: Initial urinary catecholamine metabolite concentrations and prognosis in neuroblastoma. Pediatrics 62:77-83, 1978.
89. Juan D: Pheochromocytoma: Clinical manifestations and diagnostic tests. Urology 17:1-12, 1981.
90. Peterson DD, Brown DR, Woods JW, Cole AG, Fried FA: Pheochromocytoma: recent experience with detection and management. Urology 10:133-138, 1977.
91. Bravo EL, Tarazi RC, Gifford RW, Stewart BH: Circulating and urinary catecholamines in pheochromocytoma. Diagnostic and pathophysiologic implications. N Engl J Med 301:682-686, 1979.
92. Jiang N-S, Stoffer SS, Pikler GM, Wadel O, Sheps SG: Laboratory and clinical observations with a two-column plasma catecholamine assay. Mayo Clin Proc 48:47-49, 1973.
93. Fukushima DK, Gallagher TF: Steroid production in 'non-functioning' adrenal cortical tumor. J Clin Endocrinol 23:923-927, 1963.
94. Richie JP, Gittes RF: Carcinoma of the adrenal cortex. Cancer 45:1957-1964, 1980.
95. Didolkar MS, Bescher RA, Elias EG, Moore RH: Natural history of adrenal cortical carcinoma: A clinicopathologic study of 42 patients. Cancer 47:2153-2161, 1981.
96. Sullivan M, Boileau M, Hodges CV: Adrenal cortical carcinoma. J Urol 120:660-665, 1978.
97. Drago JR, Sheikholislam B, Olstein JS, Palmer JM, Tesluk H, Link D: Virilizing adrenal cortical carcinoma with hypertrophy of spermatic tubules in childhood. Urology 14:70-75, 1979.
98. Javadpour N: The role of biologic tumor markers in testicular cancer. Cancer 45:1755-1761, 1980.
99. Javadpour N: Significance of elevated serum alpha-fetoprotein (AFP) in seminoma. Cancer 45:2166-2168, 1980.
100. Kurman RJ, Scardino PT, McIntire KR, Waldmann TA, Javadpour N: Cellular localization of alpha-fetoprotein and human chorionic gonadotropin in germ cell tumors of the testis using an indirect immunoperoxidase technique. A new approach to classification utilizing tumor markers. Cancer 40:2136-2151, 1977.
101. Wagener C, Menzel B, Breuer H, Weissbach L, Tschubel K, Henkel K, Gedigk P: Immunohistochemical localization of alpha-fetoprotein (AFP) in germ cell tumours: evidence for AFP production by tissues different from endodermal sinus tumour. Oncology 38:236-239, 1981.
102. Javadpour N: Biologic tumor markers in management of testicular and bladder cancer. Urology 12:177-183, 1978.
103. Javadpour N, Soares T, Princler GL: In vitro synthesis of alpha-fetoprotein and human chorionic gonadotropin in testicular cancer. Cancer 49:303-307, 1982.
104. Javadpour N: Management of Seminoma based on tumor markers. Urol Clin North Am 7:773-780, 1980.
105. Bosl GJ, Lange PH, Fraley EE, Goldman A, Nochomovitz LE, Rosai J, Waldmann TA, Johnson K, Kennedy BJ: Human chorionic gonadotropin and alpha-fetoprotein in the staging of nonseminomatous testicular cancer. Cancer 47:328-332, 1981.
106. Barzell WE, Whitmore WF Jr: Clinical significance of biologic markers: memorial hospital experience. Semin Oncol 6:48-52, 1979.
107. Skinner DG, Scardino PT: Relevance of biochemical tumor markers and lymphadenectomy in management of non-seminomatous testis tumors: current perspective. J Urol 123:378-382, 1980.
108. Catalona WJ, Vaitukaitis JL, Fair WR: Falsely positive human chorionic gonadotropin

136

assays in patients with testicular tumors: Conversion to negative with testosterone administration. J Urol 122:126-128, 1979.

109. Javadpour N, Soares T: False-positive and fase-negative alpha-fetoprotein and human chorionic gonadotropin assays in testicular cancer: A double blind study. Cancer 48:2279-2281, 1981.

110. Fowler JE Jr: Observations on reliability of commercial assay for alpha-fetoprotein. Urology 19:275-277, 1982.

111. Vugrin D, Whitmore WF Jr, Nisselbaum J, Watson RC: Correlation of serum tumor markers and lymphangiography with degrees of nodal involvement in surgical stage II testis cancer. J Urol 127:683-684, 1982.

112. Javadpour N, Woltering E, Soares T: Simultaneous measurement of tumor cytosol and peripheral serum levels of human chorionic gonadotropin and alphafetoprotein in testicular cancer. Invest Urol 18:11-12, 1980.

113. Javadpour N, Chen H-C: Improved human chorionic gonadotropin on concentrated 24-hour urine in patients with testicular cancer. J Urol 126:176-178, 1981.

114. Willemse PHB, Slejifer DT, Koops HS, De Bruijan HWA, Oosterhuis JW, Bruwers TM, Ockhuizen T, Marrink J: The value of AFP and HCG half lives in predicting the efficacy of combination chemotherapy in patients with non-seminomatous germ cell tumors of the testis. Oncodev Biol Med 2:129-234, 1981.

115. Vogelzang NJ, Lange PH, Goldman A, Vessela RH, Fraley EE, Kennedy BJ: Acute changes of α-fetoprotein and human chorionic gonadotropin during induction chemotherapy of germ cell tumors. Cancer res 42:4855-4861, 1982.

116. Lange PH, Vogelzang NJ, Goldman A, Kennedy BJ, Fraley EE: Marker half-life analysis as a prognostic tool in testicular cancer. J Urol 128:708-711, 1982.

117. Javadpour N: Radioimmunoassay and immunoperoxidase of pregnancy specific beta-1 glycoprotein in sera and tumor cells of patients with certain testicular germ cell tumors. J Urol 123:514-515, 1980.

118. Lange PH, Bremner RD, Horne CHW, Vessella RL, Fraley EE: Is SP-1 a marker for testicular cancer? Urology 15:251-255, 1980.

119. Javadpour N, Utz M, Soares T: Immunocytochemical discordance in localization of pregnancy specific beta-1 glycoprotein, alpha-fetoprotein and human chorionic gonadotropin in testicular cancers. J Urol 124:615-616, 1980.

120. Szymendera JJ, Zborzil J, Sikorowa L, Kaminska JA, Gadek A: Value of five tumor markers (AFP, CEA, hCG, hPL and SP_1) in diagnosis and staging of testicular germ cell tumors. Oncology 38:222-229, 1981.

121. Lieskovsky G, Skinner DG: Significance of serum lactic dehydrogenase in stages B and C non-seminomatous testis tumors. J Urol 123:516-517, 1980.

122. Johnson H Jr, Flye MW, Javadpour N: Serum β_2 microglobulin levels in patients with testicular cancer. Urology 16:522-524, 1980.

123. Uchida T, Shimoda T, Miyata H, Shikata T, Iino S, Suzuki H, Oda T, Hirano K, Sugiura M: Immunoperoxidase study of alkaline phosphatase in testicular tumor. Cancer 48:1455-1462, 1981.

124. Jeppsson A, Wahren B, Stigbrand T, Edsmyr F, Andersson L: A clinical evaluation of serum placental alkaline phosphatase in seminoma patients. Br J Urol 55:73-78, 1983.

125. Lee M, Ray PS, Sharifi R: Elevated serum calcitonin associated with an extragonadal seminoma. J Urol 128:392-394, 1982.

Editorial Comment

T. MING CHU

The author has reviewed tumor markers in genitourinary cancer in a clear and concise manner. It is heartening to note that, since Dr Gutman reported the association of acid phosphatase and metastatic prostate cancer almost five decades ago, a great deal of research on markers for genitourinary cancer has been done. An ideal marker is yet to be found. At present stage of development, AFP and HCG are the most widely accepted parameters for testicular germ cell tumors. The weakest area of investigations is perhaps renal cancer markers. Research on prostate cancer and bladder cancer has shown modest results, although much work needs to be conducted.

The greatest difficulty in searching for an ideal tumor marker, which should reveal organ site specificity and cell type specificity, is the biological heterogeneity of tumor cells. No two tumor cells are exactly alike, let alone those millions in a small mass. Compounding this problem are the non-specificity and heterogeneity, as well as poor sensitivity of immunological and biochemical reagents available to date in measurements of the putative markers.

Therefore, this review, as well as others, has re-emphasized that we must explore new approaches and techniques. It is timely and important that a few investigations on the use of monoclonal antibodies derived from recent hybridoma technology are being conducted on cancers of the prostate and bladder. Also, as the author properly points out the powerful flow cytometry in expediting the DNA analysis of exfoliated cells in bladder tumor deserves careful attention. This relatively new technique certainly is applicable to other tumor systems, including those of the genitourinary tract. An additional tool is recombinant DNA technology, which has shown changes in location, level of expression and nucleic acid sequences of certain genes in cancer cells (e.g. bladder) that are absent in their normal counterparts. It suggests the possibility of exploring the molecular approaches to the identification of tumor markers produced by malignant cells. Hopefully, these new technologies will yield a new generation of reagents and tumor markers in the not too distant future.

In the meantime, with existing markers available as reviewed in this chapter, we shall extend our utilization of these markers to patient care and management. Although these markers are not suitable for early diagnosis of genitourinary cancer, many are useful in monitor of treatment response and prognosis of disease. Another increasingly effective approach is the use of multiple markers. One advantage of a combination test is the increased detection rate. In addition, immunocytochemistry is another area which will be rewarding for urologic pathologists. Cell type and organ site specific marker with its monoclonal antibody are available, e.g. prostate antigen, which increasingly has been applied in differential diagnosis of metastasis with unknown primary origin.

6. Role of Conservative Surgery for Patients with Bilateral Kidney Tumors

STEPHEN C. JACOBS

1. INTRODUCTION

Renal cell carcinoma or renal adenocarcinoma originates in the malignant transformation of renal tubular epithelial cells. The cause of the malignant transformation is unknown. There is evidence that environmental carcinogens may be involved [1], but the incidence of renal cancer appears to be stable. Renal adenocarcinoma affects adults with an increasing incidence with age. Most series show the mean age of disease appearance in the late sixth decade and males to be affected more commonly than females. Young adults aged 20–40 develop renal adenocarcinoma less commonly, but the behavior of the cancer in young adults is essentially the same as in older adults [2].

2. ETIOLOGY OF RENAL CARCINOMA

Genetic factors definitely play a role in the development of some renal cell carcinomas. Von Hippel-Lindau syndrome is an autosomal dominant inherited disorder characterized by retinal and cerebellar angiomas. Urologic abnormalities associated with the syndrome include epididymal cysts, pheochromocytomas, renal cysts, and renal carcinoma (often multiple). Approximately one third of patients with Von Hippel-Lindau syndrome will die from renal cell carcinoma [3].

Familial renal cell carcinoma is relatively rare. Nineteen families affected with renal cell carcinoma have been reported [4–6] and 3 of these families showed a marked tendency for bilaterality and multicentricity [6–8]. Marberger recently has suggested that tumors with a hereditary background are known to behave less aggressively [9]. It is not necessarily true that familial renal cell carcinoma is less malignant. Most of the cases of familial renal cell

T. L. Ratliff and W. J. Catalona (eds), Urologic Oncology. ISBN 0-89838-628-4.
© *1984. Martinus Nijhoff Publishers, Boston. Printed in the Netherlands.*

carcinoma have died of metastatic disease. Those operated upon have reportedly done well, but this is probably primarily due to case selection and early reporting. Nephrectomy specimens have shown renal vein invasion [4, 10] and lymph nodal metastasis [5], findings usually associated with a poorer prognosis. With regard to Von Hippel-Lindau syndrome, Malek and Greene's description of 'widespread metastasis and eventually a hopeless prognosis in every instance' [3] also conflicts with any assumption that these are not malignant cancers.

Chromosomal aberrations may well play a role in the genesis of at least some renal cell carcinomas. Cohen et al. reported a fascinating family with an inherited predisposition to develop renal cancer [6]. A balanced reciprocal translocation between chromosomes 3 and 8 was found in the peripheral leukocytes in one half of the family members over 3 generations. In those family members without the chromosomal translocation, no renal cancer developed. Of those members of the family with the chromosomal translocation, one half developed renal cell carcinomas. These cancers occurred in adults of 37–59 years of age and there was a marked tendency for multicentricity and bilaterality. Fifty percent of the patients with cancer died from their disease, but 50% are alive following surgical resection of their cancers.

In this family a small deletion or mutation of a gene in chromosome 3,8 or both probably results in the predisposition to renal cancer. However, only one half of the family members affected developed the multicentric renal cancer. Therefore, a second mutation may be required to develop clinical cancer; this is in line with the Knudson's two-mutation model of cancer development [11].

Pathek et al. [5] recently described a case of familial renal cell carcinoma with translocations involving chromosomes 3 and 11 in the cancer cells. They suggest that the 3p region may be rearranged as an inherited predisposition to renal cell carcinoma.

The recurrent theme of bilaterality and multicentricity in these cases of renal cell carcinoma leads one to question the origin of all bilateral or multicentric renal cancers.

3. OCCURRENCE OF BILATERAL RENAL CARCINOMA

Bilateral renal carcinoma occurs in approximately 1.8% of patients presenting with renal carcinoma [12]. The prognosis for such patients has been felt to be very poor until recently. Patients presenting with synchronous or simultaneous bilateral renal cancers are different from those presenting with metachronous tumors. Patients with bilateral tumors may, in fact, have one renal cell carcinoma with a metastasis to the opposite kidney or 2 separately developing cancers. Metastasis to the opposite kidney from a unilateral renal cell carcinoma is unusual in autopsy series. Saitoh et al. [13] found that only 1.4% of unilateral renal cell carcinomas metastasized to the contralateral kidney as the only metastasis at death. If multiple metastases were present at death, then 4.4% of unilateral renal cell carcinomas metastasized to the opposite kidney [13]. Most renal carcinomas affecting both kidneys then have metastases present in other organs. For this reason survival should be approximately what one would find in stage IV renal cell carcinoma. Renal cell carcinoma is a very unpredictable disease and all survival data must be interpreted against a background of 5 year survival of about 10% for metastatic renal cancer [14]. If 2 renal cancers are metachronous, the length of time before the appearance of the second cancer still gives no hint as to whether this is a second primary vs a metastasis.

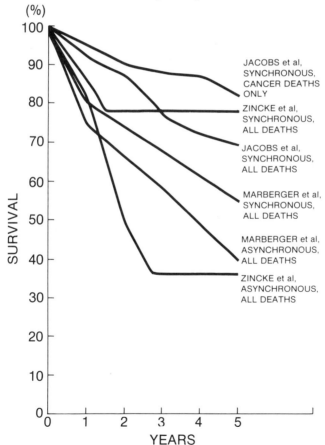

Figure 1. Comparison of survival from bilateral renal carcinomas treated surgically in three series.

Patients with synchronously appearing bilateral renal cell carcinoma appear to be suffering from a different disease. We reported in 1980 on 61 patients with synchronous bilateral renal carcinoma collected from the literature up to that time [15]. True follow-up was then obtained from the surgeons, the patients, or the families allowing the construction of a survival curve. Survival from synchronous bilateral renal carcinoma following surgical removal proved to be significantly better than one would expect from unilateral renal carcinoma (69% at 5 years). The survival data have been criticized as being based on actuarial survival. The actual 5 year survivals are as follows: 5 years had elapsed since surgery for 36 of the 60 patients. Eight of these 36 patients died of renal cancer and 6 more died of other causes. Twenty-two patients were alive and well. However, in both synchronous bilateral and in unilateral renal carcinoma, the deaths from renal cancer continue slowly even after 5 years. Recently, Zincke and Swanson [16] have reported on the Mayo Clinic series of 19 synchronous bilateral and 8 asynchronous bilateral renal carcinomas. They reported a 78% 5 year survival rate for synchronous lesions, but a 38% 5 year survival rate for asynchronous lesions. Zincke and Swanson concluded that synchronous bilateral renal cell cancer 'should be distinguished from the asynchronous form, with its dismal outcome' [16].

Recently, Marberger et al. [9] surveyed the European Intrarenal Surgical Society (EIRSS) and similarly found that 18 cases of asynchronous bilateral renal cancer did less well than 18 cases of synchronous bilateral renal cancer. They could not confirm, however, that synchronous bilateral cancer had a better prognosis than unilateral renal carcinoma. Synchronous bilateral renal carcinoma appears to be a less malignant disease with better survival rates. However, this difference may be because of a higher percentage of lower grade, lower stage cancers reported in this group when compared to a large series of unilateral renal carcinoma.

4. RENAL CARCINOMA GROWTH PATTERNS

Renal cell carcinoma grows locally by expansion. As the tumor expands it is covered by a pseudo-capsule of fibrous tissue. Adjoining renal parenchyma is resorbed to become part of the fibrous capsule as the carcinoma expands. Vermooten [17] described the process. First the tubules have collagen deposited along their basement membranes. Then connective tissue completely replaces the renal tubules. The glomeruli are affected last. They become ovoid, flattened by the expansile pressure of the tumor. then replaced by connective tissue. This capsule around the expanding renal carcinoma varies from less than 1 mm to about 3 mm in thickness. Vermooten concluded that clear cell carcinoma is not actively invasive, but rather expansile. 'It advances on a solid front and does not send out finger-like strands of cells into normal tissues.' The capsule around the tumor is thicker within the kidney than when the tumor expands into the perinephric fat. These observations hold up primarily for the grade I-II renal carcinomas. The very anaplastic or sarcomatous renal cell carcinomas actually invade tissue, but they are in a minority. It is remarkable how very rarely renal cell carcinoma invades the contiguous structures of liver, colon, small bowel, psoas muscle, and spleen. Instead, spread of renal cell carcinoma is via the lymphatic and venous systems.

Local tumor recurrence due to tumor spill at the time of surgery or incomplete resection occurs. Still, renal cell carcinoma is not a tumor with a high propensity for local recurrence. Rafla found that only 3.7% of patients died from a local recurrence [18]. These features of growth pattern characteristics and relatively low local recurrence problems would tend to make renal cell carcinoma a better candidate for local resection with slimmer margins than most cancers.

Patients with renal adenocarcinoma if left untreated die from their cancers. The tumor growth, however, is erratic and cases of relatively long survival are not rare. In fact, 4-13% of patients left untreated might be expected to survive 5 years [14, 19]. With surgical treatment survival is dependent on tumor stage and grade. Priestly showed elegantly, in 1939, that survival was directly related to tumor grade using the 4 grades of Broder's classification [20]. Forty years later Boxer et al. [21] came to the same conclusion using a 3 grade classification.

Tumor staging by the Robson [22] classification is as follows: stage I – confined to the kidney; stage II – extension to perirenal fat but within Gerota's fascia; stage III – renal vein or vena caval involvement or regional lymph node metastasis; stage IV – direct extension into adjacent organs or distant metastases. Survival for stage I and stage II are not very different. The actual extension into fat is not necessarily the feature that gives the stage II tumor a poorer prognosis. Many series have shown that tumor size is directly correlated to the presence of metastases and to survival. As renal tumors grow locally they must expand into perirenal fat. However, invasion of the renal vein does not seem to be as ominous a sign as regional lymph node metastasis. Waters and Richie found renal vein involvement does not influence survival [23]. Siminovitch et al. [24] found lymph node involvement to result in only an 11% disease-free survival despite lymphadenectomy.

Robson popularized the radical nephrectomy for renal cell carcinoma [25]. Survival rates from the disease have improved since his work by a factor of 2 [26-28]. However, it is difficult to compare survival figures from series prior to World War II with the current era. Surgeons in the 1920–1940 era were dealing with tremendous operative mortality ranging from 6–22% [29, 30]. Diagnostic modalities were crude and tumors diagnosed much later in the course of the disease. In 1929 Hunt and Hager divided their renal cell carcinomas by size: small, large or huge [30]. Today, operative mortality is in the range of 2–3% for radical nephrectomy [23, 31].

To further confound analysis, many of the principles of radical nephrectomy were established prior to World War II. Soloway in 1938 stated that 'nephrectomy, as early and as radical as possible, is the choice method of treatment'. In his description of what we today call a 'simple' nephrectomy, he stated: 'The tumor mass with the fatty capsule and the glands of the pedicle should be completely removed before metastasis has occurred' [32]. Early ligation of the vessels before any tumor manipulation was emphasized. This he felt 'reduces hemorrhage, makes it possible to remove the tumor, fatty capsule, the adrenal and regional lymph glands as well as the adherent peritoneum' [32].

Radical nephrectomy will remain the surgical treatment of choice for patients with a normal contralateral kidney. If for no other reason, it is easier to perform. However, there is room for argument as to whether radical nephrectomy is absolutely necessary. Lesser procedures which resect the tumor margins of enveloping capsule can be done with only a modest risk to the patient.

5. OPTIONS FOR TREATMENT

For patients with bilateral renal carcinoma there are currently 4 options for treatment:
1. No treatment
2. Conservative surgical excision
3. Radical bilateral excision combined with hemodialysis or
4. Renal transplantation

The results of no treatment are poor and should be reserved for the patients with prohibitive operative risk and essentially a 0% 5 year life expectancy from other diseases, age, etc. Chemotherapy and/or radiotherapy have yet to be shown to have any beneficial effect on renal cell carcinoma.

Radical bilateral nephrectomy with institution of chronic hemodialysis has been advocated for bilateral renal carcinoma. One could anticipate a respectable survival rate from cancer death. In a review in 1980 we pointed out that 4 of 6 patients so treated were cured of their cancers [15]. Unfortunately, 3 of these 4 patients died on dialysis from seizures and malnutrition. Marberger et al. [9] have pointed out that hemodialysis in Europe is no better. In his collection of 6 patients treated by bilateral nephrectomy and hemodialysis, 1 died of cancer and 4 died of typical dialysis complications. Only a 40–50% 5 year survival could be anticipated for a group of patients on chronic hemodialysis if they were cured of their cancers [33]. Management of bilateral renal cancer by bilateral nephrectomy and hemodialysis could then be expected to accomplish a 20–30% patient salvage at 5 years. If the poor quality of life for those on dialysis is added, this becomes a very poor alternative.

The addition of renal transplantation, however, is more encouraging. There have been a number of advocates of this option [34, 35]. To date 6 patients with synchronous bilateral renal carcinoma have undergone renal transplantation [15, 16, 35, 36]. Three of the 6 are alive and well without evidence of the cancer. Two of the 6 died, but not from renal cancer and 1 patient died from metastastic renal cancer. In contrast to this rather favorable experience stand those patients transplanted for asynchronous bilateral renal cancer. Four of 7 such patients died of metastatic cancer and 1 of the 7 died of sepsis [36]. Only 2 of the 7 were alive and free of renal cancer. In Penn's review of transplantation for all patients with all types of renal malignancies, he concluded that patients who waited on dialysis at least 15 months did significantly better than those who were immediately transplanted [36]. Furthermore, patients whose renal cancers were incidentally removed in preparation for transplantation and whose renal failure was caused by other diseases did very well [36].

6. CONSERVATIVE SURGICAL THERAPY

Conservative surgical excision has rapidly become the treatment of choice for patients with bilateral renal adenocarcinoma or unilateral renal cancer in a solitary function kidney. The goal of therapy is the removal of all carcinoma while still preserving enough renal tissue to support life without dialysis. Partial nephrectomy has been performed from 1882 in horseshoe kidneys but partial nephrectomy was not regularly performed in patients with 2 kidneys until 1936 when Lowsley popularized a number of techniques to control postoperative bleeding from the cut edges of the renal parenchyma [37]. These techniques included using ribbon gut through the renal capsule to compress the bleeding parenchyma and incorporating fat in the nephrotomy closure. Today many technical advances have made partial nephrectomy a safer procedure [38]. Study of the segmental renal blood supply, better suturing material, and improvements in blood banking have made partial nephrectomy safer. But it is the techniques developed for the care of end stage renal disease patients that have really made a difference in the increased popularity and availability of partial nephrectomy. Back-up temporary dialysis brought a cushion to protect patients postoperatively. The techniques of renal preservation gave surgeons a chance to do careful, delicate procedures on the kidney including extracorporeal tumor resection and autotransplantation.

Krumbach and Ansell [8] in 1952 performed a radical nephrectomy on one side and a partial nephrectomy on the other for synchronous bilateral renal carcinoma, the first such operative procedure. The patient survived 10 years only to die from a brain metastasis from his cancer. Over 100 patients with bilateral synchronous renal cancer have now undergone surgical treatment. I would like to review some of the conservative surgical alternatives in these patients.

With synchronous bilateral renal carcinoma the discussion as to which side to operate on first merits some debate. The most common operation done has been a radical nephrectomy for the more involved side and a partial nephrectomy in situ on the less involved side. About 50% of the time surgeons proceed to operate on both kidneys at the same sitting. If the operations are done at 2 sittings, then the more involved side has been done first about 50% of the time.

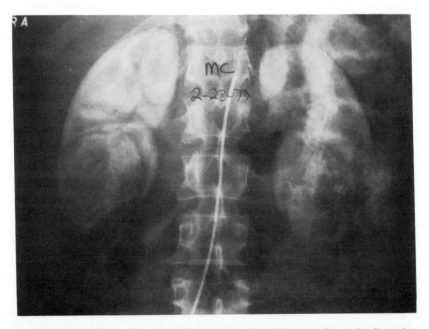

Figure 2. Arteriogram from a 39-year old female with bilateral lower pole renal cell carcinoma. This case was treated bilateral by lower pole partical nephrectomy under ischemic hypothermia in situ at separate operations 1 month apart.

Klein, Lamm and Gittes [39] studied the resistance of the dog kidney to warm ischemic damage when both kidneys were present and when only one kidney was present. They found that compensatory renal growth and resistance to ischemic injury were increased markedly if prior contralateral nephrectomy was performed. These findings should point the surgeon toward removing the larger of the two cancers with a radical nephrectomy first, before proceeding to the partial nephrectomy on the smaller tumor. However, there is a very practical reason to do the reverse. If the smaller tumor is operated on first, the small amount of remaining renal function on the more involved side is usually enough to carry the patient through the postoperative period without dialysis. Then, after complete renal recovery on the operated side, the radical nephrectomy can be performed.

Partial nephrectomy can often be done in situ and without induction of cold ischemia. However, if the renal pedicle is clamped and hypothermia established with an ice slush [40], more time can be taken to carefully dissect out the major branch renal arteries. This may allow for a segmental resection along the lines of the vascular distribution. Such resections result in much less ischemic renal tissue being left behind. The extra time and lack of bleeding under cold ischemia also allows for frozen sections of the margin of resection to be done. Before clamping the renal artery systemic heparin anti-coagulation should be given to prevent clots forming in the renal vasculature. The patient's anti-coagulation can be reversed or not after clamping the vessels.

Gibbons et al. [41] stated in 1976 that extracorporeal (workbench) surgery was over-used and associated with too many technical failures. It is true that most partial nephrectomies for renal cancer involve resection of a pole of the kidney and can be done in situ. Novick et al. found that 88% of their partial nephrectomies for tumor could be done in situ with free margins of resection [42]. Ischemic hypothermia is probably indicated or helpful in most cases.

7. SIMPLE ENUCLEATION

There has been a recent renewed interest in merely enucleating the tumors in patients with bilateral renal cell carcinomas [43–45]. The basis for attempting enucleation is found in Vermooten's description of the pseudocapsule surrounding renal cancers [17]. Developing a plane within this capsule is easy and relatively bloodless. There is no need to control the renal pedicle. Digital compression can control the bleeding and small suture ligatures and suturing of perinephric fat or gel foam into the bed of the tumor completes the hemostasis. Local recurrences do occur [43] but a true inci-

Figure 3A. Pseudo-capsule surrounding renal cell carcinoma. The compressed renal parenchyma is seen above with the pseudo-capsule being approximately 40 μm in width.

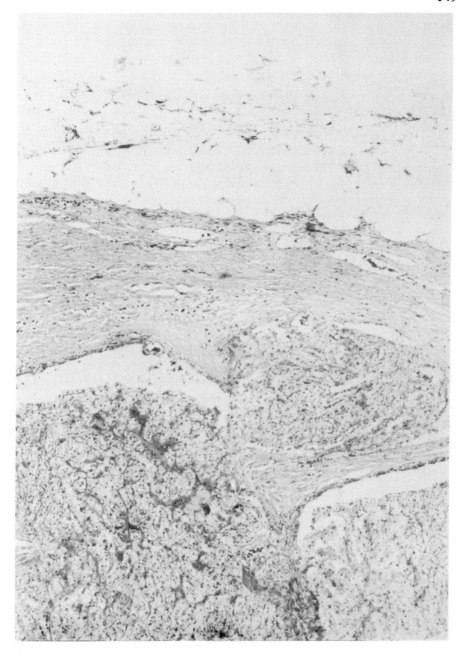

Figure 3B. Pseudo-capsule surrounding renal cell carcinoma. The perinephric fat is seen above with the pseudo-capsule being approximately 10 μm in width.

dence is not available yet. Most of the cases are not 5 year survivors as yet. It seems that the surgical margins with simple enucleations are being cut extremely thin. Certainly frozen section will not be able to determine if these margins are clear. Vermooten's description of a 1–3 mm capsule also includes the point that 'in places it is so thin that a layer of tumor cells is separated from apparently normal kidney tissue by only a few collagen fibers' [17]. Figure 3 shows the capsule Vermooten describes within the kidney compared to the capsule when the tumor expands into perinephric fat.

8. EXTRACORPOREAL PARTIAL NEPHRECTOMY

Extracorporeal partial nephrectomy, renal reconstruction, and autotransplantation of the renal remnant has become available at most medical centers. Calne [46] reported the first case in 1971 and since then more than 40 cases of renal cell carcinoma in solitary kidneys or bilateral tumors have been performed. Two recent reviews of the current status of extracorporeal surgery have appeared [47, 48]. It is important to point out the advantages and disadvantages of doing workbench surgery. The advantages are that delicate, careful, unhurried resection of the cancer can proceed in a bloodless field; the patient gets a better cancer operation. The disadvantages are

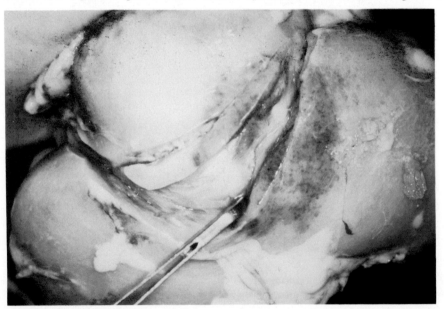

Figure 4. Extracorporeal resection of tumor occupying the mid portion of a solitary kidney (courtesy Dr R.K. Lawson).

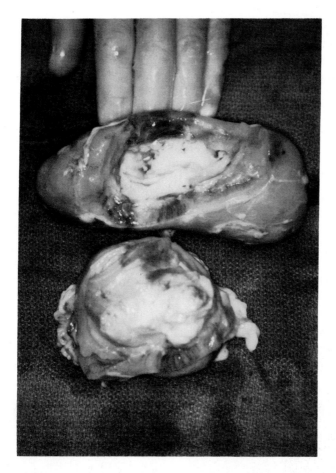

Figure 5. The renal cell carcinoma extended into the fat around the collecting system. After frozen sections demonstrated the margins to be tumor-free, this kidney was reconstructed and autotransplanted with excellent functional recovery (courtesy Dr R.K. Lawson).

the increased chances for renal injury with possible renal loss on a technical basis and the potential risk of spill of tumor cells during the cold ischemia time. A number of enthusiastic surgeons have reported on the advantages of extracorporeal surgery in the management of selected cases or renal carcinoma. However, proper selection of patients is mandatory. Patients should have a large tumor in a solitary kidney or bilateral renal carcinoma. The tumors should be large or in the mid-portion of the kidney. Extracorporeal resection will then allow for surgical margins superior to what would be accomplished with in situ resection. In cases of bilateral synchronous renal carcinoma the rate of local recurrence with extracorporeal resection appears to be lower (6%) than with in situ resection (14%) [15]. Obviously, renal reconstruction on the workbench is superior to reconstruction in situ.

Some surgeons have recommended injecting the branches of the renal artery with methylene blue to determine the proper line of segmental resection [49]. Clearly, ex vivo arteriography presents a grave risk to renal function [50] unless it is done carefully and with the right agents [51]. Some surgeons have been successful in using ex vivo renal arteriography [51, 52] to determine the completeness of tumor resection. Obtaining multiple frozen sections of the margins of resection is a safer method of being certain that all of the tumor has been removed. Still local recurrence of renal carcinoma has occurred in autotransplanted kidneys [53, 54]. In these cases the recurrences have been resected in situ [53] or on the workbench again [54].

Pulsatile cold perfusion of the kidney with cryoprecipitated plasma during the extracorporeal surgery may enhance renal preservation. However, these perfusion units recirculate the venous effluent as well as cells liberated by the resection. Gittes and McCullough have recommended that cold preservation be established immediately with Sack's or Collin's solution, but that continuous pulsatile perfusion be withheld until after the tumor resection is completed [49].

After resection of the cancer, repair of the collecting system and suture ligation of open parenchymal vessels, repair of the renal veins and arteries must be accomplished before actually dealing with the autotransplantation and the ureter. In cases in which the renal artery or the renal vein are

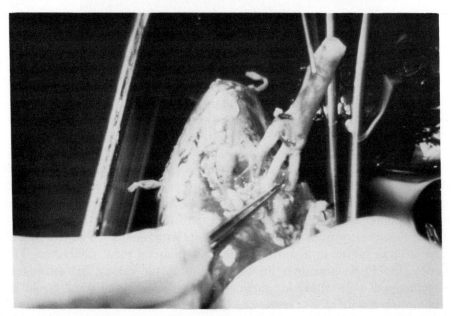

Figure 6. Reconstruction of main renal artery with hypogastric artery segment. Hypogastric artery branches are anastomosed end to end to the renal artery branches (reprinted from Lawson RK, Hodges CV: Urology 4:532-539, 1974, by permission of the publisher).

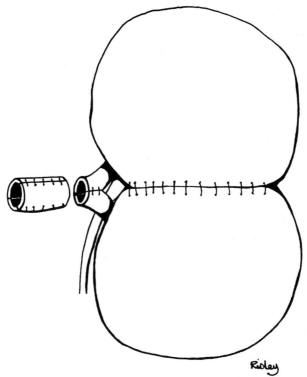

Figure 7. Reconstruction of main renal vein with saphenous vein segments.

destroyed by the resection or are insufficient for anastomosis to the pelvic vessels, substitute vessels must be constructed. The hypogastric artery is a good substitute for the main renal artery [51, 55]. Its branches can often be anastomosed end to end to the renal artery branches. Vein substitution can be more difficult. By splitting a segment of saphenous vein open longitudinally, segments of vein can be cut that can be sewn side to side to produce a large diameter vein adequate for substitution as a main renal vein. Spinal suture of saphenous vein around an appropriate sized catheter can also be used to create a renal vein substitute.

In order to perform extracorporeal surgery it is not always necessary to divide the ureter. Resection of lower pole tumors can lead to damage to the ureteral blood supply from above. Ureteral transection with ensuing ureteroneocystostomy will then lead to ureteral necrosis and this has been seen in patients with bilateral renal cancers subjected to extracorporeal surgery [34]. Whitsell et al. [56] showed in dogs and then in a human that the ureter could be left intact the kidney turned upside down and autotransplanted to the ipsilateral iliac fossa. Gittes and McCullough [49] and Berg et al. [10] have similarly advocated the technique in patients with bilateral renal car-

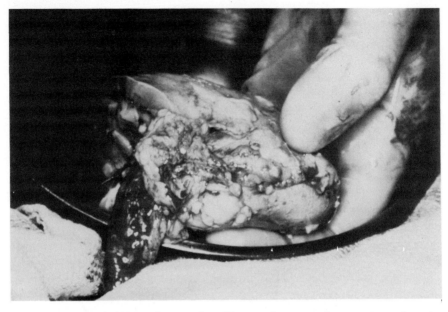

Figure 8. Cold ischemic kidney after resection of lower pole tumor prior to autotransplantation. The ureter and the ureteral blood flow are intact (courtesy Dr S.I. Berg).

cinoma (Figures 8 and 9). Ureteral drainage is then first cephalad before turning and going to the bladder. The blood supply to the ureter from below remains intact and both the potential for ureteral necrosis and the need to ureteroneocystostomy are eliminated. However, the ureteral blood supply is intact during cold ichemia and care should be taken not to allow this to cause warm ischemic injury. Patients with intact ureters during extracorporeal surgery may suffer temporary postoperative renal failure [10, 49]. A bulldog clamp across the ureter should stop this ureteral blood flow temporarily.

9. CONCLUSIONS

Synchronous bilateral or multicentric renal cell carcinoma is a malignant disease which has a prognosis approximately the same as the worst of the individual tumors.

Synchronous bilateral renal cell carcinoma clearly has a better prognosis than asynchronous renal cell carcinoma and probably patients do as well or better than patients with a unilateral renal cancer.

Bilateral nephrectomy and chronic hemodialysis is a very poor alternative therapy though renal transplantation may become an acceptable alternative therapy.

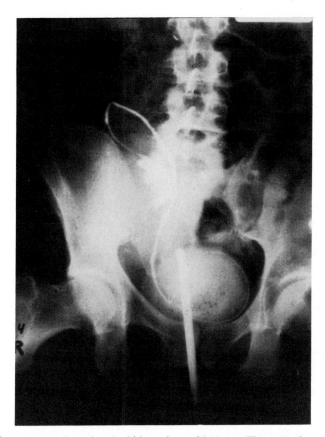

Figure 9. After autotransplantation the kidney sits upside down. The ureteral course is cephalad before gently coursing down toward the bladder (reprinted from Berg SI et al.: J Urol 126:313-315, 1981, by permission of the publisher).

Surgical resection of all cancer is the treatment of choice. This can usually be done with conservation of some functioning renal parenchyma.

Most surgical resections can be done in situ and the addition of ischemic hypothermia is helpful for careful resections. Simple tumor enucleation cannot as yet be considered adequate.

Extracorporeal resection of the cancers should be reserved for large tumors or those occupying the central portion of the kidney.

Because partial nephrectomy is a less than perfect cancer operation, local recurrences will be slightly more common and patients should be followed closely to detect recurrence early so that repeat surgery can be performed.

REFERENCES

1. Kantor AF: Current concepts in the epidemiology and etiology of primary renal cell carcinoma. J Urol 117:415-417, 1977.

156

2. Lieber MM, Tomera FM, Taylor WF, Farrow GM: Renal adenocarcinoma in young adults: Survival and variable affecting prognosis. J Urol 125:164-168, 1981.
3. Malek RS, Greene LF: Urologic aspects of Hippel-Lindau syndrome. J Urol 106:800-801, 1971.
4. Goldman SM, Fishman EK, Abeshouse G, Cohen JH: Renal cell carcinoma diagnosed in three generations of a single family. South Med J 72:1457-1459, 1979.
5. Pathek S, Strong LC, Ferrell RE, Trindade A: Familial renal cell carcinoma with a 3:11 chromosome translocation limited to tumor cells. Science 217:939-941, 1982.
6. Cohen AJ, Li FP, Berg SI, Marchetto DM, Tsai S, Jacobs SC, Brown RS: Hereditary renal-cell carcinoma associated with a chromosomal translocation. N Engl J Med 301:592-595, 1979.
7. Franksson C, Berstrand A, Ljungdahl I, Magnusson H, Nordenstrom H: Renal carcinoma (hypernephroma) occurring in 5 siblings. J Urol 108:58-61, 1972.
8. Krumbach RW, Ansell JS: Partial resection of the right kidney and radical removal of the left kidney in a patient with bilateral hypernephroma. Surgery 45:585-592, 1959.
9. Marberger M, Pugh RCB, Auvert J, Bertermann H, Constantini A, Gammelgaard PA, Petterson S, Wickham JEA: Conservative surgery of renal carcinoma: The EIRSS experience. Br J Urol 53:528-532, 1981.
10. Berg S, Jacobs SC, Cohen AJ, Li L, Marchetto D, Brown RS: The surgical management of hereditary multifocal renal carcinoma. J Urol 126:313-315, 1981.
11. Knudson AG Jr: Mutation and human cancer. Adv Cancer Res 17:317-352, 1973.
12. Vermillion CD, Skinner DG, Pfister RC: Bilateral renal carcinoma. J Urol 108:219-222, 1972.
13. Saitoh H, Hida M, Nakamura K, Shimbo T, Shiramizu T, Satoh T: Metastatic processes and a potential indication of treatment for metastatic renal adenocarcinoma. J Urol 128:916-918, 1982.
14. DeKernion JB, Ramming KP, Smith RB: The natural history of metastatic renal cell carcinoma: A computer analysis. J Urol 120:148-152, 1978.
15. Jacobs SC, Berg SI, Lawson RK: Synchronous bilateral renal cell carcinoma: Total surgical excision. Cancer 46:2341-2345, 1980.
16. Zincke H, Swanson SK: Bilateral renal cell carcinoma: Influence of synchronous and asynchronous occurrence on patient survival. J Urol 128:913-915, 1982.
17. Vermooten V: Indications for conservative surgery in certain renal tumors: A study based on a growth pattern of the clear cell carcinoma. J Urol 64:200-208, 1950.
18. Rafla S: Renal cell carcinoma. Natural history and results of treatment. Cancer 25:26, 1970.
19. Patel NP, Lavengood RN: Renal cell carcinoma: Natural history and results of treatment. J Urol 119:722-726, 1978.
20. Priestly JT: Survival following removal of malignant renal neoplasms. JAMA 113:902-906, 1939.
21. Boxer RJ, Waisman J, Lieber MM, Mampaso FM, Skinner DG: Renal carcinoma: Computer analysis of 96 patients treated by nephrectomy. J Urol 122:598-601, 1979.
22. Robson CJ, Churchill BM, Anderson W: The results of radical nephrectomy for renal cell carcinoma. J Urol 101:297-301, 1969.
23. Waters WB, Richie JP: Aggressive surgical approach to renal cell carcinoma: Review of 130 cases. J Urol 122:306, 1979.
24. Siminovitch JO, Montie JE, Straffon RA: Lyphadenectomy in renal adenocarcinoma. J Urol 127:1090, 1982.
25. Robson CJ: Radical nephrectomy for renal cell carcinoma. J Urol 89:37-42, 1963.
26. Mintz ER: Renal cancer. End results in 105 consecutive cases. N Engl J Med 218:329-337, 1938.

27. Humphreys GA, Foot NC: Survival of patients (235) following nephrectomy for renal cell and transitional cell tumors of the kidney. J Urol 83:815-819, 1960.
28. Rubin P: Current concepts in genitourinary oncology: A multidisciplinary approach. J Urol 106:315-338, 1971.
29. Bergendal S: To the clinical study and prognosis of tumours of the kidney. Acta Chir Scandinav 77:563-625, 1936.
30. Hunt VC, Hager BH: A review of 271 cases of malignant renal neoplasms. Surg Clin North Am 9:149-159, 1929.
31. Schiff M Jr, Glazier WB: Nephrectomy: Indications and complications in 347 patients. J Urol 118:930-931, 1977.
32. Soloway HM: Renal tumors. A review of one hundred thirty cases. J Urol 40:477-490. 1938.
33. Bryan FA: Sixth annual report. The National dialysis registry, Research triangle institute report no. AK-5-67-1387: Cancer, facts and figures, October, 1974.
34. Evans DB, Calne RY: Renal transplantation in patients with carcinoma. Br Med J 4:134-136, 1974.
35. Spees EK, Light JA, Smith EJ, Mostofi FK, Oakes DD: Transplantation in patients with a history of renal cell carcinoma: Long-term results and clinical considerations. Surgery 91:282-287, 1982.
36. Penn I: Transplantation in patients with primary renal malignancies. Transplantation 24:424-434, 1977.
37. Lowsley OS: Modern renal surgery with particular reference to heminephrectomy. NY State J Med 36:591-601, 1936.
38. Montie JE: Management of stage I, II and III renal adenocarcinoma. In: Principles and management of urologic cancer. Javadpour N (ed). Baltimore: Williams and Wilkins, 2nd ed, pp 00-00, 1983 (in press).
39. Klein TW, Lamm D, Gittes RF: Renal autotransplantation: Influence of contralateral nephrectomy on the damaging effect of warm ischemia during transplantation. Invest Urol 15:256-261, 1977.
40. Marberger M, Stackl W: Renal hypothermia in situ. In: Current trends in urology (Resnick MI (ed). Baltimore: Williams & Wilkins, pp 70-89, 1981.
41. Gibbons RP, Correa RJ Jr, Cummings KB, Mason JT: Surgical management or renal lesions using in situ hypothermia and ischemia. J Urol 115:12-17, 1976.
42. Novick AC, Stewart BH, Straffon RA, Banowsky LH: Partial nephrectomy in the treatment of renal adenocarcinoma. J Urol 118:932, 1977.
43. Beraha D, Block NL, Politano VA: Simultaneous surgical management of bilateral hypernephroma: An alternative therapy. J Urol 115:648-650, 1976.
44. Graham SD Jr, Glenn JF: Enucleative surgery for renal malignancy. J Urol 122:546-549, 1979.
45. Pearson JC, Weiss J, Tangho EA: A plea for conservation of kidney in renal adenocarcinoma associated with Von Hippel-Lindau disease. J Urol 124:910-912, 1980.
46. Calne RY: Tumour in a single kidney: Nephrectomy, excision and autotransplantation. Lancet 2:761-762, 1971.
47. Lawson RK: Extracorporeal renal surgery. J Urol 123:301-305, 1980.
48. Stewart BH, Banowsky LH, Hewitt CB, Straffon RA: Renal autotransplantation: Current perspectives. J Urol 118:363-368, 1977.
49. Gittes RF, McCullough DL: Bench surgery for tumor in a solitary kidney. J Urol 113:12-15, 1975.
50. Corman JL, Girard R, Fiala M, Gallot D, Stonington O, Stables DP, Taubman J, Starzl TE: Arteriography during ex vivo renal perfusion. Urology 2:222-226.

158

51. Novick AC: Extracorporeal renal surgery and autotransplantation. In: Vascular Problems in Urologic surgery, Novick AC, Straffon RA (eds). Philadelphia: WB Saunders Company, pp 305-328, 1981.
52. Palmer JM, Swanson DA: Conservative surgery in solitary and bilateral renal carcinoma: Indications and technical considerations. J Urol 120:113-117, 1978.
53. Gittes RF, Blute RD Jr: Repeat bench surgery on a solitary kidney. J Urol 127:530-532, 1982.
54. Gelin LE: Extracorporeal surgery for renal problems. Surg Ann 9:351-379, 1977.
55. Lawson RK, Hodges CV: Extracorporeal renal artery repair and autotransplantation. Urology 4:532-539, 1974.
56. Whitsell JC III, Goldsmith EI, Nakamura H: Renal autotransplantation without ureteral division: An experimental study and case report. J Urol 103:577-582, 1970.

Editorial Comment

ANDREW C. NOVICK

1. INTRODUCTION

The addition of ultrasonography and CT scanning to the diagnostic armamentarium for evaluating patients with suspected or proven renal neoplasms has enhanced the detection of bilateral renal carcinomas. The preceding chapter by Dr Jacobs offers an excellent review of the etiology, occurrence and growth patterns of this disease along with appropriate methods of treatment when bilateral renal occurrence is observed. The purpose of the ensuing commentary is to amplify on selected issues from this chapter and also to present an alternate viewpoint on certain areas of controversy that remain unresolved.

2. CLINICAL FEATURES

The incidence of bilateral renal carcinoma at the Cleveland Clinic has been 2.4% with an approximately equal number of synchronous and asynchronous presentations. In such patients, the issue of whether the second cancer represents a metastasis or a new primary neoplasm is indeed intriguing, particularly with asynchronous bilateral tumors. In the latter category, features that may suggest metastasis are lack of tumor encapsulation in the first kidney, a multiplicity of tumors in the second kidney, histologic similarity of the two renal tumors, and a short interval between the presentation of the two lesions. Unfortunately, there are currently no conclusive data to confirm these intuitive clinical impressions rendering it impossible to resolve this dilemma when such patients are evaluated.

There are emerging data which support a difference in the prognosis for patients with synchronous and asynchronous bilateral renal carcinoma. Marberger et al. [1] and Zincke and Swanson [2] noted diminished survival in the latter category, although the difference was not statistically significant. We recently reviewed our long-term results following partial nephrectomy in 23 patients with localized renal carcinoma occurring either bilaterally or in a solitary kidney [3]. The overall actuarial five-year patient survival rates for unilateral renal carcinoma ($n = 12$), bilateral synchronous renal carcinoma ($n = 4$), and bilateral asynchronous renal carcinoma ($n = 7$) were 71%, 71%, and 38%, respectively. This apparently reduced survival in asynchronous bilateral carcinomas may be due to an advanced local tumor stage in such cases when they are detected. Another possible explanation is that appearance of the second renal tumor in these patients represents the initial manifestation of metastatic disease. As initially noted by Jacobs et al. [4], the prognosis for patients with localized synchronous bilateral renal carcinoma appears to

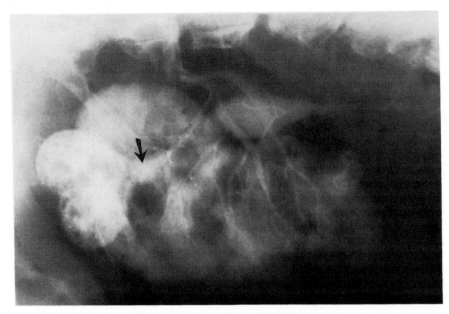

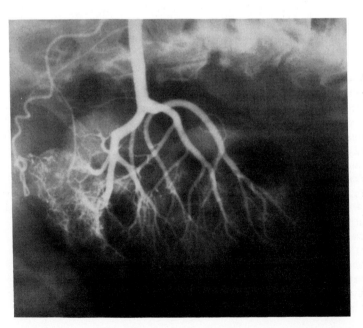

Figure 1. (A) Selective right renal arteriogram shows upper pole carcinoma in a solitary right kidney. (B) On the nephrogram phase, the margins of the tumor are smooth and discrete throughout, except inferiorly (arrow) where a 'finger-like strand' extends into adjacent parenchyma. A partial nephrectomy was done which revealed this to be a grade I stage I clear cell carcinoma.

be at least equal to and possibly better than that for patients with unilateral renal carcinoma, perhaps due to a lower tumor stage at the time of diagnosis in the former category.

Regarding the growth patterns of renal carcinoma, tumor spread occurs predominantly by lymphatic and hematogeneous routes. Both Gerota's fascia and a surrounding local tumor capsule provide natural barriers against direct tumor extension into adjacent anatomic structures which is indeed uncommon. While it is true that many renal carcinomas are completely enveloped by a pseudo-capsule of fibrous tissue, Vermooten's statement that clear cell carcinoma 'advances on a solid front and does not send out finger-like strands of cells into normal tissues' [5] is not always true even for low grade low stage tumors (Figure 1). This issue assumes clinical significance when enucleative surgery is considered as a possible method of treatment for discrete circumscribed renal carcinomas. Fortunately, in most cases, the combination of renal arteriography and CT scanning allows accurate delineation of the local extent of such tumors.

3. SURGICAL TREATMENT

Although radical nephrectomy must still be considered optimum curative therapy for patients with localized unilateral renal carcinoma and a normal opposite kidney, partial nephrectomy has become the treatment of choice for localized bilateral renal carcinoma. In such patients, partial nephrectomy offers the opportunity for complete surgical excision of the primary tumor while preserving sufficient renal parenchyma to avoid the need for renal replacement therapy. This approach is gaining in acceptance and popularity due both to surgical advances that have extended the technical feasibility of this option to encompass patients with large complex tumors, and accumulating data indicating that long-term cancer-free survival can be accomplished in a high percentage of patients [1-4]. Local tumor recurrence following partial nephrectomy has been reported in only 13 % of patients [1, 3, 4] and some of these recurrences can be surgically excised [6]. CT scanning is currently the most accurate diagnostic method for detecting such local recurrences and should be done every six months postoperatively to ensure early recognitioin of these lesions. As a corollary of this, it is wise to avoid the use of metal clips at the time of tumor excision since these will cause scatter on subsequent CT scans which limits their interpretation.

Most patients who present with synchronous bilateral renal carcinomas are in the fifth or sixth decade, are otherwise healthy, and have a life expectancy of at least ten to twenty years if they remain free of malignancy. We believe that operative therapy in such cases should be oriented toward preserving as much tumor-free renal parenchyma as possible to guard against either a renal-threatening surgical compliation or the development later in life of a disorder that impairs renal function. Therefore, our approach is currently to perform bilateral partial nephrectomies if these are technically feasible. In most cases, it is more prudent to stage these operations (Figure 2) although if both kidneys are involved with relatively small tumors, particularly ones that are amenable to simple enucleation, bilateral simultaneous renal surgery may safely be done. When one of the involved kidneys is extensively replaced by tumor, then a radical nephrectomy on that side and a contralateral partial nephrectomy are indicated. Our current preference in these cases is to perform both operations simultaneously provided there are no major intraoperative complications and the patient's condition under anesthesia remains stable. We acknowledge the pathophysiologic principles that favor staging these operations to minimize the need for postoperative dialysis. Nevertheless, we have yet to experience failure of a partial nephrectomy from ischemic renal injury and, even if a short period of dialysis is necessary, this is preferable to subjecting the patient to a second major operation. We also believe that partial nephrectomy carries a greater potential for operative morbidity than does radical nephrectomy and that, therefore, bilateral simultaneous performance of these two operations does not measurably increase the risk of a partial nephrectomy alone.

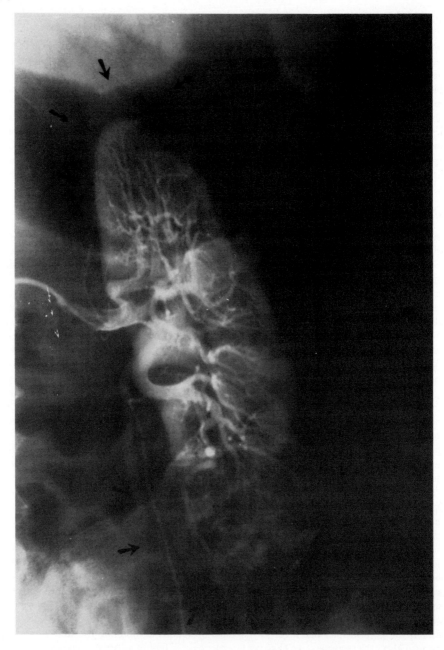

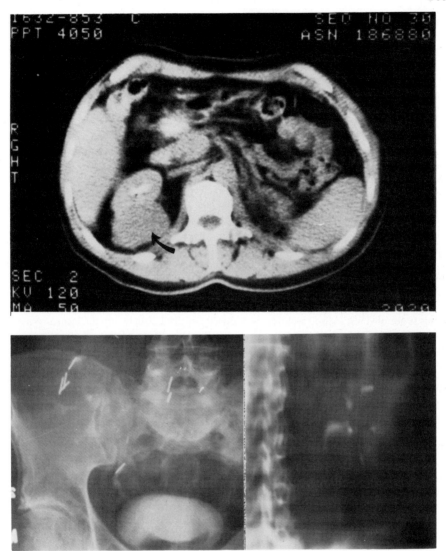

Figure 2.. (A) Selective left renal arteriogram demonstrates two carcinomas (arrows) involving the upper and lower pole segments. (B) CT scan in the same patient also demonstrates a large posterior and central carcinoma involving the right kidney (arrow). (C) This patient underwent staged in situ left partial nephrectomy followed by extracorporeal right partial nephrectomy and autotransplantation. Postoperative intravenous pyelography demonstrates excellent function of both renal remnants.

3.1 *In situ partial nephrectomy*

In the majority (75 to 80%) of patients undergoing conservative surgery for bilateral renal carcinoma, the tumors are located at either renal pole or on the lateral mid-aspect of the kidney enabling partial nephrectomy to be done in situ employing a variety of surgical techniques [7]. In patients with discrete well-encapsulated tumors, simple enucleation allows relatively avascular tumor excision with maximal conservation of renal tissue. This technique involves circumferentially incising the parenchyma around the tumor, identifying a plane between the pseudocapsule and adjacent uninvolved parenchyma, and then bluntly 'shelling-out' the lesion. It is unnecessary to occlude the renal artery and the few small bleeding points at the base of the enucleation can simply be suture ligated. There have been relatively few reports of enucleative surgery for renal carcinoma and these have generally referred to small numbers of patients with short follow-up intervals [8, 9]. From 1977 to 1983, simple enucleation has been performed in 15 patients with renal carcinoma at the Cleveland Clinic. The tumor size in these cases ranged from 1.8 to 7.0 cm in diameter. The postoperative follow-up currently ranges from three months to six years. All 15 patients are alive with stable renal function and have remained free of malignancy. These initial data suggest that simple enucleation offers an effective parenchymal-sparing technique for selected patients with renal carcinoma.

In patients with renal carcinoma confined to the upper or lower pole of the kidney, partial nephrectomy can be performed by isolating and ligating the segmental apical or basilar arterial branch while allowing unimpaired perfusion to the remainder of the kidney from the main renal artery. An ischemic line of demarcation will usually outline the segment to be removed however, if this is not obvious, indigo carmine can be directly instilled distally into the ligated segmental artery. The involved renal segment is then excised at the observed line of demarcation and frozen sections are obtained to confirm complete tumor removal.

In situ partial nephrectomy for non-encapsulated tumors that encompass more than one renal segment is best performed under local hypothermia following temporary occlusion of the renal artery. Renal arterial occlusion in such cases not only limits intraoperative bleeding but, by reducing renal tissue turgor, also improves access to intrarenal structures. In general, normothermic renal ischemia may not exceed 30 minutes if permanent damage to the kidney is to be avoided. Since the anticipated period of arterial occlusion in patients undergoing partial nephrectomy for renal carcinoma usually is > 30 minutes, additional protection from postischemic renal injury is necessary and local hypothermia currently offers the most effective technique [10]. The most popular methods of in situ renal hypothermia have involved surface cooling with ice slush packed around the kidney, various kinds of bags with cold saline solution and ice, a plastic pouch perfusion system, and advanced cooling coils. All of these techniques allow safe tolerance of at least three hours of renal arterial occlusion with no resulting permanent kidney damage. The relative ease and simplicity of ice slush cooling have made this the most commonly employed method of surface renal hypothermia in this country. In our experience, systemic anti-coagulation prior to temporary renal arterial occlusion is unnecessary in the absence of existing vascular or parenchymal disease involving the tumor-free portion of the kidney.

Another approach to local renal hypothermia following arterial occlusion has been to perfuse the kidney with a cold solution via the renal artery. This has been accomplished either by direct intraoperative needle puncture of the renal artery or by preoperative transfemoral insertion of a balloon catheter in the renal artery [11, 12]. Depending upon the composition of the perfusate and the rate of administration, the fluid has been allowed to drain either via the renal vein into the systemic circulation or directly into the operative field through a short proximal renal venotomy. Although this is an effective renal preservation technique, we have been reluctant to employ this in patients underoing partial nephrectomy for renal carcinoma because of the potential for intraoperative distant and/or local dissemination of tumor cells.

3.2 *Extracorporeal partial nephrectomy*

Extracorporeal partial nephrectomy represents an important surgical advance which now enables removal of large central renal tumors that were previously considered inoperable [13]. This technique involves increased operative time with greater potential morbidity and should therefore be reserved for the relatively small number of patients with complex tumors that are not amenable to in situ excision. The advantages of an extracorporeal approach in such cases include optimum exposure, a bloodless surgical field, the ability to perform a more precise operation with maximal conservation of renal parenchyma, greater protection of the kidney from prolonged ischemia, and a diminished risk of tumor spillage.

Extracorporeal partial nephrectomy and renal autotransplantation are generally performed through an anterior subcostal transperitoneal incision combined with a separate lower quadrant transverse semi-lunar incision. For non-obese patients, a single midline incision may alternatively be used. There is certainly a valid theoretical basis for leaving the ureter intact in such cases to preserve its distal collateral vascular supply, particularly with large hilar or lower renal tumors where complete excision may unavoidably compromise the blood supply to the pelvis and/or ureter. If the ureter is left attached, it must be temporarily occluded to prevent retrograde blood flow to the kidney during the extracorporeal operation. Although autotransplantation of the kidney 'upside down' is certainly acceptable, it is equally satisfactory to place the renal remnant into the ipsilateral iliac fossa in its normal orientation; although the intact ureter will follow a redundant course to the bladder, normal ureteral peristalsis will continue to provide effective drainage of urine from the kidney (Figure 3).

Despite the advantage of not dividing the ureter, in actual practice it is usually quite cumbersome to work on the abdominal wall with the ureter attached unless the patient is quite thin allowing unrestricted movement of the kidney outside the abdomen. We have found it preferable in most cases to divide the ureter and place the kidney on a separate workbench. This generally provides better exposure for the extracorporeal operation and allows a second surgical team to be simultaneously preparing the iliac fossa for autotransplantation. If concern exists regarding the adequacy of ureteral blood supply, the risk of postoperative urinary extravasation can be diminished by restoring urinary continuity through direct anastomosis of the renal pelvis to the retained distal ureter.

It is best to perform extracorporeal partial nephrectomy under surface hypothermia with the removed flushed kidney simply immersed in a basin of ice slush saline solution. When the resection is completed, tumor-free margins can more safely be verified by frozen sections than by extracorporeal arteriography. The latter carries the risk of intrarenal crystallization or cold-induced precipitation of contrast agents with resulting parenchymal damage. This can be obviated by employing iothalamate contrast material and by immediately reflushing the kidney with a cold electrolyte solution. Regarding vascular reconstruction of the renal remnant, we have yet to encounter a case where it was necessary to employ a vascular graft. In most cases, the main renal vessels are easily dissected away from the tumor and involved segmental branches may simply be reanastomosed if necessary. Multiple main renal arteries can be managed either by an extracorporeal conjoined or end-to-side anastomosis [14]. Certainly, if a vascular substitute is needed, autogenous hypogastric artery or saphenous vein are the materials of choice.

Following excision of the tumor and repair of the renal vessels under surface hypothermia, pulsatile perfusion of the renal remnant may then be safely performed with no risk of recirculating tumor cells. This measure is of particular advantage in enabling precise suture ligation of remaining potential bleeding points. Toward this end, the kidney is alternately perfused via the renal artery and the renal vein to facilitate both arterial and venous hemostasis. Following this, the defect created by the partial nephrectomy should be closed by suturing the kidney upon itself to ensure a watertight repair, providing that this may be done without producing obstruction of the vascular supply or collecting system. It is also generally wise to leave a nephrostomy tube

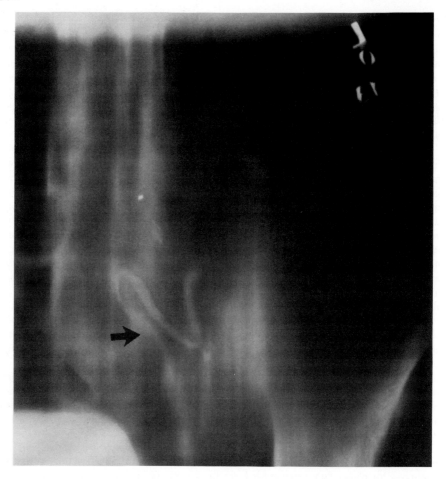

Figure 3. Postoperative intravenous pyelogram following renal antotransplantation in which the renal vessels were anastomosed to the iliac vessels with the kidney in its normal orientation and leaving the ureter attached. There is no hydronephrosis and the ureter (arrow) simply follows a redundant course to the bladder.

and ureteral stent indwelling following autotransplantation to protect against urinary extravasation, particularly when an extensive hilar dissection may have compromised ureteral or renal pelvic blood supply.

From 1976 to 1983, extracorporeal partial nephrectomy and autotransplantation have been performed in 15 patients with bilateral or solitary renal carcinoma at the Cleveland Clinic. All of these patients presented with extensive centrally-located renal carcinomas that were not considered amenable to in situ excision. Operative complications included temporary dialysis for acute tubular necrosis in four patients, urinary extravasation in four patients, and ureteral obstruction from clot in one patient. All of these problems resolved completely with appropriate treatment. Currently, 11 patients (73%) are alive, tumor-free, and have stable renal function with follow-up of three months to seven years. The four deaths were due to metastatic disease in two patients, myocardial infarction in one patient and hemorrhage in one patient. There have been no cases of postoperative local tumor recurrence in the renal remnant. In our follow-up of patients undergoing in situ partial nephrectomy for renal carcinoma, the incidence of local recurrence has been 15% [3]. Jacobs also found a diminished rate of local recurrence following extracorporeal resection (6%) compared to in situ resection (14%) in patients with bilateral synchronous renal carcinoma [4]. These findings are of particular interest since extracorporeal excision is generally done for larger more complex tumors which might be expected to yield a higher local recurrence rate. Although these observations require substantiation with greater numbers of patients they suggest that extracorporeal partial nephrectomy may diminish the risk of local tumor recurrence.

4. OTHER THERAPEUTIC OPTIONS

In patients with locally extensive but non-metastatic bilateral renal carcinoma where partial nephrectomy is not technically possible, bilateral nephrectomy with initiation of chronic dialysis offers the only possibility for curative treatment. Patients who remain tumor-free on dialysis for a minimum period of 15 months may then undergo renal transplantation with an acceptably low risk of tumor recurrence [15]. Although initial reports indicated discouraging survival rates for patients managed in this fashion, there is currently reason for renewed optimism with this approach particularly in patients <60 years of age who generally fare better on dialysis and who may then be candidates for transplantation if they remain tumor-free for a sufficient interval of time. Refinements in hemodialysis techniques along with the advent of continuous ambulatory peritoneal dialysis have significantly improved the longevity for patients on chronic dialysis [16], although the quality of life remains suboptimal for many patients. Of greater relevance perhaps are the significantly improved patient and graft survival rates currently being obtained following renal allotransplantation, particularly in recipients of cadaver kidneys. This has resulted from more conservative use of existing immunosuppressive agents, preliminary blood transfusion regimens, improved histocompatibility matching, and the advent of more effective immunosuppressive drugs such as anti-lymphocyte globulin and cyclosporine [17, 18, 19]. Currently, bilateral nephrectomy with chronic dialysis, hopefully followed by subsequent renal allotransplantation, is a viable therapeutic option for patients with bilateral renal carcinoma who are <60 years of age, free of metastases, with no significant extrarenal disease, and in whom partial nephrectomy cannot be done for technical reasons.

Other treatment modalities that have been employed in patients with bilateral renal carcinoma include hormonal therapy, chemotherapy, radiotherapy, and segmental renal arterial embolization [20, 21, 22]. There have been occasional reports of extended survival following nonoperative therapy in such patients which no doubt reflect the unpredictable natural history of this disease. Nevertheless, although these methods have helped to prolong survival in some patients, the results have generally been disappointing and surgical removal remains the only curative therapy available for this type of neoplasm.

REFERENCES

1. Margerber M, Pugh RCB, Auvert J, Betermann H, Costantini A, Gammelgaard PA, Petterson S, Wickham JEA: Conservative surgery of renal carcinoma: the EIRSS experience. Br J Urol 53:528, 1981.
2. Zincke H, Swanson SK: Bilateral renal cell carcinoma: Influence of synchronous and asynchronous occurrence on patient survival. J Urol 128:913, 1982.
3. Topley M. Novick AC, Montie JE: Long-term results following partial nephrectomy for localized renal adenocarcinoma (in press).

168

4. Jacobs SC, Berg SI, Lawson RK: Synchronous bilateral renal cell carcinoma: Total surgical excision. Cancer 46:2341, 1980.
5. Vermooten V: Indications for conservative surgery in certain renal tumors: A study based on the growth pattern of the clear cell carcinoma. J Urol 64:200, 1950.
6. Gittes RF, Blute RD: Repeat bench surgery on a solitary kidney. J Urol 127:530, 1982.
7. Novick AC, Stewart BH, Straffon RA, Banowsky LH: Partial nephrectomy in the treatment of renal adenocarcinoma. J Urol 118:932, 1977.
8. Graham SD, Glenn JF: Enucleative surgery for renal malignancy. J Urol 122:546, 1979.
9. Pearson JC, Weiss J, Tanagho EA: A plea for conservation of kidney in renal adenocarcinoma associated with von Hippel-Landau disease. J Urol 124:910, 1980.
10. Novick AC, Magnusson MO: Extracorporeal and in situ renal preservation. In: Vascular problems in urologic surgery, Novick AC, Straffon RA (ed). Philadelphia: WB Saunders Company, 1982.
11. Farcon EM, Morales P, Al-Askari S: In vivo hypothermic perfusion during renal surgery. Urology 3:414, 1974.
12. Marberger M, Georgi M, Guenther R, Hohenfellner R: Simultaneous balloon occlusion of the renal artery and hypothermic perfusion in in-situ surgery of the kidney. J Urol 119:463, 1978.
13. Novick AC: Extracorporeal renal surgery and autotransplantation. In: Vascular problems in urologic surgery, Novick AC, Straffon RA (ed). Philadelphia: WB Saunders Company, 1982.
14. Novick AC, Magnusson M, Braun WE: Multiple-artery renal transplantation: Emphasis on extracorporeal methods of donor arterial reconstruction. J Urol 122:731, 1979.
15. Penn I: Transplantation in patients with primary renal malignancies. Transplantation 24:424, 1977.
16. Paganini EP, Vidt DG: Renal replacement therapy utilizing hemodialysis and peritoneal dialysis. Urol Clin North Am 10:347, 1982.
17. Banowsky LHW: Current results and future expectations in renal transplantation. Urol Clin North Am 10:337, 1983.
18. Novick AC, Streem SB, Braun WE, Steinmuller D, Goormastic M, Cunningham R: Prophylactic antilymphoblast globulin, low-dose prednisone, and antilymphocyte globulin for first rejection: A steroid-sparing approach to immunosuppressive therapy. Transpl Proc 15:599, 1983.
19. Flechner SM: Cyclosporine: A new and promising immunosuppressive agent. Urol Clin North Am 10:263, 1983.
20. Johnson DE, Von Eschenbach A, Sternberg J: Bilateral renal cell carcinoma. J Urol 119:23, 1978.
21. Wickham JEA: Conservative renal surgery for adenocarcinoma. Br J Urol 47:25, 1975.
22. Soo CS, Chuang VP, Wallace S, Charnsangavej C, Bowers TA: Segmental renal artery embolization in solitary renal carcinoma. Urology 18:420, 1981.

7. BCG Therapy for Superficial Bladder Cancer

DAVID R. KELLEY and WILLIAM J. CATALONA

1. INTRODUCTION

Many recurrent superficial bladder cancers cannot be controlled with current standard therapies. Transurethral resection of superficial bladder tumors is curative in only 30 to 40% of cases. Adjuvant topical chemotherapy for superficial tumors may increase the cure rate to 60%. Whether topical chemotherapy can prevent the progression of these lesions to higher grades and stages is yet to be determined. There remains a significant percentage of patients (40%) who will suffer from recurrent tumors and possible cancer progression.

Immunotherapy. Experimental studies have shown that there are cell membrane-associated tumor antigens on transitional cell carcinoma cells. However, host recognition of these antigens may be diminished or absent. The degree of impairment of the host immune response appears to parallel the stage of the disease.

Although the potential beneficial effects of non-specific immunostimulants on the host immune system has been known since the 1950s, it is only in the past decade that intensive investigations have been performed using bacillus Calmette-Guerin (BCG) for cancer therapy. At present BCG immunotherapy for recurrent superficial bladder cancer represents the most successful form of immunotherapy in man [4, 7, 10, 13–15].

2. HISTORICAL BACKGROUND

In 1974, Zbar and Rapp [28] studied the effects of intralesional BCG therapy on intradermal inocula of hepatoma cells in guinea pigs. They noted that certain factors must be present if BCG therapy is to be effective: 1) close contact between the tumor cells and BCG; 2) immunocompetence of

T. L. Ratliff and W. J. Catalona (eds), Urologic Oncology. ISBN 0-89838-628-4.
© *1984. Martinus Nijhoff Publishers, Boston. Printed in the Netherlands.*

the host, i.e., the ability of the host to mount a delayed cutaneous hypersensitivity response to the mycobacterial antigens; 3) limited tumor burden; and 4) an adequate number of viable BCG organisms. In 1975, Bloomberg and associates [4] studied effects of BCG injections into the bladder of PPD-sensitized and non-sensitized dogs. They noted a profound, predictable inflammatory reaction characterized by histiocytes and leukocytes in the bladder mucosa of sensitized dogs after BCG injection. Although these animals did not have bladder tumors, a potential non-specific immunopotentiating effect of BCG in the treatment of bladder cancer was postulated.

In 1976, Morales [19] and associates published the first clinical trial on the use of intravesical BCG therapy in patients with recurrent superficial bladder cancers. They studied two groups of patients. Group I (5 patients) had a history of recurrent superficial bladder tumors treated with transurethral resections and had no gross evidence of tumor at the time of the study. Group II (4 patients) had a history of recurrent superficial bladder tumors, but resection of the tumor was incomplete. All patients had tumors that were considered to be stage T_0 or T_1. BCG was administered both intradermally and intravesically weekly for six weeks. Using a multiple puncture technique, 5 mg of BCG was injected intradermally into the upper thigh. A 50 cc saline solution containing 120 mg of BCG vaccine was instilled into the bladder and retained for not less than two hours. Cytoscopy was performed on each patient four to six weeks after their last BCG treatment. All patients exhibited a delayed cutaneous hypersensitivity response to mycobacterial antigens.

Prior to BCG therapy, a total of 22 tumor recurrences had occurred in these nine patients during 77 patient-months. After BCG treatment, only one recurrence was noted during 41 patient-months. The one reported recurrence was a squamous cell carcinoma. In five patients, having 25 patient-month periods of observation both before and after BCG treatment, there were 12 recurrences before BCG therapy and none after BCG therapy.

3. BCG PROPHYLAXIS

Based on these encouraging preliminary results, the National Cancer Institute and the Veterans Administration funded two prospective randomized clinical trials of intravesical BCG using Morales' regimen. One of these studies was reported by Camacho and associates [7, 12] in abstract form. They studied 86 patients with multiple recurrent superficial bladder tumors. The patients were either randomized to receive bladder tumor fulguration alone (43 patients) or bladder tumor fulguration plus intravesical BCG (43 patients). Before BCG treatment, the tumor recurrence rate per patient-month was 2.97 for the control group and 3.60 for the BCG group. At the completion of therapy, the control group had a recurrence rate of 2.37 tumors per patient-month while the BCG group had only 0.7 tumors per patient-month. This difference was statistically significant. The time to relapse for the TUR group (median nine months) was much shorter than the BCG group (median 36 months). The side effects of BCG treatment were reported to be mild and similar to those noted by Morales and associates. Granulomatous prostatitis was reported to occur in one patient.

Lamm and associates [13–16] conducted the other prospective, randomized clinical trial of intravesical BCG therapy and reported similar findings. Their patient population was comprised of 57 patients, all of whom had either a primary tumor or a recurrent tumor within three years of the study. They followed the protocol of Morales and associates [18] and used the same (Pasteur) strain of BCG. For the 26 controls and 28 BCG-treated patients the follow-up varied from 3 to 30 months. The two patient groups were similar with a mean age of 66 for both groups, a mean tumor grade of 2.0 for both groups and a mean number of recurrences of 1.3 for the control group and 1.2 for the BCG group. In an earlier report [14] they stated that the mean tumor stage for the control group was actually slightly lower than that of the BCG group. Delayed hypersensitivity responses to PPD, *Candida,* and *Trichophyton* antigens were tested at the beginning of the study and then at three to six month intervals. The leukocyte migration inhibition assay was used to assess the cellular immune response to PPD antigens. Only one complication (hydronephrosis) was reported in patients receiving intravesical BCG. Of those patients with superficial disease, BCG immunotherapy produced only minor side effects. Irritative bladder symptoms such as dysuria and frequency were reported in 96% of the cases and were directly related to therapy. These symptoms usually subsided within 48 hours (see Table 1). Other reported side effects were mild hematuria (34% of the patients), fever less than 101 °F (in all the patients with superficial bladder tumors), nausea (in 14%), chills and malaise (in 3%).

Table 1. Side effects in patients with superficial bladder cancer who received BCG immunotherapy [13–16].

Dysuria	96%
Frequency	86%
Mild hematuria	34%
Fever	21%
Nausea	14%
Chills	3%
Malaise	3%

Follow-up cystoscopic examinations were performed at regular three to six month intervals for both groups. Fifty percent of the control group (13 of 26) had subsequent tumor recurrences as compared with 21% of the BCG-treated patients (6 of 28). There also was a significant difference in the time to recurrence for the two groups. Sixteen months was the mean time of recurrence for the control group as compared with 29 months for the BCG treatment group. Positive cystoscopic findings for tumor occurred in 28 of 117 (24%) for the control group versus 12 of 118 (10%) for the BCG treatment group ($p = 0.005$, chi-square).

The results of PPD skin testing prior to BCG therapy revealed only six patients to be PPD-positive. Three of these six patients subsequently developed recurrent tumors after therapy. However, only one out of 17 patients whose PPD test converted from negative to positive had tumor recurrence after therapy. This suggests that the best candidates for BCG immunotherapy may be patients without prior *Mycobacterium tuberculosis* exposure, who develop a positive PPD skin test after therapy.

Lamm and associates [15] also reported on the presence of A, B, or H antigens on the resected tumors, using a mixed red cell adherence assay. The test was performed on tumors resected from 21 control patients and 22 BCG-treated patients. It was noted that ABH-negative tumors had less of a tendency to recur than the ABH-positive tumors. This tendency appeared to be independent of the mode of therapy given.

In a limited study, Antonaci and associates [3] evaluated the in vitro cytotoxic capacity of lymphocytes of patients with superficial bladder tumors. They compared two groups of patients: 1) those treated with endoscopic fulguration alone (6 patients); and 2) those treated with endoscopic fulguration plus postoperative BCG therapy (6 patients). Both systemic and intravesical BCG (Pasteur strain) was given on the 6th and 7th postoperative day. Scarification with 75 mg of BCG was performed on an upper extremity and an equivalent amount was diluted in 50 cc of normal saline and instilled into the bladder. Patients were instructed to retain the BCG for a minimum of 2 hours. Using T-24 bladder cancer target cells, lymphocyte cytotoxicity was tested 4 days prior to surgery and 12 days after surgery. Preoperatively, lymphocytes from both groups showed higher levels of cytotoxicity against target cells derived from bladder tumors than from colon tumors. The control group showed a marked depression in their cytotoxicity after surgery, while the BCG-treated patients had no depression in their level of cytotoxicity. Thus, BCG therapy when administered early in the postoperative period appeared to negate the immunosuppressive effects of surgical stress. These results support the contention of Morales and associates' that early postoperative BCG therapy is desirable.

In 1980, Martinez-Pineiro [18] reported on his experience with BCG for non-infiltrating papillary tumors of the bladder. Twenty-nine patients were treated prophylactically with BCG after endoscopic resection of the bladder tumor(s). All patients had superficial tumors (stage O, A, or B_1). Also before the institution of BCG therapy, PPD-negative patients were sensitized with intradermal injections of BCG. Fourteen patients were treated for primary tumors and 15 were treated for recurrent tumors. There were three treatment groups. Group I (10 patients) received cutaneous scarification with 150 mg of BCG vaccine. A total of 10 scarifications, each 5 cm in length, was administered weekly for the first month, then monthly for one year, and finally every three months for another year. Group II (12 patients) received intravesical BCG instillations. A 50 cc solution containing 150 mg of BCG was instilled into the bladder on a weekly basis for one month, and then monthly for a minimum of one year. Group III (7 patients) received both cutaneous scarification and intravesical instillation of BCG. The patients in this group received both intravesical BCG and BCG scarification on the same day following the same treatment schedules as group I and II. Two different strains of BCG were used in this study. Seven patients in group I were treated with the Pasteur strain [17] and the remaining 22 were treated with 'immuno-BCG Pasteur' vaccine. The patients were followed with urine cytology and cystoscopic examinations at the following intervals: six weeks, 12 weeks, every three months the first year, and every six months thereafter. The range of follow-up was between five and 42 months (mean 15.1 months). No tumor recurrences were noted in the 14 patients who received adjuvant BCG therapy after resection of their primary tumor(s). Of the 15 patients who received adjuvant BCG therapy after resection of a recurrent bladder tumor, six (40%) had recurrent tumors. Unfortunately, because of the low number of patients with recurrent disease, the inclusion of patients with muscle-invading tumor, and the combined fashion in which the results were reported, it is difficult to conclude which route of vaccine administration is best.

In 1981, Flamm and Grof [9] published unfavorable results on the use of adjuvant intravesical BCG therapy with endoscopic resection of superficial bladder tumors. A total of 45 patients were treated. The Connaught strain of BCG was used. There were two different doses of vaccine (60 mg and 120 mg) tested. The vaccine was diluted in 50 cc of normal saline and administered intravesically. Systemic sensitization to BCG via intradermal injections was performed on only two patients. Both of these patients reportedly had severe ulcerative skin reactions. Two different treatment series were tested. A single treatment series consisted of six weekly intravesical instillations of either 60 or 120 mg of BCG vaccine. A double treatment series consisted of the above plus a six week follow-up period, then an additional six weekly instillations of 120 mg of vaccine. Their results after a two to five year follow-up period were reported in a combined fashion. Persistent tumor was found in 36% of the patients and recurrent tumors were found in 59%. There was no significant difference between the single and double treatment series. Because the results were published in a combined fashion, it is not possible to determine any difference between the two dosages of vaccine tested. Although systemic BCG sensitization alone has been reported to have no effect on tumor recurrence [27], perhaps a protocol including both systemic sensitization plus intravesical BCG would have improved their results.

Netto Jr and Lemos [23] compared BCG therapy with conventional therapy (i.e. endoscopic resection and topical chemotherapy) for prophylaxis of recurrent superficial bladder tumors. However, unlike previous BCG protocols, they administered the BCG orally. They studied 55 patients, all with stage O or A transitional cell carcinoma of the bladder. Therapy was assigned on a rotational basis to one of three categories. Group I consisted of 22 patients treated with endoscopic resection alone. Group II included 17 patients treated by endoscopic resection plus postoperative intravesical Thiotepa. Group III included 16 patients treated with endoscopic resection plus oral BCG vaccine postoperatively. Follow-up cytologic and cystoscopic examinations were performed at three month intervals for the first year, six month intervals for the next two years, and on an annual basis thereafter. Topical chemotherapy consisted of 60 mg of Thiotepa in a 60 cc saline solution, which was instilled into the bladder and retained for two hours. Instillation of Thiotepa was started on the second postoperative day then on a daily basis for one week, then monthly for three months, then every three months for one year, then semi-annually for two years, and finally yearly for two years. A complete blood count, including a platelet count, was obtained prior to each series of Thiotepa instillations. If a patient developed a recurrent tumor, therapy was discontinued and the patient again started the protocol from the beginning.

The oral BCG vaccine (Moreau strain) was administered according to the patient's dermal reaction to injections of dinitrochlorbenzene and croton oil. Gradations of the skin response were designated either as none, moderate or marked. BCG dosages of 800, 400, and 200 mg were given for none, moderate, and marked skin reactions, respectively. The oral vaccine was given three times a week, indefinitely. The dosage was altered according to changes in skin test results, which were performed every three months.

The results showed 80% of patients (16 of 20) treated with endoscopic resection alone suffered tumor recurrences. Some prophylaxis was afforded by topical Thiotepa postoperatively for group II in whom 42.9% (6 of 16) had recurrences. Oral BCG vaccine administered postoperatively provided the best prophylaxis; only 6.2% of these patients had recurrences. A significantly lower recurrence rate was noted in patients treated with oral BCG as compared with the other two groups. Tumor recurrences per patient-year were as follows: group I – 0.5, group II – 0.45, and group III – 0.03. Netto Jr and Lemos [23] reported that, although the metabolism and absorption of BCG is not completely understood, oral BCG caused no significant adverse side effects. This low morbidity may make oral therapy the preferred route of administration if these observations are confirmed in other studies. These investigators are currently performing a prospective study comparing oral and intravesical BCG therapy.

Based on their prior encouraging experimental results, Adolphs and Bastian [1] conducted a study on chemoimmune prophylaxis of superficial bladder tumors. They treated a total of 90 patients, all of whom had either primary or recurrent stage pTa or pT_1 tumors. Requirements for all patients before the initiation of therapy were: absence of residual tumor, sterile urine, and positive skin testing to PPD and/or dinitrochlorbenzene. Intravenous cyclophosphamide (700 mg/M^2) was administered two weeks after *total* transurethral resection of the tumor. Two weeks later the patients received both systemic and intravesical BCG (Connaught strain). A suspension of 120 mg of BCG in 50 cc of saline was instilled into the bladder and retained for a minimum of one hour. Cutaneous administration of BCG (dosage not given), was also performed at the same time. Intravesical BCG and cutaneous administration was repeated five times at weekly intervals. At the completion of therapy, patients were monitored at regular three monthly intervals with urine cytology and cystoscopy. Liver function profiles, complete blood count, erythrocyte sedimentation rate, and serum creatinines also were monitored at 6 and 12 months after therapy. Although this clinical trial was neither a prospective nor randomized, the authors compared their results with those observed in a historical control group of 65 patients. The BCG treatment group had a follow-up period which ranged from 3 to 48 months (median 13.3 months). There were eight tumor recurrences (9%) noted in the BCG treatment group over this follow-up period. In comparig these results with the historical controls, BCG-treated patients had significantly fewer tumor recurrences. It was further noted that 26 patients in the BCG treatment group who were followed for 18 months postoperatively had no tumor recurrences.

Table 2. Side effects of cyclophosphamide and BCG therapy [1].

Dysuria	79%
Urinary frequency	60%
Fever	28%
Allergy	1%
Epididymitis	1%

The side effects associated with this treatment regimen were generally mild and well tolerated, and subsided at the completion of therapy (Table 2). There were no abnormal laboratory studies reported at 6 and 12 months post-therapy. Normalization of urinary cytology usually occurred at two to three months after the last BCG treatment. The authors did not include control groups receiving cyclophosphamide alone or BCG alone. Therefore, further studies will be necessary to determine which components of this regimen are most important in producing these favorable results.

4. INTRAVESICAL CHEMOTHERAPY VS INTRAVESICAL BCG

A study comparing intravesical Thiotepa with intravesical BCG for recurrent superficial bladder cancer was conducted by Brosman in 1982 [5]. In this prospective, randomized clinical trial, there were a total of 49 patients of whom 22 were randomized to receive intravesical Thiotepa and 27 were randomized to receive intravesical BCG. In addition, 12 patients who were Thiotepa failures and who were not a part of the randomized study also were treated with intravesical BCG.

The BCG treatment protocol differed from that used in previous studies in the strain used, the amount of vaccine instilled per treatment, and the treatment schedule. Brosman used 6×10^8 organisms (approximately 60 mg) of the Tice strain diluted in 60 cc of saline, which was retained in the bladder for one and one half to two hours. No intradermal BCG vaccine injections were given. BCG was instilled weekly for six weeks, then every two weeks for three months, and then monthly over a 24 month total treatment period. Thiotepa (60 mg) was diluted in 60 cc of saline and was instilled using the same treatment schedule as the BCG group. The patients underwent cystoscopic examinations at regular time intervals. Six and 12 weeks after the clinical trial was started, PPD skin tests were performed.

After two years of follow-up nine of 19 patients (40%) who completed the Thiotepa therapy developed recurrent tumors, while no recurrences were noted in the 27 randomized patients or in the 12 non-randomized patients who received BCG therapy. A three year follow-up was also reported on seven of the patients who received BCG therapy, and there were no recurrences. In a subsequent oral presentation, Brosman [6] reported seven percent later had tumor recurrences.

There were more adverse side effects noted with Brosman's BCG protocol. Irritative bladder symptoms occurred in all of the patients, and the majority experienced fever and malaise. Most patients became symptomatic within four hours after therapy, but the symptoms subsided within 48 hours. Severe toxic side effects were noted in 11 patients (28%). Isoniazid was given to six patients who had marked irritative symptoms along with anorexia, fever, and chills. Triple drug therapy consisting of Isoniazid, Rifampin and Ethambutol was given to four patients who developed pulmonary infections and aberrant liver profile studies. BCG therapy was effective in treating residual tumors in 10 of 12 patients who had failed Thiotepa therapy.

In the BCG group, 13 of the 16 patients who initially had negative PPD skin tests converted to positive at six weeks and all 16 were positive at 12 weeks. Therefore, systemic sensitization to BCG occurred with intravesical vaccine instillation alone. The tumor recurrence rate using Brosman's protocol is substantially lower than that using Morales' protocol (7% versus 22%) and the toxicity appears to be greater despite the fact that Brosman's protocol calls for half the dosage of BCG (60 mg versus 120 mg). The other differences between these two treatment protocols are that Brosman used the Tice strain of BCG while Morales used the Pasteur strain and that Brosman employed monthly maintenance therapy while Morales did not. These results are open to several different interpretations: either the Tice strain of BCG is more effective (and perhaps more toxic) than the Pasteur strain or maintenance therapy is important in preventing tumor recurrences (but may also be associated with more toxicity). Further studies will be required to distinguish among these possibilities.

5. BCG THERAPY FOR CARCINOMA IN SITU

In 1980, Morales and associates [20] published favorable results on the treatment of carcinoma in situ of the bladder with systemic and intravesical BCG therapy. They used the Pasteur strain of BCG and the treatment protocol used was the same as described in their previous study. Seven patients underwent BCG therapy. They were followed at regular three month intervals with cystoscopy, biopsies, and urinary cytology. The follow-up period ranged from 12 to 33 months (mean 22.2). Of the six patients who completed the BCG therapy, five were found to be tumor-free, with a mean follow-up of 22.6 months. Again, the side effects from this treatment protocol were mild and self-limited.

Lamm and associates [16] reported on twelve patients which carcinoma in situ treated with BCG therapy. They followed the same BCG protocol as described by Morales and associates. Ten of their twelve patients (83%) had complete resolution of their disease. The two patients, who failed therapy had inoperable invasive residual tumor in addition to carcinoma in situ.

In 1983, Herr and associates [10, 11] reported on the effect of BCG therapy on carcinoma in situ of the bladder. Their study is a continuance of the randomized prospective trial previously reported by Camacho and associates [7] in 1980. Their BCG protocol was the same as that described by Morales and associates [19] in 1976. They treated a total of 69 patients with superficial bladder tumors. Thirty-five patients were randomized to group I, the control group, and treated with transurethral resection alone. The 34 remaining patients were randomized to group II, the BCG group, and were treated with transurethral resection plus adjuvant BCG therapy postoperatively.

Of the 69 patients treated, 41 patients (59%) had pathological documentation of carcinoma in situ on more than two occasions at least three months apart. Twenty-four of these patients were randomized to the control group and 17 were randomized to the BCG group. The patients in both groups were similar as regards sex, age, voiding symptoms, stage and number of associated papillary tumors. The criteria for complete response to therapy included all of the following: cystoscopic improvement of the bladder mucosa, negative urinary cytology, absence of disease on biopsy and improvement of any voiding symptoms by three months post therapy. Follow-up evaluation for all patients was at least one year, in which time at least four cystoscopic examinations had been performed. The results at the end of one year follow-up revealed that only two of the 24 control patients (8%) were without evidence of CIS, while 11 of the 17 BCG-treated patients (65%) were tumor-free. The BCG-treated patients who responded to therapy usually showed improvement at the time of their first follow-up cystoscopy which was performed six to eight weeks after therapy. Only three of the eleven patients (27%) with irritative voiding symptoms in the control group had improvement of symptoms post-therapy. This is in sharp contrast to the BCG group in which eight out of the nine patients (89%) had dramatic improvement of irritative voiding symptoms by their fourth to sixth treatment. Symptomatic improvement proved to be a good indicator of early therapeutic effectiveness.

Local or systemic progression of disease was noted in 12 patients (50%) in the control group and seven (41%) in the BCG treatment group. All 12 patients in the control group who showed progression of disease eventually required a cystectomy, wheras only two patients in the BCG group underwent radical surgery because of CIS involvement of the prostatic urethra or prostatic ducts. Both of these patients showed complete resolution of CIS in their bladder. This observation is consistent with the experimental observation made by Zbar and Rapp [27] that close contact between tumor cells and BCG is required for successful therapy. All 12 patients in the control group who did not have disease progression had either cytologic and/or pathologic evidence of carcinoma in situ at 18 months follow-up.

Side effects of BCG therapy were noted to be mild and well tolerated.

Table 3. BCG therapy for carcinoma in situ.

	Total no. of patients	Resolution	Percentages
Morales and associates [20][a]	7	5	71%
Lamm and associates [16][a]	12	10	83%
Herr and associates [10, 11][a]	17	11	65%
Brosman [4][b]	7	5	71%
Total	43	31	72%

[a] Protocol described by Morales and associates.
[b] Protocol described by Brosman.

None of the patients in the BCG treatment group had toxic side effects that warranted interruption of therapy.

Herr and associates [10] noted that superficial papillary tumors recurred in 9 of 24 (38%) of control patients and 6 of the 17 (35%) of the BCG-treated patients. Recurrent papillary tumors were noted to recur even in some patients who had favorable responses in terms of control of carcinoma in situ.

Using the Tice strian with monthly maintenance therapy Brosman [4] treated seven patients with carcinoma in situ. A 60 mg dose of BCG was administered intravesically on a weekly basis. No intradermal BCG injections were given. Follow-up bladder biopsies were performed every six weeks. After 18 weeks of therapy, five of the seven patients (71%) showed resolution of cellular atypia (Table 3).

Taken together, results from these four studies show that about two thirds of the patients treated with intravesical BCG therapy had resolution of in situ carcinoma.

6. BCG THERAPY FOR RESIDUAL BLADDER TUMOR

Regression of existing bladder tumors with BCG therapy was reported by Douville and associates [8] in 1978. They used the same BCG strain (Pasteur) that was used by Morales and associates. Their protocol, which was similar to the protocol used by Morales and associates in 1976, involved abdominal scarification with 5 mg of BCG and instillation of 120 mg BCG in 50 cc of saline, which was retained in the bladder for two hours. Treatments were given on a weekly basis for six weeks. A follow-up cystoscopy was performed at four to six weeks after therapy. Four of the six patients (67%) had no residual tumors noted on follow-up. The four patients who responded to therapy had variable degrees of adverse side effects, while the two non-responders experienced no toxic side effects.

In 1981, Morales and associates [21] presented their results on the treatment of partially resected bladder tumors with systemic and intravesical BCG. They treated 17 patients with persistent non-infiltrating tumor with the same BCG protocol as described in their prior study. Particular importance was placed on the time interval between the bladder tumor resection and the initiation of BCG therapy. They advocated that BCG therapy be started within 10 days of the bladder tumor resection to allow for close contact between the vaccine and the disrupted bladder mucosa. Four to six weeks after the treatment had been completed, cystoscopic examinations were done and urine was collected for cytology. These examinations were repeated at three to six month intervals thereafter. In addition to random bladder biopsies at four preselected sites, any persistent tumor or previous tumor site was also biopsied. Complete residual tumor regression was noted in ten patients (59%). Tumor regression occurred in all patients with grade II tumors, but in only 17% of those patients with higher grade tumors. The side effects of BCG therapy reported by Morales and associates were generally mild and similar to those noted in their prior clinical trial. Irritative bladder symptoms, low grade fever and malaise were common. One of the 17 patients required Isoniazid for toxic systemic effects.

In 1982, Lamm and associates [15] reported on the use of BCG therapy for residual bladder tumors. They treated 10 patients who had stage B bladder cancer, and who either refused radical surgery or who were not operative candidates. The Pasteur strain of BCG was employed, and the treatment protocol as described by Morales and associates was followed. Six of these 10 patients were found to be tumor-free at an average follow-up of 14 months post-immunotherapy. An additional patient who had recurrent tumors at nine months post-treatment has remained tumor-free with maintenance BCG therapy. The three remaining patients had residual tumor three months after starting BCG therapy and required other treatments.

Table 4. BCG therapy for residual bladder tumor(s).

Clinical study	Total number of patients	Number of patients without residual disease post-therapy	Percentage
Douville and associates [8][a]	6	4	67%
Morales and associates [21][a]	17	10	59%
Lamm and associates [15][a]	10	6	60%
Brosman [5][b]	12	10	83%
Total	45	31	68%

[a] Protocol described by Morales and associates.
[b] Protocol described by Brosman.

Also in 1982, Brosman [4] reported on intravescial BCG therapy in 12 patients who had multiple superficial bladder tumors. These patients had been treated previously with endoscopic tumor resections and topical chemotherapy. All 12 patients had documented residual disease present at the beginning of BCG therapy. Using the Tice strain of BCG, weekly intravesical instillations (60 mg) of the BCG vaccine were given. Cystoscopic examinations were performed at six week intervals after therapy. After six months of maintenance BCG therapy, 10 of the 12 patients (83%) were without clinical evidence of disease (Table 4).

7. DISCUSSION

According to the present United States Cancer Statistics [25], there will be 38,500 new cases of bladder cancer diagnosed in 1983. Over 80% of these patients will have local and potentially curable tumors. Using conventional therapy, i.e., transurethral resection and adjuvant topical chemotherapy, over 12,500 patients will suffer recurrent tumors. This large annual patient population who are destined to fail standard therapy demonstrates a need for investigating potentially new and better treatments for bladder cancer.

The efficacy of adjuvant BCG therapy for superficial bladder tumors is now well documented in prospective, randomized clinical trials. However, clinical experience with this treatment is still limited and long-term followup is lacking. There remain many questions to be answered. These questions concern the preferred BCG preparation to be used, the optimal dose schedule and route of administration of BCG, and the value of maintenance therapy. Experimental studies in animals have shown that different strains of BCG have different immunogenicity. Lamm and associates showed in an animal model that the Tice and Pasteur strains of BCG were more effective as immune adjuvants than the Glaxo strain.

A variety of dosages and routes of administration of BCG have been employed by different investigators. For instance, Brosman [4] used a 60 mg dose, Morales, Lamm, and Herr used 120 mg while Netto Jr and Lemos [23] used 200 to 800 mg of BCG. Also various routes of administration have been used. Brosman used intravesical BCG only. Morales, Lamm, and Herr used both intravesical and intradermal BCG while Netto Jr and Lemos used oral BCG. Finally, the necessity of maintenance therapy remains an open question. Brosman maintained patients on monthly BCG instillations while Morales, Lamm, and Herr did not.

The toxic responses to BCG therapy also have varied. Somewhat paradoxically the toxicity reported by Brosman using 60 mg seemed to be greater than that observed by Morales, Lamm, and Herr using 120 mg. Virtually no toxicity was reported by Netto Jr and Lemos using 200 to 800 mg of BCG administered orally. Concern has been expressed about dissemination of BCG infection and the possibility of the development of bladder contractures and/or ureteral strictures as can occur with chronic tuberculosis of the urinary tract. In this regard, there have been no reports of bladder contractures in patients treated with BCG therapy. Histologic studies demonstrate that the granulomatous changes within the bladder subside with time.

Another potential limitation of BCG therapy is the occurrence of carcinoma in situ extravesically. Herr and associates recently reported that 36% of patients who initially responded favorably to BCG therapy subsequently developed carcinoma in situ either in the distal ureters or the prostatic urethra. With the exception of one patient, all were without clinical evidence of bladder involvement.

Attempts have been made to identify patients most likely to respond favorably to BCG therapy. Although a variety of different immunologic parameters have been monitored, information is conflicting about the correlation between host immune reactivity and the eventual therapeutic response. Lamm and associates reported that patients who convert PPD skin tests from negative to positive have a very high incidence (94%) of favorable responses to BCG therapy. Other investigators have excluded from treatment patients who were PPD-negative before therapy. This exclusion may have eliminated some of the best candidates for BCG therapy. Finally, little is known about the underlying mechanism of action of BCG therapy in bladder cancer patients.

In conclusion, adjuvant BCG therapy has been shown to be safe and effective as a means of prophylaxis for patients with superficial bladder tumors, and in the treatment of non-infiltrating bladder tumors including diffuse carcinoma in situ. Further study will be required to determine the optimal treatment protocol, patient selection, and mechanism of action.

REFERENCES

1. Adolphs H, Bastian H: Chemoimmune prophylaxis of superficial bladder tumors. J Urol 129:29, 1983.
2. Adolphs HD, Bastian HP: Chemoimmune prophylaxis of superficial bladder tumors. Results after treatment of more than 130 patients in four years. Abstract 347. Americal urological association, seventy-eight annual meeting, Las Vegas, Nevada, April, 1983.
3. Antonaci S, Piccinno A, Lucivero G, Miglietta A, Piccininno A, Bonoma L: Effect of BCG immunotherapy on cell mediated cytotoxicity in bladder cancer patients following surgical treatment. Tumori 67:177, 1981.
4. Bloomberg SD, Brosman SA, Hausman MS, Cohen A, Battenberg JD: The effect of BCG on the dog bladder. Invest Urol 12:423, 1975.

5. Brosman SA: Experience with bacillus Calmette-Guerin in patients with superficial bladder cancer. J Urol 128:27, 1982.
6. Brosman SA: Experience with bacillus Calmette-Guerin in patients with superficial bladder cancer. Presented at National Bladder Cancer Conference, Sarasota, Florida, January, 1983.
7. Camacho F, Pinsky CM, Kerr D, Whitmore WF Jr, Oettgen H: Treatment of superficial bladder cancer with intravesical BCG. Abstract C-160, Proc Am Assoc Cancer Res and Am Soc Clin Oncol 21:359, 1980.
8. Douville Y, Pelouze G, Roy R, Charrois R, Kibrite A, Martin M, Dionne L, Coulonval L, Robinson J: Recurrent bladder papillomata treated with bacillus Calmette-Guerin: A preliminary report (phase I trial). Cancer Treat Rep 62:551, 1978.
9. Flamm J, Grof F: Adjuvant local immunotheraphy with bacillus Calmette-Guerin (BCG) in treatment of urothelial carcinoma of the urinary bladder. Wien Med Wochenschr 131:501, 1981.
10. Herr HW, Pinsky CM, Whitmore WF Jr, Oettgen HF, Melamed MR: Effects of intravesical bacillus Calmette-Guerin (BCG) on carcinoma in situ of the bladder. Cancer 51:1323, 1983.
11. Herr HW, Pinsky CM, Whitmore WF Jr, Oettgen HF, Melamed MR: Intravesical bacillus Calmette-Guerin (BCG) therapy of superficial bladder tumors. Abstract 307. American Urological Association, Seventy-eight annual meeting, Las Vegas, Nevada, April, 1983.
12. Herr HW, Whitmore WF Jr, Logsini PC, Pinsky CM: Extravesical carcinoma in situ after intravesical bacillus Calmette-Guerin (BCG). Abstract 346. American Urological Association, Seventy-eighth annual meeting, Las Vegas, Nevada, April, 1983.
13. Lamm DL, Thor DE, Harris SC, Reyna JA, Stogdill VD, Radwin HJ: Bacillus Calmette-Guerin immunotherapy of superficial bladder cancer. J Urol 124:38, 1980.
14. Lamm DL, Thor DE, Winters WD, Stogdill VD, Radwin HM: BCG Immunotherapy of bladder cancer: Inhibition of tumor recurrence and associated immune responses. Cancer 48:82, 1981.
15. Lamm D, Thor DE, Stogdill VD, Radwin H: Bladder cancer immunotherapy. J Urol 128:931, 1982.
16. Lamm DL, Stogdill VD, Radwin HM: The current status of BCG in the treatment of human bladder cancer. Abstract 345. American Urological Association, Seventy-eighth annual meeting, Las Vegas, Nevada, April, 1983.
17. Martinez-Pineiro JA, Muntanola P: Non-specific immunotherapy with BCG vaccine in bladder tumors. Eur Urol 3:11, 1977.
18. Martinez-Pineiro JA: BCG vaccine in the treatment of non-infiltrating papillary tumors of the bladder. In: Bladder tumors and other topics in urological oncology, Pavone-Macaluso M, Smith PH, Edsmyr F (eds). New York: Plenum Press, p 175, 1980.
19. Morales A, Eidinger D, Bruce AW: Intracavitary bacillus Calmette-Guerin in the treatment of superficial bladder tumors. J Urol 116:180, 1976.
20. Morales A: Treatment of carcinoma in situ of the bladder with BCG. A phase II trial. Cancer Immunol Immunother 9:69, 1980.
21. Morales A, Ottenhof P, Emerson L: Treatment of residual, non-infiltrating bladder cancer with bacillus Calmette-Guerin. J Urol 125:649, 1981.
22. Morales A: Long-term results and complications of intravesical BCG therapy for cancer. Abstract 344. American Urological Association, Seventy-eighth annual meeting, Las Vegas, Nevada, April, 1983.
23. Netto NR Jr, Lemos GC: A comparison of treatment methods for prophylaxis of recurrent superficial bladder tumors. J Urol 129:33, 1983.
24. Shapiro A, Kadmon D, Catalona WJ, Ratliff TL: Immunotherapy of superficial bladder cancer. J Urol 128:891, 1982.

184

25. Silverberg E, Lubera JA: A review of American Cancer Society estimates of cancer cases and deaths. Cancer 33:2, 1983.
26. Sparks FC: Hazards and complications of BCG immunotherapy. Med Clin North Am 60:499, 1976.
27. Stober U, Peter HH: BCG-Immunotherapie zur Rezidivprophylaxe beim Harnblasenkarzinom? Therapiewoche 30:6067, 1980.
28. Zbar B, Rapp HJ: Immunotherapy of guinea pig cancer with BCG. Cancer 34:1532, 1974.

Editorial Comment

DONALD L. LAMM

The authors have comprehensively reviewed the world's literature on BCG immunotherapy of bladder cancer and conclude that BCG is effective in the prevention of bladder tumor recurrence and the treatment of superficial transitional cell carcinoma and carcinoma in situ. The authors also conclude that BCG is a relatively safe therapy for bladder cancer. My experience certainly supports these conclusions, but we must withold judgment on the long-term safety of BCG until further experience is gained. The widespread usage of BCG, variations in BCG strains, increased dosage and frequency of treatments, and increased variation in the route of administration might be expected to increase the observed toxicity of BCG.

Some simple points should be stressed to avoid unnecessary toxicity. First, BCG should never be injected into the skin. While many authors have reported that '5 mg' is administered percutaneously using a multiple puncture technique, in fact, a very small (and undetermined) fraction of that amount is actually delivered through the skin. Intradermal injection of 5 mg of BCG will cause local necrosis and ulceration as documented by Flamm and Groff[3]. Percutaneous inoculation can be accomplished by applying 5 mg of the vaccine to the skin and puncturing the area several times with a 27 gauge needle. This technique provides good systemic immunization and avoids the scarring inherent in the skin scarification procedure. Secondly, while we have observed beneficial responses from intralesional injection of BCG in experimental animals [6], it should be stressed that intralesional injection is very dangerous. At least three deaths have occurred following direct injection of BCG into tumors [10]. Life-threatening anaphylactoid or septic reactions may occur. Reactions typically occur in a patient who has been previously sensitized to BCG. After a latency period of 1 to 12 hours, high fever, chills, hypotension, oliguria, and respiratory distress followed by intravascular coagulopathy may occur. Prophylactic administration of acetaminophen, diphenhydramine and Isoniazid may reduce the incidence of these reactions. When such reactions occur, vigorous resuscitation with intravenous fluids, parenteral Isoniazid, diphenhydramine, mannitol, vasopressors and corticosteroids may be necessary.

The review very correctly points out that the optimal protocol for BCG immunotherapy remains to be developed. Strains that have demonstrated efficacy in the treatment of human bladder cancer include the Pasteur strain, the Institut Armand Frappier preparation, the Tice strain, the Connaught strain, and the Moreau strain. It is remarkable that wide doses, variation in treatment schedules, and routes of administration have been effective. Many early investigators assumed, based on the animals studies [12], that local administration of BCG would be necessary and perhaps sufficient for optimal response. The remarkable response observed by Brosman with Tice BCG administered only by the intravesical route might suggest that systemic sensitization is not necessary. However, as noted by the authors, systemic immunity as demonstrated by PPD skin test conversion did occur in these patients. In animal experimentation [1], local inflammatory reaction was increased in dogs with systemic immunity. In chemically induced bladder tumors, we observed an antitumor response from intralesional injection only in animals previously sensitized to BCG [6]. It is of interest to note that while intravesical Tice

BCG resulted in PPD skin test conversion of 13 of 16 patients in Brosman's study, Pasteur strain from Institut Armand Frappier, has resulted in no skin test conversion in our 7 PPD-negative patients given intravesical BCG. The importance of systemic response to BCG is further emphasized by Netto and Lemos' observation [9] of a dramatic reduction in tumor recurrence in patients given BCG by the oral route alone. Intradermal BCG alone, however, was found to be ineffective in preventing tumor recurrence [11].

In our experience, the addition of percutaneous BCG administration has resulted in more effective systemic immunity and a lower incidence of tumor recurrence than administration by the intravesical route alone. Twenty percent of patients given intravesical and percutaneous BCG had tumor recurrence compared with a 40% recurrence rate in 10 patients given only intravesical BCG. Patients who converted PPD skin test from negative to positive have had only a 4.5% (1/22) incidence of tumor recurrence. However, Herr and associates [4] have had different results. They observed no reduction in antitumor activity in patients who received the same strain and dose of BCG by the intravesical route. These conflicting results might be due to the higher incidence of pre-existing immunity to PPD in their population. The morbidity of percutaneously administered BCG is so slight that its continued use would certainly appear to be justified at this time in patients who are PPD skin test-negative.

Since patients with bladder cancer have a continued diathesis for tumor recurrence, and the immunostimulation induced by BCG tends to diminish with time, it is reasonable to assume that maintenance immunotherapy, like maintenance chemotherapy, would further reduce the rate of tumor recurrence. Indeed, the only common factor in the two reported studies with the lowest rate of tumor recurrence is the use of a maintenance schedule of BCG immunotherapy. In Brosman's study, no tumor recurrences were seen in 39 patients followed for a minimum of 2 years [2]. Tice strain BCG was given by the intravesical route in that study on a monthly maintenance schedule. In Netto's study [9], only 0.03 recurrences per patient-year occurred in patients given the Moreau strain by the oral route on a maintenance schedule of 3 times a week. In our experience, maintenance intravesical and percutaneous BCG at 3 to 6 month intervals has decreased the incidence of tumor recurrence from 20% to 9% and the rate of tumor recurrence from 19/100 patient-months to less than 5/100 patient-months.

The remarkable efficacy of BCG in the treatment of carcinoma in situ is well documented and offers an excellent therapeutic option to this high risk group of patients. The observation of a 36% incidence of subsequent development of carcinoma in situ in the distal ureters or prostatic urethra [5] is certainly worrisome. One of our 14 patients with carcinoma in situ has developed urethral CIS. I have approached this problem by administering systemic as well as intravesical BCG and by routinely instilling BCG in the urethra in patients with CIS. If oral BCG is as effective in treating carcinoma in situ as it appears to be in preventing tumor recurrence, it could become the treatment of choice for CIS since the location of the disease should be irrelevant.

The mechanism of action of BCG is best described as non-specific and the authors are correct in concluding that, while the efficacy of BCG cannot be denied, its mechanism of action in bladder cancer is undetermined. There is some evidence that BCG may share antigenic determinants with a variety of tumors [8]. BCG has long been recognized as a potent immune adjuvant and has numerous actions including stimulation of the reticuloendothelial system resulting in hyperplasia and increased phagocytic and cytolytic activity of macrophages, and augmentation of delayed cutaneous hypersensitivity. BCG administration has been associated with increased resistance to bacterial and viral infection, enhanced humoral immunity, and increased interferon production. Intravesical BCG administration results in an intense inflammatory cell infiltration, but it is unlikely that this is the sole mechanism of action since the potent inflammatory agent DNCB has no antitumor activity in the bladder [7], and oral BCG has been reported to be effective in the prevention of tumor recurrence without causing irritative vesical symptoms [9]. Elucidation of the mechanisms of action of BCG, which are in all likelihood immune in nature, could provide rationale for the selection of patients, and permit tailoring of the treatment protocol to the individual patient. An understanding of the mechanisms involved could also result in the development of new and more effective immune modulating agents.

While improvement in the management of superficial bladder cancer using BCG immunotherapy is a significant accomplishment, invasive transitional cell carcinoma represents a much greater challenge. Several patients with invasive disease have unexpectedly responded to BCG treatment, but, in general, clinical observations support the animal data which suggest that response to BCG is limited to hosts with very small tumor burdens. In my opinion, it is preferable to make every effort to transurethrally resect bulky superficial lesions, even if multiple operations are necessary, before initiating BCG immunotherapy. Cystectomy remains the treatment of choice for most patients with tumor invading muscle. The primary reason for failure in patients with invasive disease treated with cystectomy is the existence of occult distant metastases. If systemic BCG is effective in eradicating microscopic disease, as suggested by the reported response to oral BCG immunotherapy, immunotherapy might be a useful adjunct to cystectomy.

After a somewhat shaky beginning, it now appears that immunotherapy has established itself as a legitimate, effective modality in the management of at least one human malignancy. We look forward to the development of new and more effective immunotherapy modalities in the treatment of bladder cancer, and the further application of immunotherapy to other urologic malignancies.

REFERENCES

1. Bloomberg SD, Brosman SA, Hausman MS, Cohen A, Battenberg JD: The effect of BCG on the dog bladder. Invest Urol 12:423, 1975.
2. Brosman SA: Experience with bacillus Calmette-Guerin in patients with superficial bladder cancer. J Urol 128:27, 1982.
3. Flamm J, Grof F: Adjuvant local immunotherapy with bacillus Calmette-Guerin (BCG) in treatment of urothelial carcinoma of the urinary bladder. Wien Med Wochenschr 131:501, 1981.
4. Herr HW, Pinsky CM, Whitmore WF Jr, Oettgen HF, Melamed MR: Intravesical bacillus Calmette-Guerin (BCG) therapy of superficial bladder tumors. Abstract 307. American Urological Association, Seventy-eighth annual meeting, Las Vegas, Nevada, April, 1983.
5. Herr HW, Whitmore WF, Jr, Logsini PC, Pinsky CM: Extravesical carcinoma in situ after intravesical bacillus Calmette-Guerin (BCG). Abstract 346. American Urological Association, Seventy-eighth annual meeting, Las Vegas, Nevada, April, 1983.
6. Lamm DL, Reichert DF, Harris SC, Lucio RM: Immunotherapy of murine transitional cell carcinoma. J Urol 128:1104-1108, 1982.
7. Lamm DL, Harris SC, Gittes RF: Bacillus Calmette-Guerin and dinitrochloride benzene: Immunotherapy of chemically-induced bladder tumors. Invest Urol 14:369, 1977.
8. Minder P: Shared antigens between animal and human tumors and microorganisms in BCG in cancer immunotherapy. In: Jamoureux G, Turcotte R, Portleance V (eds). New York: Grune and Stratton, pp 73-81, 1976.
9. Netto NR Jr, Lemos GC: A comparison of treatment methods for prophylaxis of recurrent superficial bladder tumors. J Urol 129:33, 1983.
10. Robinson JC: Risks of BCG intralesional therapy: An experience with melanoma. J Surg Oncol 9:587-593, 1977.
11. Stober U, Peter HH: NCG-Immunotherapy zur Rezidivprophylaxe beim Harnblasenkarzinom? Therapiewoche 30:6067, 1980.
12. Zbar B, Rapp HJ: Immunotherapy of guinea pig cancer with BCG. Cancer 34:1532, 1974.

8. Differentiation in Teratocarcinoma: Its Implications in Therapy

PERINCHERY NARAYAN and WILLIAM C. DEWOLF

1. INTRODUCTION

Testes cancer is the most common solid tumor affecting males 20–34 years of age. Recent epidemiologic evidence suggests a growing incidence in the United States and Europe. For example, in the USA from 1935–39, testicular cancer represented 13% of all cancers in the 15–34 age group; whereas in 1975–76, the proportional incidence increased significantly to 19% [1]. In addition to its increasing prominence in clinical oncology, testes cancer has demonstrated several unique features that has attracted the attention of researchers from several fields. Specifically, the teratocarcinoma model has assumed an important role in fundamental research involving not only mechanisms of malignant transformation but also development of the embryo and fetus. This perhaps is not unexpected because teratocarcinoma is a tumor of germ-line origin with the capacity to produce differentiated cell types representing derivatives of the primary germ layers and, therefore, potentially represents a direct link between malignancy and development.

The fundamental importance of the relationship between fetal cells and malignancy is based on the hypothesis that cancer cells represent a disordered form of the genetic regulation involving early embryonic cells. After initial division, such cells continue to proliferate because of lack of proper genetic controls. There are several lines of evidence for this reasoning (discussed herein). In a practical sense, it has been found that teratocarcinoma cells can exhibit their properties of malignancy and differentiation in vitro as well as in vivo. Therefore, the availability of large numbers of cultured teratocarcinoma cells has allowed laboratory analysis of a number of fundamental mechanisms in early embryonic and fetal development as well as malignant transformation of these cells. For example, the murine teratocarcinoma (MT) model, which has been studied extensively, can form in vivo

T. L. Ratliff and W. J. Catalona (eds), Urologic Oncology. ISBN 0-89838-628-4.
© *1984. Martinus Nijhoff Publishers, Boston. Printed in the Netherlands.*

tumors and also participate (under appropriate experimental conditions) in the formation of a normal mouse embryo by contributing to cells and tissues derived from all three primary germ layers in the resultant adult mouse [for review see Ref. 2, 3].

A fundamental drawback of the in vitro MT model, however, is that its origin may be different from human teratocarcinoma. For example, most murine teratocarcinomas studied are derived from manipulated embryonic cells that have been induced to form teratocarcinomas by explanting them to an extra-uterine site. The relationship then, between MT, which is embryo derived and human embryonal carcinoma which is germ cell derived is somewhat tenuous, and the two are not identical as is sometimes implied. Spontaneous germ cell tumors in the mouse occur very rarely. Only in one strain, 129J, does the frequency of testicular tumors approximate the frequency with which these tumors occur in humans [4, 5]. Additionally several studies have shown human teratocarcinomas to be distinct from murine teratocarcinomas in several of its properties [6-8]. These studies suggest that in order to understand human testes cancer we cannot fall back on the more extensively studied murine teratocarcinoma model since, at this time, it is unclear whether those findings are applicable to the human tumor.

Human teratocarcinoma (HT) * on the other hand, has been studied less extensively than MT. There is evidence, however, that in vitro cultured HT cells can recapitulate early events in embryonic development similar to MT cells. For example, one HT cell line HT-H (2061H) differentiates from an adherent monolayer to a non-adherent aggreagete which closely resembles the preimplantation embryo (embryoid body) [9]. Additionally, in vitro HT cells also produce substances such as AFP and HCG which are also products of fetal cells. The HT model is now being developed to answer important questions concerning: 1) a definition and understanding of the stem cell origin of HT; although no current definition exists recent clinical evidence suggests at least 2 types of stem cells are present in non-seminomatous germ cell tumors, e.g., those that are nullipotent (will not differentiate) and those that are multipotent; 2) new methods to identify additional and better tumor markers to help in early detection and management of patients with germ cell tumors; 3) a better understanding of normal human spermatogenesis and germ cell development, especially with respect to defining the origins of teratocarcinoma; 4) development of a model that represents early embryonic events to better understand embryonic development and cell differentiation. The recent availability of cultured HT cells should now sti-

---

* HT will refer to an investigative term indicating all tumors having embryonal carcinoma, alone or with other elements, and exclude pure seminoma and pure choriocarcinoma.

mulate more and rapid progress in this field. This chapter will address these points and their therapeutic implications.

2. BACKGROUND

2.1 *Relationship between embryonic – fetal cells and cancer*

The hypothesis that fetal cells and cancer cells are related is a recurrent theme in cancer research and is at least 100 years old [10]. The theory behind this hypothesis is that malignancy is a result of abnormal gene regulation manifested by diminished or disordered cell differentiation. This is usually thought to involve the 'stem cell' and differentiative events which normally occur during embryogenesis and early development rather than in the adult [11]. This view of malignant conversion of a stem cell population that ultimately enlarges with an associated impairment in its ability to differentiate has received appreciable attention and has led Pierce and Cox to refer to some neoplasms as 'caricatures of tissue renewal' [12]. The occurrence of fetal products in certain tumors is consistent with this interpretation.

The association between malignant and fetal–embryonic tissues is further emphasized by several unique biologic properties that are shared. For example: (a) invasiveness is a prime characteristic of the trophoblast as well as tumor cells; one of the contributing factors is thought to be due to secretion of a protease, plasminogen activator, which has been isolated from both trophoblast and malignant cells [13, 14]; (b) metastasis is another shared event because it may be likened to specific cell migration during fetal–embryonic development [15]; (c) similar changes in malignant and embryonic cell membranes can also occur as evidenced by changes in lectin binding properties [16, 17]; (d) tumors have long been known to produce a factor which stimulates the host to provide a blood supply; this angiogenesis factor is also found in the placenta [18]; (e) tumors containing many tumor-specific and fetal antigens can escape destruction by the host immune response; since this is also a characteristic of fetal tissues which are known to induce antibodies in the mother, a common escape mechanism has been suggested for both fetal and neoplastic tissues [19, 20]; (f) there is extensive literature on isoenzyme homology between fetal and malignant tissue [21]; (g) there is a rapidly increasing number of embryonic and fetal antigens found to be associated with neoplastic tissue. The most extensively studied example is alpha-fetoprotein produced by hepatocellular carcinomas and embryonal cell carcinoma of the ovaries and testis (discussed in Chapter 6).

The MT model represents one of the most unique systems for the study of the correlation between embryonic and malignant gene expression. This is true because cells from in vitro and in vivo MT lines and from the developing mouse embryo may be interchanged without loss of biologic potential. That is to say, MT cells from in vitro or in vivo tumor lines may be injected into a murine blastocyst and the MT contribution will partake in normal embryonic and fetal development [22–24]. The converse is also true; normal embryo cells can be cultured to produce MT cell lines [25, 26]. This experimental relationship, therefore, poses the two most fundamental questions regarding the fetal–cancer relationship. 1) Do 'transformed' cells continue proliferation in the undifferentiated state because neoplastic conversion has reduced their efficiency of response to the normal signals of differentiation? 2) Is it possible that embryonal carcinoma cells are not transformed but rather represent a selected population of completely normal embryonic cells that are programmed to divide until they receive the appropriate signals for differentiation? When the cells are in an extra-embryonic site, the signals they receive are apparently not conducive to completely normal embryogenesis. The answers to these questions are unknown.

The HT model is less well characterized compared to its murine counterpart, however, it has an inherent advantage of being 'human' oriented. At least four lines of evidence illustrate the importance of HT towards understanding the malignant and fetal–embryonic relationship.

2.2 Human teratocarcinoma forms in vivo and in vitro 'embryoid bodies'

A feature of MT cells that has allowed considerable understanding of mechanisms of early embryonic events has been the ability of MT cells to form in vivo and in vitro embryoid bodies [27]. These structures are similar to preimplantation embryos in several aspects. Although human embryoid bodies have been reported in vivo in tumors [28], until recently, in vitro human-derived embryoid bodies were unavailable for study. We have recently characterized an embryoid body formed by the spontaneous differentiation in culture of human teratocarcinoma cell line HT-H (2061H) [9]. On the basis of electron microscopy and immunosurgery, we have analyzed the different cell subsets of this multicellular structure and have determined that these bodies resemble the normal mouse preimplantation embryo even more than the MT-derived embryoid body.

2.3 Human teratocarcinoma cells react with antisera which identify mouse stage-specific embryonic antigens

The F9 cell line is a stable MT mouse embryo-derived line which expresses cell surface antigens in common with male germ cells and early cleavage stage embryos [29]. After day 10 of development, F9 antigens are detectible only on spermatogenic cells [30, 31]. On this basis, F9 antigens have been termed stage-specific embryonic antigens. Following reports that F9 stage-specific embryonic antigen was present on MT, similar investigations were performed on HT. The results indicated that some HT cell lines reacted with F9 heteroantisera [32, 33]. In addition, HT cells were found to express either HLA or F9 (or an antigen cross-reactive with F9) but not both, similar to mouse F9 carcinoma cells [32]. More recently, the relationship between human teratocarcinoma and early mouse embryonic development has been further defined with the aid of two informative monoclonal antibodies. The first is stage-specific embryonic antigen-1 (SSEA-1) defined by reactivity with a monoclonal antibody prepared by immunization of syngeneic mice with F9 teratocarcinoma [34]. The antigen determinant is probably a glycolipid present on late but not early cleavage stage mouse embryos and, additionally, is present on human teratocarcinoma. SSEA-3 is another stage-specific embryonic antigen defined by reactivity with a monoclonal antibody prepared by immunization of a rat with 4-to-8 cell stage mouse embryos. The antigenic determinant, present on oocytes becomes restricted first to the inner cell mass at the blastocyst stage and later to primitive endoderm [35]. It is interesting that murine teratocarcinoma stem cells (and other random tumor lines) do not react with this antibody whereas in vitro and in vivo human teratocarcinoma stem cells are SSEA-3-positive [6, 8]. This data provides some of the best evidence to date that human teratocarcinoma may represent a unique model for the study of embryonic and oncofetal antigens by expressing embryonic antigens not shared by mouse teratocarcinoma.

2.4 *Antibodies in human pregnancy allosera cross-react with human teratocarcinoma*

The characterization and use of human allosera has proven to be highly successful in unraveling specific problems of immunogenetics, for example, as related to HLA and blood group antigens. Although the specificity and affinity of selective allosera may not be as good as heteroantisera or monoclonal antibodies, their use in defining new tissue antigens and allospecificities has proven invaluable. Such allosera are usually collected from screened women with a history of pregnancy. The basis for the formation of such antibodies is derived from the fact that during pregnancy fetal cells 'leak' into the maternal blood stream by 15 weeks gestation, and the maternal host responds immunologically by the production of antibodies against histocompatibility antigens and antigens associated with fetal–embryo development [19, 20].

This concept was supported experimentally in a recent report providing evidence that murine pregnancy is associated with the production of antibodies recognizing fetal antigens on F9 and PYS-2 MT cell lines [36]. Antigens expressed by F9 and PYS-2 include F9 and endo which are also found on preimplantation mouse embryos and sperm [31]. The functional presence of fetal antigens during pregnancy has been suggested by experiments demonstrating that pregnancy can confer some protection against subsequent tumor challenge [37]. Specifically mice immunized with 11-day old fetal cells protect against Meth-A transplanted sarcoma [38]. The inverse is also true, that is female mice preimmunized with F9 MT will have reduced fertility [39]. Other studies that implicate a close relationship between fetal and tumor antigens are numerous. For example, normal Wistar multiparous rats have cytotoxic antibodies reactive against 13–15-day syngeneic embryonic tissue [40] and these same rats produce antibodies specific for 1, 2 dimethylhydrazine-induced colon carcinoma cells [41].

Human experimentation has produced similar findings. In our laboratory, 1076 sera from patients with a history of pregnancy or infertility and 30 sera from a normal control production were screened for reactivity to teratocarcinoma by complement-mediated cytotoxicity (CMC) and immunofluorescence (IF) assays. 121/1076 (11%) of allosera and 0/30 normal control sera were found to react with HT. Twenty-six of them (based on relatively good reactivity and larger amounts available) were further tested. Extensive absorption analysis showed the reactivity was non HLA, non blood group and was probably shared by all HT lines. Further analysis of one of these sera using Western blot technique has revealed at least 3 proteins p80, p55, and p40 which were variably expressed on 3 HT lines and human germ cells but not expressed on human lymphocytes or spermatozoa. We feel that one or more of these proteins may represent new oncofetal antigens and have potential clinical application as tumor markers.

2.5 Human teratocarcinoma studies and its relevance to germ cell research

Since teratocarcinoma arises from germ cells, it is not unreasonable to assume that certain antigens may be shared between teratocarcinoma and male germ cells. This was demonstrated experimentally when Artzt et al. reported that 129/SV-CP mice immunized against syngeneic primitive teratocarcinoma cells produce antiserum that reacts with sperm and early cleavage stage embryos [29]. A more recent example is SSEA-1, an antigen present on mouse germ cells and morulae and detected by a monoclonal antibody which also reacts with human sperm and HT [34]. The potential importance of these findings with respect to spermatogenesis and contraception is suggested by several other recent experimental observations. For example, antibodies to mouse F9 teratocarcinoma cells cause significant inhibition of spermatogenesis in syngeneic (129/SV inbred mouse strains) allogeneic (Balb/c mice) and xenogeneic (guinea pigs) immunization experiments [42]. Also, Hamilton and Anderson [36] have demonstrated that immunization of female 129/TER-SV mice with irradiated F9 teratocarcinoma cells significantly interfered with pregnancy. No implantation sites were observed and their data strongly suggests that local anti F9 antibody in the female reproductive tract interferes with conception or gestation prior to implantation. Thus teratocarcinoma cells express functionally important antigens involved in normal spermatogenesis, fertilization and embryonic development. Furthermore, they may have potential for use as immunologic contraceptives. Studies in our laboratory have also shown that there are at least 2 lines of evidence implicating shared antigens between human germ cells and human teratocarcinoma. On the basis of two-dimensional electrophoresis, we have found a group of proteins (p94/5.7) that are shared between human round spermatids and human teratocarcinoma. Secondly, we have found that human pregnancy allosera have antibodies that recognize antigens on HT and human germ cells (as described herein). Since the embryo has alloantigens of paternal origin as well as stage-specific embryonic antigens, it is not unreasonable to expect sera from multiparous women to contain antibodies that may react with human germ cells and HT. These alloantisera have identified several proteins (p80, p55, p40) variably expressed on 3 HT lines and human germ cells but are not on normal lymphocytes. Thus HT may be a new tool to advance our understanding of male human germ cell development.

In trying to understand the disordered genetic regulation behind carcinogenesis, several associations between the major histocompatibility complex (MHC), spermatogenesis and teratocarcinoma have become evident. A temporal association between tumor-associated fetal and embryonic antigens (TAFEA) and MHC antigens was first suggested by observations of an inverse relationship between the quantitative expression of these determinants on the malignant cell surface [43–45] and on the developing mouse embryo [31]. Further studies supporting a physical linkage between TAFEA and MHC antigens was shown by immunochemical and co-capping studies of these determinants [46, 47]. For example, Evans has demonstrated common anti-TAFEA antibodies in serum from either multiparous, methylcholanthrene tumor-immune or Maloney sarcoma virus tumor-bearing rats (NSB). The TAFEA was characterized as a 10 000 dalton glycoprotein and was found to be physically associated with NSB histocompatibility antigens at the cell surface as demonstrated by co-capping experiments [48, 49]. Further relationships between tumor antigens and MHC products have also been described in terms of cross-reactivity of tumor antigens with allogeneic H-2 determinants [50, 51]. For example, protection against chemically induced tumor growth can be provided by previous exposure to allogeneic grafts of 9–19-day old fetal cells [52]. An exact understanding of these phenomena is not yet available. Its importance relative to teratocarcinoma, however is based on two related facts. 1) Extensive investigation of the murine MHC region has shown that genes affecting embryonic differentiation, spermatogenesis and organogenesis are linked to the MHC, approximately 14 crossover units to the left of the H-2 [53, 54]. These differentiation genes are known as the T/t complex because they were discovered as a result of abnormalities in the animals tails. One of the genes of the T/t complex, t^{+12}, controls the expression of F9 antigen present on morulae, spermatozoa and teratocarcinoma of both mouse and human origin [30, 31]. Another T/t complex gene, Tcp-1, controls the expression of another cell surface antigen p63/6.9 [55] found principally on germ cells. 2) The genetic control of two mouse teratocarcinoma transplantation antigens (Gt-1, Gt-2) is controlled by loci flanking the MHC [56]. Because their identification is based on histocompatibility and tumor rejection, speculation exists that they represent embryonic histocompatibility antigens as part of the mouse T/t complex in its role in embryonic development. Because teratocarcinoma is a tumor of germ-line origin involving cells preparatory for embryogenesis, it seems reasonable that genes affecting the expression of teratocarcinoma should be within the T/t complex region and therefore be MHC linked. Evidence for a relationship between HT and MHC in humans has been found in a study showing a significantly higher frequency of HLA-Dw7 in men with teratocarcinoma than would be expected by chance ($p < 0.01$) [57]. At least 2 possible mechanisms exist to account for this association: (a) HLA-Dw7 may act as a marker for a teratocarcinoma 'determinant' similar to the TL antigen in mice controlled by an MHC-linked locus; (b) Dw7 may cross-react with a teratocarcinoma antigen.

3. CLINICAL IMPLICATIONS

Current therapy of testes cancer consists of surgery for low stage tumors (stage I, II a, b) and chemotherapy followed by cytoreductive surgery for residual disease in high stage tumors (stage IIc, III) [58, 59]. The survival for patients with stage I is 95–100% while in stage II and III it is in excess of 80% [58, 59]. The success of therapy, however, is based on proper histologic diagnosis and accuracy of staging both of which can be affected by our understanding of differentiation and its effect on the presence of tumor markers.

3.1 Histology of the primary tumor
Histologic diagnosis is of major importance in testes tumors because it directly influences whether treatment is radiation or surgery, with or with-

out chemotherapy. Histologically, these tumors may present as single cell type neoplasms (60%) or as a mixture of cell types (40%) [60]. Also, the histology of tumor metastases or recurrences of germ cell neoplasms, vary from the original cell type. Both these features are important to the clinician.

Primary testes tumors may broadly be classified as seminomas or non-seminomatous tumors (NSGCT). Seminomas are radiosensitive while NSGCT require surgical extirpation. It is important to search all primary tumors that appear to be pure seminomas for any evidence of non-semino-matous elements. The presence of NSGCT tumor markers such as AFP, is conclusive evidence of NSGCT elements in any tumor [61]. A patient with 'pure' seminoma and elevated AFP in the serum should be treated as NSGCT. Recently, the use of antibodies to AFP and immunoperoxidase staining techniques has been successful in the detection of AFP producing cells in many 'pure' seminomas [62]. This technique is now commonly used to confirm the presence of suspected NSGCT elements in seminomas and may detect the AFP producing cells even when the serum level of AFP is not sufficiently elevated to be detected in the peripheral blood. More about these subjects are given in Chapter 6.

3.2 Histology of metastasis and recurrences

Because of the multipotent nature of teratocarcinoma cells, it is not uncommon to find that the histology of metastatic or recurrent tumor varies widely from the original tumor. A metastasis from 'pure' seminoma that does not respond to radiation therapy as expected should be treated as an NSGCT tumor, even if tumor markers are not elevated. There is also evidence that those patients with seminoma and syncytiotrophoblastic giant cells in their primary tumors accompanied by elevated HCG (10% of patients) may be likely to have non-seminomatous metastases. For example, Braunstein and associates found that 38% of all patients with metastatic seminoma had elevated HCG levels [63]. This is especially important considering 35% of all patients dying of metastatic seminomas have non-sem-inomatous disease [64].

The phenomenon of differentiated metastasis from primary embryonal cell carcinoma of the testes is not new [65, 66]. However, it is being recognized more often and its incidence may be increasing [59, 67–70]. Recent reports estimate 30% or more of all recurrences following treatment of NSGCT to contain differentiated teratomas [59, 70]. The most logical explanation for this recent increase relates to the chemotherapeutic interventions that are currently used in the treatment of NSGCT presumably because chemotherapy preferentially affects rapidly dividing 'undifferentiated' cells compared to differentiated mature cells. This explanation is supported by two facts: (a) there is a two-fold increase in the incidence of differentiated teratomas among metastases in patients following chemotherapy compared to untreated patients [65–70]; (b) Oosterhuis et al. have found that among chemotherapy-treated patients with differentiated teratoma in their residual metastases, 90% (11/12) have differentiated elements in their primaries. Conversely, when differentiated elements are absent in the primary, only 12% (1/8) of treated patients and none (0/10) of the untreated patients had differentiated teratoma in their metastasis [70]. These findings also suggest that chemotherapy alone is unlikely to induce teratocarcinoma cells to differentiate and that the presence of differentiated elements in the metastasis appears to be an inherent property of the tumor in which the differentiated elements are less affected by chemotherapy. Additional data to support this concept is that (a) chemotherapy is less effective in producing complete remission in patients with teratocarcinoma than in patients with pure embryonal carcinoma [72, 73], and (b) pure teratoma appears to be non-responsive to chemotherapy [74].

The increased occurrence of differentiated teratoma metastasis has required modifications in therapy. It has been established for residual abdominal disease following chemotherapy that complete excision is necessary for cure [59]. Since these residual tumors have revealed changes varying from cystic or necrotic areas to frankly malignant areas, sample biopsies do not reveal the full extent of the disease. In the case of lung metastasis, the role of surgery versus chemotherapy is still evolving. With the excellent responses to present regimens of chemotherapy, it would seem prudent to employ chemotherapy initially for these metastatic lesions and restrict surgery to those patients non-responsive to chemotherapy.

A reasonable hypothesis that would account for all these facts is to assume that the so-called pure embryonal carcinoma (EC) is actually a mixture of EC cells with variable potency. For example, one subset of cells has the ability to differentiate and form teratoma (multipotent EC) and some EC cells are nullipotent without the ability to differentiate. Teratocarcinomas would then contain the EC stem cells that are more likely to differentiate since some of them already have formed teratoma in the primary itself. If the EC stem cell population actually represents a heterogeneous population, it is reasonable to suppose their differential susceptibility to chemotherapy, thus explaining why TC has a different success rate following chemotherapy compared to EC, i.e. TC is made up of a different stem cell population than pure EC. This would also explain why some 'pure' EC also metastasize to form differentiated teratomas. It should also be considered that the relative increase in frequency of these metastases recently observed may just be a manifestation of the increased number of patient survivals since the advent of newer chemotherapy. However, until such time as more is known about the stem cells of human teratocarcinoma and the influence of chemotherapeutic agents and environmental factors on differentiation and metastases, these questions will remain unanswered.

3.3 Staging and tumor markers

The accuracy of staging and the success of therapy in testes cancers relies heavily on the production of tumor markers by these cancers. The two best characterized are alpha-fetoprotein (AFP) and beta chain of human chorionic gonadotropin (HCG).

AFP is a glycoprotein of 70 000 molecular weight. Its normal level in the serum is < 3 ngs/ml and it is elevated in 70 % of NSGCT patients. In these tumors it is produced by the embryonal carcinoma and yolk sac elements [75, 76]. It is also elevated in several other conditions apart from NSGCT. These include patients with primary hepatic cancer, ovarian teratocarcinoma, ataxia telangectasia and some patients with pancreatic, biliary, gastric and other gastrointestinal neoplasms. AFP is also elevated in patients with non-malignant liver disease in which active hepatic regeneration is occurring and a few patients with non-gastrointestinal tumors metastatic to the liver. To the clinician who is managing a patient with testes cancer these other conditions rarely pose a problem because of the younger age of the patients with testes cancer and because many of the conditions may be excluded by simple liver function tests [75, 77, 78].

The beta subunit of human chorionic gonadotropin (HCG) is a glycoprotein of 45 000 molecular weight and is elevated in 60–70 % of patients with NSGCT and in 10 % of seminomas. HCG is synthesized by the syncytiotrophoblast giant cells in testes tumors. Both markers are elevated in 80–90 % of patients with NSGCT [77, 79], and therefore are very useful in the management of patients with testes cancer and may also be of some predictive value in the prognosis of these patients. They are further discussed in Chapter 6.

3.4 Current research on new tumor markers

Because of the relationship between teratocarcinoma and fetal cells, the potential for teratocarcinoma cells to produce informative oncofetal antigens is great. Since the inaccuracy of staging in testes cancer is about 20–40 % [80], there is a need for new markers to improve the diagnostic and staging accuracy in this disease. Up to now the search for new markers has been restricted to hormones of pregnancy. Two that have shown early promise include pregnancy-specific protein (SP-1) and placental alkaline phosphotase (PLAP) [79, 81]. We are using an entirely new approach to identify unique teratocarcinoma antigens by using selective allosera. Based on the assumption that (a) antigens on embryonic or reproductive cells are sequesterd and, therefore, foreign (and immunogenic) to the immune system and (b) teratocarcinoma cells express antigens of both reproductive and embryonic origin, an investigation was begun to determine if allosera with the potential to recognize fetal embryonic antigens would react with human teratocarcinoma. These alloantisera have identified at least 3 proteins, one or more of which may represent new oncofetal antigens and have potential clinical application as tumor markers (described in pages 194, 195).

Recently, monoclonal antibodies to HCG have been utilized in early detection of recurrent testes cancer [82, 83]. The technique (radioimmuno-localization) consisted of injecting radiolabeled mouse monoclonal antibodies to HCG into patients and then localization of HCG production by tumors with external scanners. The advantage of the technique is in detecting extremely small recurrences well before they can be picked up by conventional techniques. The disadvantage is that only small amounts of antibody can be used and with repeat injection, the patient may develop serum sickness or anaphylaxis.

3.5 Implications in germ cell reserach, contraceptive vaccines

Recent advances in isolation and purification of human germ cells has facilitated the biochemical analysis of normal male human germ cell antigens. Studies show at least one group of proteins (p95/5.8) that are shared between human round spermatids (haploid) and human teratocarcinoma cells and are not present on human pachytene spermatocytes (diploid) [84]. These studies may lend important insight into fundamental questions of origin of human teratocarcinoma in relation to spermatogenesis. In addition, several marker proteins of human germ cell development have been identified such as p45/5.2 a marker of human pachytene germ cells. Studies are underway to determine if antibodies to these marker proteins will help unravel their function and ultimately to determine their role in fertility.

Immunologic methods of contraception is currently being explored in several animal species as a means of safe, effective long-term means of contraception. Advances such as monoclonal antibody production and the discovery of new fetal and embryonic antigens has given new impetus to these studies. The prerequisites for immunologic contraceptive vaccines for use in humans are a specificity for the reproductive target and a function in fertilization that can be blocked by an antibody. Reproductive hormones, germ cells, embryonic and fetal antigens have the potential to qualify as contraceptive vaccines. Antibodies to HCG have been used in baboons and in humans with limited success [85, 86]. LDH-C4 (a mitochondrial isoenzyme of lactate dehydrogenase found only in male germ cells) has been especially effective in preventing pregnancies in primates, and its effects are reversible and without side effects [87].

The future of human teratocarcinoma research is promising. Understanding the teratocarcinoma model may ultimately prove beneficial not only to the patient with testes cancer, but also to those investigators dealing with problems in basic cell biology. Because of its germ-line origin, human teratocarcinoma studies may provide a window into the process of both cell differentiation and malignant transformation.

ACKNOWLEDGEMENTS

Perinchery Narayan is an American Urologic Association Scholar. William C. DeWolf is a recipient of Research Cancer Development Award AI00406. This work was supported by the American Cancer Society Grant IM246A and NIH Grant CA28611. We would like to acknowledge the excellent assistance of Ms Karen Dowell in the preparation of this manuscript.

REFERENCES

1. Schottenfeld D, Warshauer M, Sherlock S, Zauber A, Leder M, Payne R: The epidemiology of testicular cancer in young adults. Am J Epidemiol 112:232-246, 1980.
2. Martin G: Teratocarcinoma and mammalian embryogenesis. Science 209:768-776, 1980.
3. Stevens LC: Genetic influences on teratocarcinogenesis and parthenogenesis. In: Mammalian Genetics and Cancer, Russell ES (ed). New York: Alan R Liss, pp 93-104, 1981.
4. Stevens LC, Hummel KP: A description of spontaneous congenital testicular teratoma in strain 129 mice. J Natl Cancer Inst 18:719-747, 1957.
5. Stevens LC, Little CC: Spontaneous testicular teratomas in an inbred strain of mice. Proc Natl Acad Sci USA 40:1080-1087, 1954.
6. Caroll P, DeWolf WC: Immune properties of human teratocarcinoma I. Human teratocarcinoma targets distinguish between natural killer and activated killer cells. J Immunol 131:1007-1010, 1983.
7. Carroll P, DeWolf WC: Immune properties on human teratocarcinoma II. Sensivity to AK mediated cytolysis is differentiation dependent (submitted).
8. Damjanov I, Fox N, Knowles BB, Solter D, Lange P, Fraley EE: Immunohistochemical localisation of murine stage specific antigens in human testicular germ cell tumors. Am J Pathol 108:225-230, 1982.
9. Ducibella T, Anderson D, Aalberg J, DeWolf WC: Cell surface polarization, tight junctions and eccentric inner cells characterize human teratocarcinoma embryoid bodies. Dev Biol 94:197-205, 1982.
10. Cohnheim JF: Lectures on General Pathology. London, 1889.
11. Mintz B, Fleischman RA: Teratocarcinomas and other neoplasms as developmental defects in gene expression. Adv Cancer Res 34:211-278, 1981.
12. Pierce GB, Cox WF Jr: In: Cell differentiation and neoplasia, Saunders GF (ed). New York: Raven Press, pp 57-66, 1978.
13. Pollack R, Risser R, Conlon S, Rifkin D: Plasminogen activator production accompanies loss of anchorage regulation in transformation of primary rat embryo cells by simian virus 40. Proc Natl Acad Sci USA 17:4792-4796, 1974.

14. Sherman MI, Strickland S, Reich E: Differentiation of mouse embryonic and teratocarcinoma cells in vitro: plasminogen activator production. Cancer Res 36:4208-4216, 1976.
15. Coggin JH, Anderson NG: Cancer differentiation and embryonic antigens: some central problems. Adv Cancer Res 19:105-165, 1974.
16. Burger M, Noonan KD: Restoration of normal growth by covering of agglutinin sites on tumor cell surface. Nature 228:512-515, 1970.
17. Mascona AA: Embryonic and neoplastic cell surfaces. Availability of receptors for concanavalin A and wheat germ agglutinin. Science 171:905-907, 1971.
18. Folkman J: Antiangiogenesis: New concept for therapy of solid tumors. Ann Surg 175:409-446, 1972.
19. Tuffery M, Bishun NP, Barnes RD: Porosity of the mouse placenta to maternal cells. Nature 221:1029-1030, 1969.
20. Sinkovics JG, DiSiaia PJ, Rutledge FN: Tumor immunology and evolution of the placenta. Lancet 2:1190-1191, 1970.
21. Stein G, Stein J, Thompson J: Chromosomal proteins in transformed and neoplastic cells. Cancer Res 38:1181-1201, 1978.
22. Mintz B, Illmensee K: Normal genetically mosaic mice produced from malignant teratocarcinoma cells. Proc Natl Acad Sci USA 72:3585-3589, 1975.
23. Brintser RL: The effect of cells transferred into mouse blastocyst on subsequent development. J Exp Med 140:1049-1056, 1974.
24. Papaioannou VE, McBurney MW, Gardner RL, Evans MJ: Fate of teratocarcinoma cells injected into early mouse embryos. Nature 250:70-73, 1975.
25. Martin G: Isolation of a pluripotent cell line from early mouse embryos cultured in medium conditioned by teratocarcinoma stem cells. Proc Natl Acad Sci USA 78:7634-7638, 1981.
26. Evans MJ, Kaufman MH: Establishment in culture of pluripotential cells from mouse embryos. Nature 292:154, 1981.
27. Stevens LC: Embryology of testicular teratomas in strain 129 mice. J Natl Cancer Inst 23:1249-1261, 1959.
28. Dixon FJ, Moore RA: In: Atlas of Tumor Pathology, Section 8, Fasc 32b and 32. Washington, DC: Armed Forces Institute of Pathology, 1952.
29. Artzt K, Dubois P, Bennett D, Condamine H, Babinet C, Jacob F: Surface antigens common to mouse cleavage embryos and primitive teratocarcinoma cells in culture. Proc Natl Acad Sci USA 70:2988-2992, 1973.
30. Gachelin G, Fellous M, Guenet JL, Jacob F: Developmental expression of an early embryonic antigen common to mouse spermatozoa and cleavage embryos and to human spermatozoa: its expression during spermatogenesis. Dev Biol 50:310-320, 1976.
31. Jacob F: Mouse teratocarcinoma and embryonic antigens. Immunol Rev 33:3-32, 1977.
32. Hogan B, Fellous M, Avner P, Jacob F: Isolation of a human teratoma cell line which expresses F9 antigen. Nature 270:515-518, 1977.
33. Holden S, Bernard O, Artzt K, Whitmore W Jr, Bennett D: Human and mouse embryonal carcinoma cells in culture share an embryonic antigen (F9). Nature 270:518-520, 1977.
34. Solter D, Knowles BB: Monoclonal antibody defining a stage specific mouse embryonic antigen (SSEA-1). Proc Natl Acad Sci USA 75:5565-5569, 1978.
35. Shevinsky LH, Knowles BB, Damjanov I, Solter D: Monoclonal antibody to murine embryos defines a stage specific embryonic antigen expressed on mouse embryos and human teratocarcinoma cells. Cell 30:667-670, 1982.
36. Hamilton M, Anderson DJ: Antibodies to antigens on teratocarcinoma cells are associated with parity in mice. Biol Reproduction 27:104-109, 1982.
37. Moon RC: Relationship between previous reproductive history and chemically induced mammary cancer in rats. Int J Cancer 4:312-317, 1969.

38. Castro JE, Hunt R, Lace EM, Medawar P: Implications of the fetal antigens theory for fetal transplantation. Cancer Res 34:2055-2060, 1974.
39. Hamilton MS, Beer AE, May RD, Vitetta ES: The influence of immunization of female mice with F9 teratocarcinoma cells on their reproductive performance. Transpl Proc 11(1):1067-1072, 1979.
40. Baldwin RW, Vose BM: The expression of a phase specific fetal antigen on rat embryo cells. Transplant 18(6):525-530, 1974.
41. Bansal SR, Mark R, Rhoads JE, Bansal SC: Effect of embryonic tissue immunization on chemically induced gastrointestinal tumors in rats I: Can embryonic antigens act as rejection antigens? J Natl Cancer Inst 61:189-201, 1978.
42. Vojtiskova M, Pokorna Z, Draber P: Autoimmune damage to spermatogenesis in rodents immunized with mouse F9 embryonic carcinoma cells. Proc Natl Acad Sci USA 80:459-461, 1983.
43. Haywood GR, McKhaun CF: Antigenic specificities on murine sarcoma cells. Reciprocal relationship between normal transplantation antigens (H-2) and tumor specific immunogenicity. J Exp Med 133:1171-1187, 1971.
44. Cikes M, Friberg S, Klein G: Progressive loss of H-2 antigens with concomitant increase of cell surface antigen(s) determined by Moloney leukemia virus in cultured murine lymphomas. J Natl Cancer Inst 50:347-362, 1973.
45. Tsakraklides E, Smith C, Kersey JH, Good RA: Transplantation antigens (H-2) or virally and chemically transformed Balb/3T3 fibroblasts in culture. J Natl Cancer Inst 52:1499-1504, 1974.
46. Callahan GH, Allison JP, Pellegrino MA, Reisfeld RA: Physical association of histocompatibility antigens at tumor cell surfaces. J Immunol 122:70-74, 1979.
47. Schrader JW, Cunningham BA, Edelman GM: Functional interaction of viral and histocompatibility antigens at tumor cell surfaces. Proc Natl Acad Sci USA 72:5066-5070, 1975.
48. Flaherty L, Rinchik E: No evidence for foreign H-2 specificities on the EL4 mouse lymphoma. Nature 273:52-53, 1978.
49. Fox RI, Weissman IL: Maloney virus induced cells surface antigens and histocompatibility antigens are located on distinct molecules. J Immunol 122:1697-1704, 1979.
50. Invernizzi G, Parmiani G: Tumor associated transplantation antigens of chemically induced sarcomata cross reacting with allogeneic histocompatibility antigens. Nature 254:713-714, 1975.
51. Martin JW, Gipson TG, Rice JM: H-2ᵃ associated alloantigen expressed by several transplacentally induced lung tumors of C3H mice. Nature 265:738-739, 1977.
52. Parmiani G, Lembo R: In: Embryonic and Fetal Antigens, Anderson NG, Loggin JH, Cole E (eds). Springfield VA: National Technical Information Service, p 159, 1972.
53. Artzt K, McGormick P, Bennett D: Gene mapping within the T/t complex of the mouse I. t lethal genes are non-allelic. Cell 28:463-470, 1982.
54. Artzt K, Shin HS, Bennett D: Gene mapping within the T/t complex of the mouse II. Anomalous position of H-2 complex in t haplotypes. Cell 28:471-476, 1982.
55. Silver L, Artzt K, Bennett D: A major testicular celle protein specified by a T/t complex gene. Cell 17:275-284, 1979.
56. Shedlovsky A, Clipson L, Vandeberg J, Dove WF: Strong teratocarcinoma transplantation loci Gt-1 and Gt-2, flank H-2. Immunogenetics 7:103, 1978.
57. DeWolf WC, Lange PH, Emarson M, Yunis EJ: HLA and testicular cancer. Nature 277:216-217, 1979.
58. Fraley EE, Lange PH, Kennedy BJ: Germ cell testicular cancer in adults. New Engl J Med 301:1420-1426, 1979.

59. Donohue JP, Einhorn LH, Williams SD: Cytoreductive surgery for metastatic testes cancer. Consideration of timing and extent. J Urol 123:876-880, 1980.
60. Mostofi FK, Price EB Jr: In: Tumors of the Male Genital System, Mostofi FK, Price EB Jr (eds). Washington, DC: Armed Forces Institute of Pathology, Fasc, 8, pp 68-71, 1973.
61. Lange PH, Nochomovitz LE, Rosai J, Fraley EE, Kennedy BJ, Bosl G, Brisbane J, Catalona WH, Cochran JS, Comisarow RH, Cummings KB, DeKernion JB, Einhorn LH, Hakala TR, Jewett M, Moore MR, Scardino PT, Streitz JM: Serum alpha fetoprotein and human chorionic gonadotropins in patients with seminoma. J Urol 124(4):472-478, 1980.
62. Kurman RJ, Scardino PT, McIntire KR, Waldman TA, Javadpour N: Cellular localizations of alpha fetoproteins and human chorionic gonadotropins in germ cell tumors using an indirect immunoperoxidase technique. A new approach to classification using tumor markers. Cancer 40:2136-2151, 1977.
63. Braunstein GD, Vaitukaitis JL, Carbone PP, Ross GT: Ectopic production of chorionic gonadotropins by neoplasms. Ann Intern Med 78:39-45, 1973.
64. Mostofi FK, Price EB Jr: In: Tumors of the Male Genital System, Mostof FK, Price EB Jr (eds). Washington, DC: Armed Forces Institute of Pathology, Fasc 8, p 74, 1973.
65. Smithers DW: Maturation in human tumors. Lancet 2:949-952, 1969.
66. Snyder RN: Completely mature pulmonary metastases from testicular teratocarcinoma: Case report and review of the literature. Cancer 24:810-819, 1969.
67. Willis GW, Hajdu ST: Histologically benign teratoid metastases of testicular embryonal carcinoma. Am J Clin Pathol 59:338-343, 1973.
68. Merrin C, Baumgartner G, Wajsman Z: Benign transformation of testicular carcinoma by chemotherapy. Lancet 1:43-44, 1975.
69. Hong WK, Wittes RE, Hadju ST, Cvitkovic E, Whitmore WF, Golbey RB: The evolution of mature teratoma from malignant testicular tumors. Cancer 40:2987-2992, 1977.
70. Oosterhuis WJ, Suurmeyer AJ, Sleyfer DT, Koops HS, Oldhoff J, Fleuren G: Effects of multiple drug chemotherapy on the maturation of retroperitoneal metastases of non-semi- nomatous germ cell tumors of the testes. Cancer 51:408-416, 1983.
71. Bracken RB, Johnson DE, Frazier OH, Logothetis CJ, Trindade A, Samuels ML: Role of surgery following chemotherapy in stage III germ cell neoplasms. J Urol 129(1):39-43, 1983.
72. Einhorn LH, Donohue J: Cis-diamminedichloroplatinum, vinblastine and bleomycin com- bination chemotherapy in disseminated testicular cancer. Ann Intern Med 87:293-298, 1977.
73. Vugrin D, Cvitkovic E, Whitmore WF, Cheng E, Golbey RB: VAB4 combination chemo- therapy in the treatment of metastatic testes tumors. Cancer 47:833-839, 1981.
74. Carr BI, Gilchrist KW, Carbone PP: Variable transformation in metastases from testicular germ cell tumors: Need for selective biopsy. J Urol 126 (1):52-54, 1981.
75. Abelev GI: Alpha-fetoprotein as a marker of embryo specific differentiation in normal and tumor tissue. Transplant Rev 20:3-37, 1974.
76. Abelev GI, Assecritova NA, Kraevesky NA: Embryonal serum alpha globulin in cancer patients: diagnostic value. Int J Cancer 2:551-558, 1967.
77. Lange PH, Fraley EE: Serum alpha-fetoprotein and human chorionic gonadotropin in the treatment of patients with testicular tumors. Urol Clin North Am 4:393-406, 1977.
78. Scardino PT, Cox HD, Waldman TA, McIntire RK, Mittemeyer B, Javadpour N: Value of serum markers in the staging and prognosis of germ cell tumors of the testes. J Urol 118:994-999, 1977.
79. Rosen SW, Javadpour N, Calvert I, Kaminska J: Pregnancy specific beta 1, glycoprotein (SP-1) is increased in certain non-seminomatous germ cell tumors. J Natl Cancer Inst 62:1439-1441, 1979.

80. Donohue JP, Einhorn LD, Williams SD: Is adjuvant chemotherapy following retroperitoneal node dissection for non-seminomatous cancer necessary? Urol Clin North Am 7:747-756, 1980.
81. Lange PH, Millan JL, Stigbrandt T, Vessella RL, Ruoslahti E, Fishman WH: Placental alkaline phosphatase as a tumor marker for seminoma. Cancer Res 42:3244-3247, 1982.
82. Ballou B, Levine G, Hakala T, Solter D: Tumor location detected with radioactively labelled monoclonal antibody and external scintigraphy. Science 206:846-847, 1979.
83. Goldenberg DM, Kim EE, vanNagell JR Jr, Javadpour N: Radioimmunodetection of cancer using radioactive antibodies to human chorionic gonadotropin. Science 208:1284-1286, 1980.
84. Narayan P, Scott BK, Millette CF, DeWolf WC: Human spermatogenic cell marker proteins detected by two-dimensional electrophoresis. Gamete Res 7:227-239, 193.
85. Stevens VC: The current status of antipregnancy vaccines based on synthetic factions of HCG. In: Immunological Aspects of Reproduction and Fertility Control, Hearn JP (ed). Baltimore: University Park Press, p 203, 1980.
86. Talwar GP, Das C, Tanden A, Sharma MG, Salahuddin M, Dubey SK: Immunization against hCG: Efficacy and teratological studies in baboons. In: Non-human Private Models for Study of Human Reproduction, Anand Kumar TC (ed). Basel: Karger, p 190, 1980.
87. Goldberg E, Wheat TE, Powell JE, Stevens VC: Reduction of fertility in female baboons immunized with lactate dehydrogenase C_4. Fertil Steril 35:214-217, 1981.

Editorial Comment

WENDELL C. SPEERS

Drs Narayan and DeWolf have very nicely summarized the diverse, complex and extensive literature on teratocarcinoma differentiation and discussed its clinical relevance. I would like simply to emphasize a couple of points and indulge myself in some speculation on a future therapy for these germ cell neoplasms.

Much of what we think we know about human teratocarcinomas is derived from observations and studies of the teratocarcinoma system of strain 129 mice developed by Stevens. Histologically, both murine and human tumors are composed of a chaotically arranged, heterogeneous mixture of cell types usually representative of all three embryonic germ layers. Kleinsmith and Pierce [1] demonstrated by cloning experiments that this diverse set of tissues was derived by the process of differentiation from a stem cell population termed embryonal carcinoma (EC). Histologically similar cells are present in human teratocarcinomas and are also termed EC. Recent studies have suggested that the murine EC cells are analogous to the inner cell mass cells of the developing embryo and their differentiation represents recapitulation of embryonic germ layer formations [2].

Pierce et al. [3] performed transplantation experiments which strongly suggested that the differentiated cellular elements derived from the EC stem cells were biologically benign. That is, the malignancy of the tumor depended on the presence of the undifferentiated EC stem cells. One implication of these observations was that manipulation of the differentiated state of the cell might allow control of the malignant phenotype.

In the early 1970s several groups succeeded in obtaining tissue culture lines of murine teratocarcinomas. This allowed isolation and experimental manipulation of the EC stem cells. The stem cell nature of the EC and the benignity of the differentiated cells was reaffirmed in the classic blastocyst injection experiments. More recently, various types of chemical agents have been found capable of inducing differentiation of the EC cells. The F9 line of EC was originally considered to be 'nullipotent' or incapable of differentiation. However, when treated with retinoic acid (RA), extensive differentiation into endoderm was obtained [4].

Using the F9 system and dietary RA, Strickland and Sawey [5] were able to demonstrate induction of differentiation in vivo. Using direct intratumor injections of RA and dimethylacetamide, Speers [6] showed that not only could EC be induced to differentiate in vivo, but that when the differentiation was complete, the biological nature of the tumor was distinctly altered. The differentiated tumors grew more slowly, tumor-bearing hosts survived longer, and histologically the tumors resembled benign teratomas (see Figure 1). The tumor cells appeared to follow a relatively normal developmental sequence in their differentiation, at least in the neuroepithelial elements. These studies indicated that: 1) a failure of the biological mechanisms controlling cellular differentiation may in part be responsible for the malignant phenotype; 2) manipulation

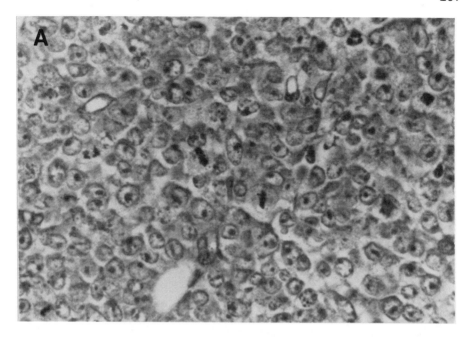

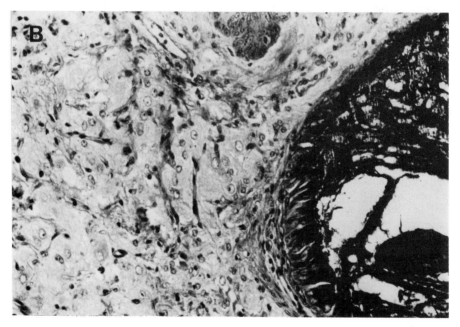

Figure 1. (A) Undifferentiated murine embryonal carcinoma tissue section from a transplantable tumor. Note high nucleus to cytoplasm ratio and numerous mitotic figures. Hosts bearing such tumors generally succumb within 14–28 days after the tumor has become palpable. (×625). (B) A tumor similar to that in (A) was treated with retinoic acid and dimethylacetamide for 10 days. The tumor decreased in growth rate and its host was healthy when sacrificed 86 days after treatment of the palpable tumor was begun. This section shows histologically benign, mature brain tissue (left) and an endodermal cyst containing secretion material (right). (×250).

of the differentiated state of the cell is possible with pharmacological agents; and 3) such manipulation, indeed, alters the biological potential of the cells. In summary, a malignant tumor can be converted to a benign tumor by induction of differentiation.

A murine EC cell within a tumor has three possible fates. It can die; it can divide and produce two EC cells; or it can differentiate. EC differentiation appears to be a multistep process in which cell division continues, but at a decreasing rate [6] until in some cell types (e.g., neurons) it ceases completely. Inducing agents increase the probability of differentiation. When that probability reaches one hundred percent, the tumor is benign, unless some additional transformation event occurs. The authors have correctly pointed out the unique nature of the murine EC system in that most of these original tumors were not spontaneous, but embryo-derived. Such an origin does not obviate the fact that these cells produce rapidly growing, highly malignant tumors which can kill their hosts in a matter of days.

We have a relatively good understanding of the murine teratocarcinoma system. If the human teratocarcinoma system is biologically similar, we would expect that clinical manipulation of differentiation might be therapeutically beneficial in human tumors having an abundant EC stem cell population. As the authors point out, however, it is not established that human EC is analogous to murine EC. Although there are distinct morphologic similarities between the two, there are serological and functional differences. Limited differentiation of human EC cells has been observed in vitro, but definite trilineal differentiation and maturation has not been described. If human EC cells are not the stem cells of the teratocarcinoma, what are they? First, as suggested by the authors, they may be 'nullipotent EC', perhaps genetically degenerate forms incapable of differentiation. Our lessons from the F9 murine system suggest that even 'nullipotent' cells may under appropriate circumstances be induced to differentiate. Alternatively, human EC may represent an early differentiated cell in the yolk sac and/or trophoblast lineage. Alpha-fetoprotein and human chorionic gonadotropin are found in human EC tumors. Perhaps these are markers of the EC cells themselves, as well as the better differentiated, histologically obvious, extra-embryonic tissues. If this is the case, then we may still need to look for the true stem cell of the human teratocarcinoma. The finding of 'mature metastases', especially after chemotherapy, has suggested to some that perhaps the agents used were inducing differentiation of the tumors. The authors rightly point out that in this context selection for differentiated elements by these agents is more likely than induction of differentiation. Such mature elements imply that stem cells do exist, but they do not prove that what we call EC is that stem cell population. A third possibility is that the entity termed EC is really a mixture of two or more morphologically similar cell types, including stem cells and early differentiated cells.

Remarkable progress has been made over the past decade in the treatment and clinical management of human germ cell neoplasms. This has been brought about largely by improvements in chemotherapeutic agents, but also by an improved understanding of the differentiation of neoplastic tissues. The next step might very well be the clinical manipulation of the differentiated state by pharmacological agents, 'differentiation therapy', as an adjunct to the current therapeutic modes. Before this will become a reality, much basic research on *human* teratocarcinomas will be required. The lessons learned from the murine system should prove to be a valuable foundation for these studies.

REFERENCES

1. Kleinsmith LJ, Pierce GB Jr: Multipotentiality of single embryonal carcinoma cells. Cancer Res 24:1544–1552, 1964.
2. Martin GR, Wiley LM, Damjanov I: The development of cystic embryoid bodies in vitro from clonal teratocarcinoma stem cells. Dev Biol 61:230–244, 1977.

3. Pierce GB, Dixon FJ, Verney EL: Teratocarcinogenic and tissue-forming potentialities of cell types comprising neoplastic embryoid bodies. Lab Invest 9:583–602, 1960.
4. Strickland S, Mahdavi V: The induction of differentiation in teratocarcinoma stem cells by retinoic acid. Cell 15:393–403, 1978.
5. Strickland S, Sawey MJ: Studies on the effect of retinoids on the differentiation of teratocarcinoma stem cells in vitro and in vivo. Dev Biol 78:76–85, 1980.
6. Speers WC: Conversion of malignant murine embryonal carcinomas to benign teratomas by chemical induction of differentiation in vivo. Cancer Res 42:1843–1849, 1982.

9. Interferon as an Antitumor Agent for Urologic Tumors

TIMOTHY L. RATLIFF, AMOS SHAPIRO and WILLIAM J. CATALONA

1. INTRODUCTION

In recent years there has been considerable interest in interferon (IFN) as a possible antitumor agent. Numerous clinical trials have been performed on tumors of diverse origins but a clear definition of the usefulness of IFN as an antitumor agent remains elusive.

Early studies on animal models have suggested that IFN may be useful as an antitumor agent. These early animal studies were limited by the scarcity of IFN and by the impurity of the IFN preparations. The same problems also have influenced early clinical trials. In most clinical studies to date patients have been treated with crude IFN preparations without sufficient knowledge of appropriate dosage or treatment schedules. These investigations suggest that IFN is biologically active, but it has not been available in sufficient quantities for adequate toxicity or pharmacology studies or for the treatment of a sufficient number of patients in a prospective, randomized, manner to determine efficacy and appropriate treatment regimens.

Recent advances in recombinant DNA technology have led to production systems capable of producing sufficient quantities of IFN for clinical studies. These advances have introduced new problems, however, such as the discovery of multiple IFN subclasses which are present, depending upon the methods of production and purification, in varying proportions in naturally produced IFN preparations. The IFN subclasses have been shown to mediate diverse biological effects, thus giving rise to questions concerning the efficacy of individual IFN subclasses and possible synergistic effects of various mixtures. Such functional diversity greatly complicates the study of IFN as an antitumor agent, but the availability of unlimited quantities of purified IFN ultimately will lead to a clear definition of its role in tumor therapy.

This review focuses on the efficacy of IFN in the treatment of urologic

T. L. Ratliff and W. J. Catalona (eds), Urologic Oncology. ISBN 0-89838-628-4.
© 1984. Martinus Nijhoff Publishers, Boston. Printed in the Netherlands.

tumors and includes a discussion of the basic biological properties of IFN. To date, the few reports describing the use of IFN as a therapeutic agent for urologic tumors have included only a few patients, and the treatment regimens have differed from study to study. Therefore, the value of IFN for the treatment of urologic tumors remains an open question.

2. GENERAL CONSIDERATIONS

Interferon (IFN), discovered in 1957 by Isaacs and Lindenmann [65], is defined biologically as a protein that reacts with normal cells and induces resistance to infection by a wide variety of viruses. IFN units are defined as the reciprocal of the dilution that protects 50% of cells from viral infection. In most reports IFN units are standardized against an International Reference Standard provided by the National Institutions of Health to help reduce unit variability between laboratories. However, considerable variability remains, and the unit described in each report should be interpreted as an approximate dose.

Although first recognized for its antiviral effects, IFN has now been implicated in the regulation of the immune response and as an antitumor agent [44, 105]. IFN is known to be composed of a heterogeneous group of proteins that may be catagorized into 3 major classes, *alpha* (leukocyte), *beta* (fibroblast) and *gamma* (immune), based on antigenic and physicochemical properties. *Alpha* (α) and *beta* (β) interferons are produced by leukocytes or fibroblasts, respectively, after stimulation by virus or by a multitude of non-viral IFN inducers [105] while *gamma* (γ) IFN is produced by immunocompetent lymphocytes in response to sensitizing antigen or mitogen stimulation [39, 116]. In mice IFN production by L929 fibroblasts after viral stimulation results in the production of a combination of IFNα and IFNβ which is designated IFNα, β. IFNα is comprised of multiple subclasses, while IFNβ and IFNγ are each apparently homogeneous [27]. The reader is referred to recent reviews for more detailed information concerning the production and properties of the interferon classes [72, 105, 115].

Throughout this chapter the abbreviation IFN, will refer to all interferon classes and subclasses. Such reference is inexact because of the diversity of class and subclass function; however, historically the biological activity of one class of IFN has been imputed to all IFN classes since by definition all classes mediate antiviral activity. Where possible, distinctions between IFN classes and subclasses will be made.

3. MECHANISM(S) OF ACTION

Two fundamental mechanisms are thought to be associated with the anti-tumor properties of IFN: direct inhibition of tumor cell proliferation and immunomodulation. We will examine the data supporting these hypotheses.

3.1 *Inhibition of tumor cell proliferation*

In 1962 Paucker et al. [92] first reported the inhibitory effect of IFN on cell multiplication. Considerable controversy arose in that it was unclear whether IFN or a contaminating substance mediated the antiproliferative activity [8]. Recent studies using electrophorectically pure [32, 50] and recombinant IFN [33] preparations have shown unequivocally that IFN is the mediator of the antiproliferative activity.

Tumors differ in their susceptibility to the antiproliferative effects of IFN. Tsuruo et al. [109] examined the susceptibility of several mouse cell lines to the antiproliferative activity of IFNα, β. IFNα, β concentrations ranging from 3.3 to 10 000 units per ml were tested in an assay in which cells were exposed to IFNα, β for 3 days and further cultured in fresh medium for 2 days. The results were reported as the concentration of IFNα, β required to inhibit cell growth by 50%. The number of units required for 50% inhibition ranged from 10.5 units for B16 melanoma to 10 000 units for a colon carcinoma designated colon 26. Several cell lines required intermediate concentrations; other cell lines were not sensitive at all to the antiproliferative effects of IFNα, β.

Human tumor cell lines also have been shown to vary in their response to IFNα. Von Hoff et al. [113] tested the inhibitory effects of IFNα on 62 tumors from a variety of origins in a soft agar clonogenic assay. Cells were exposed to 1000 units/ml IFNα which was included in the soft agar medium containing the cells. IFNα enhanced cell growth in three tumors with the enhancement ranging from 39 to 141% of controls. Others also have shown enhanced tumor growth in the presence of IFNα as well as IFNβ [106]. By the authors' criteria, in which 70% inhibition was required to designate the tumor as being sensitive to IFN, only 5 of 62 tumors were sensitive to IFNα. These were a lymphosarcoma cell leukemia, a small lung cancer, an adenocarcinoma of the lung, a breast cancer and a pancreatic cancer. The overall response varied considerably, with inhibition ranging from 0 to 90% in a series of 21 tumors for which IFNα dose response data were obtained. Of these 21, 10 were not inhibited by IFNα.

Interestingly, Epstein and Marcus [31] showed that ovarian tumors obtained from separate sites in the same patient varied in their response to IFNα. A soft agar clonogenic assay was used and cells were exposed to 300 units/ml IFNα which was incorporated into the agar. Four tumors were tested, from which both solid and ascites specimens were obtained. Three of four ascites specimens showed a reduction in tumor colony number by >25% while none of the solid tumors were IFNα-sensitive.

The sensitivity of tumor cells to the antiproliferative effects of the three classes of IFN also varies. Ludwig and Swetly [77] showed that human tumor cells differed in their sensitivities to IFNα and IFNβ. These authors tested the effects of 120 units/ml IFN on myeloma stem cells obtained from bone marrow. IFNα inhibited 50% of the tumors tested while IFNβ inhibited only 23%. Seven tumors were significantly inhibited by both IFNα and IFNβ. Of these, 4 had greater inhibition in the presence of IFNα, 1 greater inhibition with IFNβ and 2 had equivalent inhibition.

In contrast, Borden et al. [19] showed that IFNβ mediated more potent antiproliferative activity than IFNα. These investigators studied a large number of human cell lines for susceptibility to IFNα and IFNβ. The cells were continuously exposed to IFNα or IFNβ for 72 or 120 hours, counted and compared with control cultures. The sensitivity of the cell lines varied but the inhibitory effect of IFNβ was usually greater than that of IFNα.

Bradley and Ruscetti [20] evaluated the effects of IFNα and IFNβ on the proliferation of several solid and hematological tumors in a clonogenic assay. Cells were exposed continuously to IFN at 100 units/ml. All interferons showed the same magnitude and direction of inhibitory activity.

The relationship between IFNγ-mediated antiproliferative activity and that of IFNα or IFNβ also is being studied. Preliminary studies using recombinant human IFNγ showed that IFNγ did not inhibit mitogen-induced proliferation of peripheral blood lymphocytes while both IFNα and IFNβ were inhibitory [24]. Wallach et al. [114], however, suggested that human recombinant IFNγ was more effective in inhibiting the proliferation of normal fibroblasts than either IFNα or IFNβ. In this regard, Blalock et al. [16] tested partially purified human IFNγ for its antiproliferative effects against WISH and HEp-2 cells. They observed 20–100 times more inhibitory activity per antiviral unit with IFNγ when compared to IFNα or IFNβ. These results are supported by those of Zhang et al. [117]. These investigators studied both human and murine IFN and showed that the number of antiviral units required to produce 50% inhibition was lower for IFNγ than either IFNα or IFNβ for all tested cell lines. In our own studies using partially purified mouse IFNγ preparations, we observed greater inhibition of mouse bladder tumor growth by IFNγ as compared with IFNα, β in a clonogenic assay. The concentration of IFNγ required to inhibit colony formation by 50% was 67 units while 700 units IFNα, β were required to produce the same effect [67].

In contrast, Tomita et al. [108] reported that IFNγ was not effective in inhibiting proliferation of either Daudi or P3HR-1 lymphoma cells. Both IFNα and IFNβ had a 50% inhibition titer of <50 units whereas up to 1000 units IFNγ had no effect on proliferation. In addition, IFNγ did not elevate 2-5A synthetase levels while both IFNα and IFNβ did. In studies on other cell lines, these investigators observed a lack of inhibitory activity by all IFN classes against K562 cells and equivalent inhibitory activity by all IFN classes against RSa cells (50% inhibition titer 50 units for IFNα, IFNβ and IFNγ). Ankel et al. [5] showed that both IFNβ and IFNγ inhibited the proliferation of mouse leukemia L1210 cells. Moreover, IFNγ was shown to inhibit the growth of an L1210 subline that was resistant to the antiproliferative effects of IFNβ [21].

Not only do the 3 major classes of interferons differ in their antiproliferative activity but class subtypes also appear to express differential effects. Evinger et al. [32] obtained eight subspecies of IFNα during purification. All species were tested for their growth inhibitory and antiviral activity. All expressed both antiviral and antiproliferative activity, however, the ratio of growth inhibition to antiviral activity was not constant among the subtypes. These results have been confirmed with recombinant IFNα for which at least 15 distinct subtypes have been identified. Grant et al. [41] showed that IDNα$_D$ and IFNα$_A$ expressed differential antiproliferative effects on human leukemia and normal myeloid progenitor cells. For IFNα$_A$ the concentration that produced 50% reduction in colony formation was 400 and 300 units/ml for HL-60 and KG-1 leukemia cell lines, respectively, and averaged 1250 units/ml for non-leukemic bone marrow samples. IFNα$_D$ had a 50% inhibition titer of 650 and 950 units/ml for HL-60 and KG-1 while 5000 units/ml were required for non-leukemic samples.

Recent studies using xenografts of human tumors in athymic nude mice suggest that sufficient concentrations of IFN can be obtained in vivo to inhibit tumor cell division [6, 7, 25, 61]. Balkwill et al. [6] showed that human IFNα inhibited 2 of 3 human breast tumors implanted in nude mice. Inhibition was dose-dependent and required daily treatment for maximum effects. Tumor growth was inhibited but no regression was observed. Analysis of tumors after therapy showed that both IFN-treated and control tumors were histologically similar and no mononuclear infiltration was observed in the treated tumors. These investigators suggested that the inhibitory effects resulted from direct inhibition of tumor cell proliferation for two reasons. First, 2-5A synthetase was elevated in tumors treated with human IFN but not in normal mouse tissue. Secondly, in vitro studies showed that human IFNα did not augment mouse natural killer cell activity.

The mechanisms by which interferons inhibit cell multiplication are not well understood. Clearly, cell surface receptors are required. The existence of receptors was shown in ^{125}I-labeled binding experiments for IFNα and IFNγ [3, 5, 83]. IFNα and IFNβ have been shown to compete for the same binding sites [21, 83] while minimal competition for binding sites between IFNα and IFNγ has been observed [5]. These results suggest that receptor binding is required for the expression of IFN-mediated antiproliferative activity. This has been shown using L1210 cell lines sensitive (S) or resistant (R) to both IFNα and β. The L1210S line has IFNα and β receptors and its proliferation is inhibited by IFNα, β while L1210R line does not bind IFNα, β and is resistant to its antiproliferative effects [2, 49]. Interestingly, L1210R expresses receptors for IFNγ and is susceptible to its antiproliferative effects [5].

Receptor binding is required but alone is not sufficient for the expression of IFN-mediated antiproliferative activity. Mogensen et al. [83] tested several cell lines for their binding capacity for IFNα at 4 °C and compared this with binding and inhibition of cell growth at 37 °C. The most sensitive cell line to the antiproliferative activity of IFNα (Daudi) gave a complete biological response with only a fraction of its binding sites occupied while the insensitive cell line (Raji) showed no response even though receptors were expressed and fully saturated.

The inhibitory activity of IFN is not clearly cell cycle-dependent as both resting and log growth cells are inhibited equally well. Panniers and Clemens [91] studied the effects of IFNα, β on the duration of cell cycles. The results showed a prolongation of mitosis by 150%, G2 phase by 44% and S phase by 100%. Others suggest the IFNα, β inhibits cells from proceeding into the cell by shunting them into the GO loop [75].

Finally, IFNα and IFNβ do not appear to be cytolytic but IFNγ may be. IFNγ was tested against several cell lines for cytolytic activity. When cells were cultured with IFNγ at a low density, cytolysis was observed. The IFNγ-induced cytolysis decreased with increasing numbers of cells and was not apparent when more than 2×10^3 P388 cells were plated. IFNα, β was not observed to be cytolytic under any conditions [110].

Taken together the studies described above clearly show heterogeneity in the susceptibility of tumor cells to the antiproliferative activity of IFN as well as heterogeneity among the IFN classes and subclasses when directed against specific tumors. If one considers the antiproliferative effects of IFN to be of prime importance, selection of the appropriate IFN class for therapeutic use must be made for each tumor with the distinct possibility that lesions at separate sites may respond differently. Perhaps the best therapeutic modality would be to administer all three IFN classes to each patient. In this regard, preliminary studies using mixtures of murine IFNα, β and IFNγ have shown potentiation of the antitumor effect, suggesting that combinations of IFN classes are synergistic [26, 37].

3.2 Modulation of the immune response

Early studies by Gresser and associates [46, 49] using cell lines resistant to the antiproliferative effects of IFNα, β form the basis for the hypothesis that the immune response is associated with the antitumor effects of IFN. In these studies an L1210 subline, L1210R, which is resistant to the antiviral and antiproliferative effects of IFNα, β in vitro, was developed [49]. L1210R lacks cell surface receptors for IFNα, β but does respond in vitro to the antiviral and antiproliferative effects of IFNγ [2, 21]. Both the resistant and susceptible L1210 tumors are susceptible to the inhibitory effects of IFNα, β in vivo. These studies suggested that the immunomodulatory capacity of IFNα, β was responsible for the inhibition of tumor growth. More recent studies on Friend leukemia cells using the same experimental approach, i.e., IFN-sensitive and IFN-resistant cell lines, provided similar results [10, 11]. Belardelli et al. [11] attempted to identify the immune mechanism responsible for the inhibition of the IFN-resistant cell line, but were without success. In this regard, Blalock [15] has shown that direct binding of IFN may not be required for expression of antiviral activity. Instead, cell-to-cell communication may relay signals between IFN-activated and unactivated cells. Thus, an IFN-resistant cell line could be susceptible to IFNα, β in vivo through signals from the susceptible surrounding cells.

Clearly, immune parameters are modulated both in vitro and in vivo by IFN. IFN has been shown to modulate both cellular and humoral immune responses including antibody production [66, 103], cytotoxic T lymphocyte generation [34], natural killer cell activity [98] and macrophage-mediated cytotoxic activity [107]. Whether such modulation is an important mechanism in the antitumor activity of IFN remains to be established. Non-specific systemic modulation of the immune response by a variety of agents has not proven to be effective in the inhibition of tumor growth [9, 81]. Moreover, augmentation of immune parameters in clinical trials with IFNα have not correlated well with tumor responsiveness [40].

The interactions between tumors and the immune response encompass a complex series of events. Several immune mechanisms have been implicated in antitumor immunity with natural killer cells, T lymphocytes and macrophages currently considered as the most important [12, 13, 56, 59, 68, 70]. Even though the mechanisms can be demonstrated to be active against certain tumors, these tumors retain the ability to grow in vivo and kill the host [13, 38, 57, 104]. The mechanisms underlying the immunologic escape of tumors are unclear but have been attributed to modulation of recognition antigens on tumor cell surfaces [104], serum blocking factors [57], suppressor factors [38], and suppressor cells [13]. The effect of IFN administration on these components of the immune system is unclear and needs further study.

Currently, the only in vivo data available implicating the immune response in the inhibition of tumor growth by IFN is 'correlation data' which simply documents modulation of an immune response in conjunction with inhibitioin of tumor growth [14, 35, 36, 56, 70]. To more clearly understand immunologic mechanisms by which IFN inhibits tumor growth, direct relationships must be established. This is difficult with in vivo studies but can be accomplished by first characterizing the immune parameters capable of influencing tumor growth, and then characterizing the effects of IFN on those parameters.

3.3 Pharmacokinetics

The pharmacokinetics of IFNα, IFNβ and IFNγ are not well understood. This brief summary will focus on serum levels obtained after IFN injection and subsequent clearance rates, with some discussion of the role of the kidney in clearance, which may have relevance to the treatment of urologic tumors. More detailed information is available in two relatively recent reviews [17, 105].

Current data suggest that IFNα, IFNβ, and IFNγ exhibit different pharmacokinetic patterns. IFNα readily enters the bloodstream after intramuscular, intraperitoneal or subcutaneous injection while IFNβ and IFNγ do not [29, 54]. Figure 1 shows a typical serum clearance curve for patients

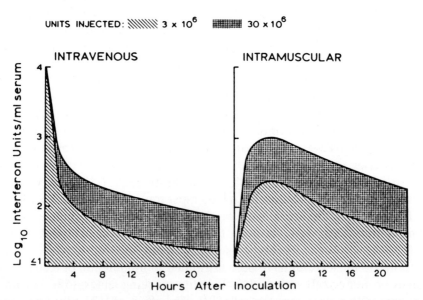

Figure 1. Blood clearance rates of IFNα after intramuscular or intravenous injection (reproduced from Ref. 2 with permission from Springer-Verlag, New York, NY).

injected either intravenously or intramuscularly with IFNα. Intravenous injection of either IFNβ or IFNγ results in a serum clearance rate similar to that described for IFNα; however, serum levels obtained after the intramuscular injection of IFNβ or IFNγ differ from that shown for IFNα. Injection of as much as 1.8×10^7 units IFNβ intramuscularly results in a serum peak of only 20 units while intramuscular injection of 9.6×10^6 units of IFNγ does not result in detectable serum IFNγ levels [30, 54]. Recent studies have shown that serum levels and clearance rates of recombinant IFNα1 and IFNαA obtained with either intramuscular or intravenous injection are similar to those obtained with naturally produced IFNα which is composed of a mixture of the IFNα subclasses [55, 96].

Of interest in the treatment of urologic tumors is the possible involvement of the kidney in the catabolism of interferon. The subject is reviewed in detail by Bocci [17].

In general, it is known that the kidney is important in the turnover of proteins of less than 50 000 daltons. IFNα, IFNβ and IFNγ are all proteins with molecular weights in the range of 18 000 to 20 000 daltons, suggesting a possible role for the kidney in IFN catabolism. IFNα clearance studies performed in rabbits with rabbit IFN also implicate the kidney in IFNα catabolism. Bilateral nephrectomy resulted in an increase in the serum half-life of rabbit IFNα. Furthermore, selective damage of tubular function by injection of maleate inhibited luminal uptake of rabbit IFNα and resulted in a substantial increase in rabbit urine IFNα levels [22, 54]. These studies have led to the hypothesis that a maximum rate of tubular uptake exists which when surpassed results in excretion of interferon in the urine.

Ho [60] also studied renal clearance of rabbit IFNα. This investigator detected urine levels ranging from 0.2–2.0% of the levels of IFNα injected intramuscularly. IFNα in the urine of humans, however, have not been observed [60]. Injection of 2×10^7 units of human IFNα did not result in detectable urine levels of IFNα in patients even when urine was collected over a 24 hr period. The reasons for the inability to detect IFN in urine of human subjects is unclear. It may result from lack of participation of the kidney in catabolism or simply from inactivation of IFNα by the urine [22].

4. CLINICAL TRIALS

4.1 General comments

Clinical trials testing the efficacy of IFN as an antitumor agent have been in progress for several years. These studies have been hampered by the limited availability of IFN and have provided inconclusive results. The list of tumor types under investigation expands each year and now includes breast cancer, melanoma, osteosarcoma, myeloma, non-Hodgkin's lymphoma, malignant melanoma, laryngeal papilloma, and squamous cell carcinoma of uterine cervix, to name only a few. The studies to date have been open-ended phase I, II trials which do not include control patients or use historical controls. The results have been suggestive but not impressive. For example, Borden et al. [18] recently reported the results of a phase II trial in which the efficacy of IFNα was studied in breast cancer. Twenty-three patients entered the study and five had objective partial responses with a mean duration of 92 days (range 14 to 176). These patients subsequently experienced relapse and disease progression. The authors stated that 'at the dose used in this trial, interferon alpha was no more active than other available single agents for metastatic breast cancer'. The same statement could be made for most of the trials reported to date. There are exceptions, the most notable of which are the reports on the treatment of squamous cell carcinoma of the uterine cervix [62, 71, 73]. In these studies IFNα was used as adjuvant therapy to surgery. IFNα was applied topically with a contraceptive pessary (2×10^6 units daily for 21 days). Of 37 patients studied, none experienced progression of disease during IFNα therapy and in a follow-up of up to 5 years only 3 have died. These studies are promising, but additional trials are needed to confirm the early uncontrolled results.

A close examination of the antitumor studies of IFN in various animal models reveals two important facts that have important implications for clinical trials. First, intralesional injection of IFN is superior to systemic administration [43, 45]. Gresser and Bourali [43] showed that intraperitoneal injection of interferon for the treatment of Ehrlich ascites tumors resulted in greater than 30 days survival of 15 of 15 mice while only 7 of 20 mice survived when given subcutaneous injections of IFN.

Secondly, only one report, which remains unconfirmed, indicates that IFN is effective in inducing complete regression of an existing tumor [69]. Most reports suggest that interferon is effective in inhibiting the outgrowth of transplanted tumors or in delaying tumor progression and therefore prolonging survival [42, 43].

The clinical data to date support the fundamental observations obtained in animal models. Thus, treating advanced cancer patients with IFN administered systemically will probably not succeed. The highest probability of success lies in treating less advanced tumors locally with IFN. Again, treatment of uterine carcinoma serves as an example. Ikic et al. [64] treated patients with precancerous states of the uterine cervix with IFNα in a prospective randomized study. Thirteen patients with CIS grade I and II (borderline) were treated with a daily dose of 10^6 units IFNα administered for 21 days in a contraceptive pessary. Eighteen patients with similar cytologic diagnoses were randomized to receive placebos. After 2 years, 7 of 13 IFNα-treated patients presented with normal cells only while none of 18 placebo patients fell into this category. Only one patient in the IFNα-treated group showed progression while 8 controls progressed. The number of patients is small and the follow-up short (only 2 years) but the design of the study lends strength to the results and suggests a need for additional trials of this type.

4.2 Urologic tumors

Few studies have been reported on the effects of IFN in patients with urologic tumors. A summary of the data now available is provided in Tables 1, 2, and 3. These tables are not all-inclusive, for other reports refer to the treatment of isolated cases of urologic tumors. These other reports, however, do not include sufficient data for evaluation of the therapeutic effects of IFN and have not been included in this discussion.

In 1978 Christophersen et al. [23] reported on the effects of IFNα on two patients with recurrent superficial transitional cell carcinoma of the bladder (Table 1). These patients were treated with an intramuscular injection of 3×10^6 units daily for 2 months followed by 4×10^6 units 3 times per week for a maximum of 1.5 years. The patients showed normalization of their bladder urothelium within a few months of IFNα therapy. Regression of papillomas smaller than 1 cm was detected while those larger than 1 cm became stationary. Osther et al. [89] subsequently studied an additional 7 patients with recurrent superficial transitional cell carcinoma of the bladder (Table 1). These patients were treated with intramuscular injections of IFNα ranging from 4 to 8×10^6 units per injection. A complete response was observed in 1 of 7 patients. This patient had a 5 year history of recurrent papillary tumors that were treated with electrocoagulation prior to the initiation of IFNα therapy. Treatment began with intramuscular injection of 4×10^6 units IFNα daily for 30 days, which was followed by administration of 4×10^6 units 3 times per week for 74 weeks. All papillomas regressed early in the treatment protocol. After 47 weeks of therapy a minor papilloma was observed which was removed by electrocoagulation. No further tumors developed, and the patient remained tumor-free 25 months after termination of therapy. A partial response was observed in 3 of 7 patients. All three of these patients relapsed during therapy and one required cystectomy. The other two were treated with a second course of IFNα. The response to the second treatment series was less than partial. Of the 3 remaining patients 2 did not respond to IFNα even when IFNα levels were elevated to 8×10^6 units per injection. The remaining patient experienced stabilization of the disease.

Aleman et al. [4] reported a complete response to IFNα treatment by 2

Table 1. Summary of the effects of IFN treatment of superficial transitional cell carcinoma of the bladder[a].

Pa-tient	Age	Sex	Tumor grade	Previous therapy	Condition bladder at therapy initiation	Method of IFN administration	Quantity and type IFN	Effects of therapy[b]	Length of follow-up or to recurrence	Remarkable side effects	Refe-rences
1.	46	F	G I	RT, TUR, CT	TUR	intramuscular[c]	10^6 units, IFNα	CR	24 months	none	97
2.	53	M	G I	TUR, CT	TUR	intramuscular[c]	10^6 units, IFNα	REC[d]	6 months	none	97
3.	57	F	G II	RT, TUR, CT	TUR	intramuscular[c]	10^6 units, IFNα	REC	18 months	none	97
4.	59	M	G I	RT, TUR, CT	MT	intramuscular[c]	10^6 units, IFNα	REC	18 months	none	97
5.	57	M	G II	TUR, CT	MT	intramuscular[c]	10^6 units, IFNα	CR	24 months	none	97
6.	55	F	G II	TUR	MT	intramuscular[c]	10^6 units, IFNα	PR	24 months	none	97
7.	57	M	G II	RT, TUR, CT	MT	intramuscular[c]	10^6 units, IFNα	PR	24 months	none	97
8.	80	F	G I	TUR	TUR	intramuscular[e]	3×10^6 units, IFNα	CR	16 months	–	88
9.	80	M	G II-III	TUR	TUR	intramuscular[e]	3×10^6 units, IFNα	CR	25 months	–	88
10.	66	F	G I-II	TUR	MT	intramuscular[e]	3×10^6 units, IFNα	CR	10 months	–	88
11.	58	M	G II	TUR, CT	TUR	intramuscular[e]	3×10^6 units, IFNα	REC	6 months	–	88
12.	60	M	G I	TUR	MT	intramuscular[e]	3×10^6 units, IFNα	PROG	8 months	–	88
13.	68	M	G II	TUR	MT	intramuscular[e]	3×10^6 units, IFNα	PROG	7 months	–	88
14.	75	M	G II	TUR	–	intramuscular[f]	$4-8 \times 10^6$ units, IFNα	PROG	–	malaise	89
15.	66	F	G II	TUR	–	intramuscular[f]	$4-8 \times 10^6$ units, IFNα	PR	8 months	fever	89
16.	48	F	G II	TUR	–	intramuscular[f]	$4-8 \times 10^6$ units, IFNα	PR	8 months	none	89
17.	45	M	G II	TUR	–	intramuscular[f]	$4-8 \times 10^6$ units, IFNα	CR	25 months	none	89
18.	58	M	G II	TUR	–	intramuscular[f]	$4-8 \times 10^6$ units, IFNα	PROG	6 months	fever	89
19.	66	F	G II	TUR	–	intramuscular[f]	$4-8 \times 10^6$ units, IFNα	STAB	4 months	none	89
20.	56	M	G II	TUR	–	intramuscular[f]	$4-8 \times 10^6$ units, IFNα	PR	21 months	malaise	89

223

Table 1. (continued).

Pa-tient	Age	Sex	Tumor grade	Previous therapy	Condition bladder at therapy initiation	Method of IFN administration	Quantity and type IFN	Effects of therapy[b]	Length of follow-up or to recurrence	Remarkable side effects	Refe-rences
21.	75	F	G II	TUR	–	intramuscular[g]	2×10⁶ units, IFNα	CR	34 months	–	63, 80
22.	53	F	G I	TUR	–	intramuscular[g]	2×10⁶ units, IFNα	unclear[h]	29 months	–	63, 80
23.	42	M	G II	TUR	–	intramuscular[g]	2×10⁶ units, IFNα	REC	4 months	–	63, 80
24.	56	F	G II	TUR	–	intramuscular[g]	2×10⁶ units, IFNα	unclear[h]	25 months	–	63, 80
25.	68	F	G II	TUR	–	intramuscular[g]	2×10⁶ units, IFNα	unclear[h]	36 months	–	63, 80
26.	65	F	G II	RT, TUR	–	intramuscular[g]	2×10⁶ units, IFNα	unclear[h]	46 months	–	63, 80
27.	54	M	G II	RT, TUR	–	intramuscular[g]	2×10⁶ units, IFNα	REC	16 months	–	63, 80
28.	52	M	G II	TUR	–	intramuscular[g]	2×10⁶ units, IFNα	unclear[h]	22 months	–	63, 80
29.	54	M	G I	TUR	–	intramuscular[i]	4×10⁶ units, IFNα	STAB	6 months	–	23
30.	46	F	G II	TUR	–	intramuscular[i]	4×10⁶ units, IFNα	STAB	7 months	–	23

a Abbreviations: RT, radiation therapy; CT, chemotherapy; TUR, transurethral resection; MT, multiple tumors; CR, complete response; REC, recurrence; PROG, progression; STAB, stabilization; PR, partial response.
b Response criteria: complete response – no tumor detectable after treatment; partial response – greater than 50% decrease in measurable tumor size with no progression; stabilization – less than 25% change in tumor burden; progression – lack of response of tumors to therapy; recurrence – reappearance of tumor(s) after interval without tumor(s).
c 10⁶ units administered every 48 hr for 6 months.
d 3×10⁶ units administered daily for 3 weeks followed by a 4 week rest.
f 4×10⁶ units administered daily for 14 weeks followed by 8×10⁶ units for 2 months.
g 2×10⁶ units injected into the tumor base or the surrounding tissue daily for 21 days. Treatment was repeated at monthly intervals until regression occurred.
h It is unclear from the data whether these patients suffered recurrences or whether they remained tumor-free at the follow-up times indicated.
i IFN administered daily for 2 months followed by 3 injections per week for 16 months.

Table 2. Summary of effects of IFN therapy on renal cell carcinoma [a].

Patinet	Age	Sex	Tumor stage	Metastatic lesion (locations)	Previous therapy	Method of IFN administration	Quantity and type IFN	Effects of therapy [b]	Length of follow-up	References
1.	49	M	IV	lungs, bone	NEPH	intramuscular [c]	escalating 10^6–10^8 units, IFNα	PR	4 months	79
2.	75	M	IV	lungs	HT, NEPH	intramuscular [d]	3×10^6 units, IFNα	PR	4 months	94
3.	60	M	IV	lungs	HT, NEPH	intramuscular [d]	3×10^6 units, IFNα	PR	4 months	94
4.	53	M	IV	lungs	NEPH	intramuscular [d]	3–18×10^6 units, IFNα	PR	9 months	94
5.	56	F	IV	lungs, bone	HT, CT, NEPH	intramuscular [d]	3–18×10^6 units, IFNα	PR	7 months	94
6.	51	M	IV	lungs	NEPH	intramuscular [d]	3×10^6 units, IFNα	PR	4 months	94
7.	46	M	IV	lungs	HT, CT, IFN, NEPH	intramuscular [d]	3–36×10^6 units, IFNα	LR	9 months	94
8.	63	M	IV	lungs	HT, CT, NEPH	intramuscular [d]	3–18×10^6 units, IFNα	LR	4 months	94
9.	57	M	IV	lungs, bone	RT, NEPH	intramuscular [d]	3–18×10^6 units, IFNα	MR	–	94
10.	54	M	IV	lungs, bone	NEPH	intramuscular [d]	3–36×10^6 units, IFNα	MR	–	94
11.	55	F	IV	lymph node	CT, RT, NEPH	intramuscular [d]	3–18×10^6 units, IFNα	MR	–	94
12.	58	M	IV	lungs	HT, NEPH	intramuscular [d]	3–36×10^6 units, IFNα	SD	6 months	94
13.	64	F	IV	lungs, bone	HT, NEPH	intramuscular [d]	3×10^6 units, IFNα	SD	5 months	94
14.	49	F	IV	lungs	NEPH	intramuscular [d]	3–36×10^6 units, IFNα	PROG	–	94
15.	74	F	IV	lungs, bone	HT, RT, NEPH	intramuscular [d]	3–18×10^6 units, IFNα	PROG	–	94

Table 2. Summary of effects of IFN therapy on renal cell carcinoma [a] (continued).

Patient	Age	Sex	Tumor stage	Metastatic lesion (locations)	Previous therapy	Method of IFN administration	Quantity and type IFN	Effects of therapy [b]	Length of follow-up	References
16.	68	M	IV	lungs, bone	NEPH	intramuscular [d]	3×10^6 units, IFNα	PROG	—	94
17.	29	M	IV	lungs	CT, NEPH	intramuscular [d]	3×10^6 units, IFNα	PROG	—	94
18.	66	M	IV	bone	RT, NEPH	intramuscular [d]	3×10^6 units, IFNα	PROG	—	94
19.	58	M	IV	lungs, bone	HT, RT, NEPH	intramuscular [d]	3×10^6 units, IFNα	PROG	—	94
20.	42	M	IV	lungs, bone	HT, RT, NEPH	intramuscular [d]	3×10^6 units, IFNα	PROG	—	94
21.	63	M	IV	—	—	intramuscular [e]	$1-10 \times 10^6$ units, IFBβ	PROG	—	82
22.	51	M	IV	—	—	intramuscular [e]	$1-10 \times 10^6$ units, IFNβ	PROG	—	82
23.	65	M	IV	—	—	intramuscular [e]	$1-10 \times 10^6$ units, IFNβ	PROG	—	82
24.	54	M	IV	—	—	intramuscular [e]	$1-10 \times 10^6$ units, IFNβ	PROG	—	82
25.	56	F	IV	—	—	intramuscular [e]	$1-10 \times 10^6$ units, IFNβ	PROG	—	82

[a] Abbreviations: NEPH, nephrectomy; HT, hormonal therapy; CT, chemotherapy; RT, radiation therapy; PR, partial response; MR, mixed response; LR, less than partial response; SD, stable disease; PROG, progression.

[b] Response criteria: partial response – greater than 50% reduction in measurable tumor size with no progression of other detectable tumors; less than partial response – greater than 25% but less than 50% reductions in tumors with no progression at other tumor sites; mixed response – regression of some tumors and progression of others; stable disease – less than 25% change in tumor size; progressive disease – continued growth of tumors.

[c] Escalating doses of recombinant IFNα2 were administered at weekly intervals.

[d] IFNα administered daily at $3-18 \times 10^6$ units and 3 times per week at $18-36 \times 10^6$ units.

[e] IFNβ administered intramuscularly at levels of 10^6 units 3 times per week for 2 weeks, 5×10^6 units 3 times per week for 2 weeks and 10×10^6 units 3 times per week for 2 weeks after which therapy was terminated.

Table 3. Summary of effects of IFN therapy on adenocarcinoma of the prostate.

Patient	Age	Tumor stage	Metastatic lesion (location)	Previous therapy	Method of IFN administration	Quantity and type IFN [a]	Effects of therapy [b]	Length of follow-up	Remarkable side effects	References
1.	62	D	disseminated	hormone, chemotherapy	intramuscular	escalating doses, 10^6–10^8 units, IFNα2	progression	–	fever, malaise	79
2.	67	D	disseminated	hormone, chemotherapy	intramuscular	escalating 10^6–10^8 units, IFNα2	progression	–	fever, malaise	79
3.	70	D	disseminated	hormone, chemotherapy	intramuscular	escalating doses 10^6–10^8 units, IFNα2	stabilization	–	central nervous system toxicity	79
4.	76	D	disseminated	hormone, chemotherapy	intramuscular	escalating doses 10^6–10^8 units, IFNα2	partial response	4 months	malaise	79

[a] Recombinant IFNα2 administered at weekly intervals in escalating doses.
[b] Response criteria: partial response – greater than 50% decrease in measurable tumor size with no progression of other detectable tumors; stabilization – less than 25% change in tumor size; progression – continued growth of tumor(s).

patients with diffuse superficial transitional cell carcinoma of the bladder. IFNα was injected intramuscularly at 3×10^6 units per injection daily for 3 weeks followed by 4 weeks rest. Both patients experienced complete remissions and remain tumor-free after 11 and 7 months, respectively (not summarized in Table 1).

Osther and Hill [88] extend the original observations of Aleman and associates to include 6 patients (Table 1). Three patients experienced complete responses and 3 did not respond to IFNα therapy. Patient 1 had TCC grade I TIS. The tumors were removed by electrocoagulation and IFN therapy (i.m. injection 3×10^6 units daily for 3 weeks followed by 4 weeks rest) was initiated. The patient remained tumor-free after a follow-up of 16 months. Patient 2 was diagnosed with TCC grade II-III, T1. Again, tumors were removed and IFNα therapy was initiated. The patient remained tumor-free after a follow-up of 25 months. The third responding patient had diffuse TCC grade I-II, stage T1 and had tumors partially removed prior to initiation of IFN therapy. The remaining tumors regressed during therapy, and the patient remained tumor-free after a follow-up of 10 months.

The tumors of the 3 non-responding patients were diagnosed as follows: (a) TCC grade I, stage T1S, (b) TCC grade II, stage T1, and (c) TCC grade II, stage T1. These patients received IFNα but recurrences were observed at 8, 6 and 7 months, respectively.

Ikic et al. [63] and Maricic et al. [80] reported the effects of intralesional injection of IFNα on recurrent superficial TCC of the bladder (Table 1). Eight patients were studied and all showed complete or partial responses to therapy. IFNα (2×10^6 units) was injected transurethrally with a surgical cystoscope daily for 21 days into the tumor base or the surrounding tissue as near the tumor as possible. Two patients were given 2×10^6 units IFNα intramuscularly simultaneously with transurethral injection. The treatment was repeated at monthly intervals until the tumors regressed. Of the patients treated one was diagnosed with grade I TCC while the remaining 7 had grade II tumors. Treatment ranged from 1 to 6 months and a complete response was observed is all patients. Two patients had the tumors removed by electrocoagulation after the first month's treatment with IFNα. All patients remain tumor-free with follow-ups ranging from 6 to 30 months.

Scorticatti et al. [97] tested the effects of IFNα on multiple superficial TCC of the bladder (grade I or II) in a total of 8 patients (Table 1). One patient, for reasons not described in the report, did not complete the treatment protocol and is not included in this discussion. IFNα (10^6 units/injection) was administered intramuscularly every 48 hours for 6 months. The patients were followed for 2 years and those that suffered recurrences were treated with a second course of IFNα. Three patients were treated with transurethral resection (TUR) immediately prior to initiation of IFNα therapy. One of these patients had no recurrences for the duration of the study (24 months), while 2 required a second IFNα treatment and are considered to have the disease under control. Two of 5 patients with tumor at the beginning of therapy experienced tumor regression and had no recurrence for the duration of therapy. The remaining 3 patients were classified as having the disease stabilized by IFNα therapy.

To date, studies of IFN therapy in bladder cancer patients have provided equivocal results, but suggest that IFN is a potentially active agent. Few patients have been studied and more importantly, the studies have not included sufficient controls. If IFN is to be considered a valuable therapeutic agent for bladder cancer, controlled studies must be performed. This is particularly important because sufficient quantities of IFN are now available and the natural history of superficial papillary bladder tumors lends itself well to randomization.

Quesada et al. [94] studied the effects of IFNα on 19 renal cell carcinoma patients (Table 2). IFNα was obtained from the State Serum Institute, Finnish Red Cross Center, Helsinki, Finland. The preparation contained approximately 10^6 IFNα units/mg protein. All patients received daily injections of 3×10^6 units intramuscularly, which was increased in some patients to 18×10^6 units daily or $18-36 \times 10^6$ units twice weekly. All patients studied had undergone nephrectomy with resection of primary tumor and all had clinical metastatic disease. IFNα treatment (3×10^6 units daily) resulted in partial responses in 5 patients (26%), objective minor responses in 2 patients (10.5%), some evidence of biological response in 3 patients (16%), stabilization in 2 patients and no evidence of response with progressive disease in 7 patinets (37%). The responses were observed early in therapy, occurring within 30–90 days. Escalation of IFNα doses did not enhance antitumor activity nor did it induce a response in those patients not responding initially to therapy. Two patients with partial responses relapsed after 6 and 9 months while the remaining responding patients continued treatments. These patients had a mean response duration of 6 months (range 4–9). It is of interest to note that all regressions occurred in lung and mediastinal metastases but that none of the regressions were complete.

Madajewicz et al. [79] reported the effects of recombinant IFNα2 on one renal carcinoma patient (Table 2). The patient had stage IV disease with lung and bone metastases, and IFNα2 was administered intramuscularly in increasing doses (10^6–10^8 units per injection) at approximately one week intervals. IFNα2 therapy resulted in the disappearance of the lung metastases. The patient has been followed for 8 months.

McPherson and Tan [82] tested the effects of IFNβ on the progression of several tumors including five renal cell carcinoma patients (Table 2). This was a phase I toxicology study in which patients were treated with intramuscular injections of 10^6 units 3 times per week for 2 weeks, followed by 5×10^6 units 3 times per week for 2 weeks and finally 10^7 units 3 times per week for 2 weeks. As indicated above, intramuscular injection of IFNβ provides marginally detectable serum IFN levels which may have influenced the therapeutic results. IFNβ treatment was terminated after the 10^7 units course and treatment with other drugs was initiated. Four of five patients appeared to have stable disease during therapy while the fifth patient experienced progressive tumor growth. All patients experienced disease progression after termination of IFNβ therapy.

The studies on IFN therapy of renal cell carcinoma, like other IFN therapy studies, are only suggestive. The patient numbers are small, follow-up times are short and although suggestive, the results are not impressive.

Madajewicz et al. [79] studied the effects of IFNα2 on 4 patients with prostatic adenocarcinoma (Table 3). All patients had metastatic disease (stage D) and had had previous hormonal therapy and chemotherapy. The injection protocol was the same as that described for renal carcinoma patients. One patient experienced a partial response in that the supraclavicular lymph nodes decreased in size by 50%. One patient experienced stabilization of disease and the remaining 2 patients did not respond to therapy. This is a very preliminary study which was designed primarily as a toxicity study. It would be premature to evaluate the effectiveness of IFN in prostate cancer based on these data.

4.3 Toxicity of IFN

Interferon administered at doses below 10^7 units has proven to be relatively non-toxic in the clinical trials performed to date. With improved production systems sufficient quantities of IFN are available for the administration of very high doses to determine toxicity levels. Early phase I trials with high doses ($> 10^7$ units) of recombinant IFNαA suggest that dose levels of IFN are limited by adverse side effects.

The side effects observed during clinical trials with low doses of IFN (an approximate maximum dose of 5×10^6 units/day) are relatively minor. They occur with both IFNα and IFNβ, are present when highly purified recombinant interferons are administered and do not appear to result from contaminants such as bacterial endotoxin [53, 86, 93, 95, 101, 102]. Side effects occurring in almost all patients receiving this approximate dose include depressed peripheral WBC, fever, headache, fatigue and anorexia. Other side effects associated with this approximate dose of interferon include chills, gastrointestinal disturbances (nausea and diarrhea), hypotension, joint pains, alopecia, myalgia, recurrent herpes simplex lesions, and inflammation at the injection site.

The side effects obtained in initial studies with crude naturally produced

IFNα were also observed with administration of similar levels of highly purified recombinant IFNαA [53, 101]. IFNαA, in doses of less than 5×10^7 units produced relatively mild side effects that mimicked those listed above. The toxic side effects became progressively more severe with doses greater than 5×10^7 units.

Smedley et al. [102] reported dose-limiting central venous system (CNS) toxicity at IFNαA doses of 2×10^7 units/m^2 daily or 5×10^7 units/m^2 three times a week. The CNS toxic effects included profound somnolence, confusion, paresthesia, signs of an upper motor neurone lesion in the legs of one patient and slow wave activity in encephalograms for all patients. The CNS toxicity of IFNαA was reversible and did not recur with additional treatments at lower doses.

The long-term side effects of maximal tolerated doses of IFN remain unclear. Animal studies indicate that long-term side effects may include an increased frequency of autoimmune disorders and glomerulonephritis. Early animal studies by Gresser and associates [52] showed that injection of murine IFN into newborn mice resulted in liver degeneration and death. In Swiss or C3H mice injected with 4×10^4 units of IFN daily for the first 8 days of life followed by 8×10^4 units daily for an additional 30 days, mice suffered from liver degeneration and had 100% mortality within 40 days. The LD$_{50}$ ranged from 5×10^3 to 1.2×10^4 units IFN per injection and required daily administration beginning the day of birth and continuing for a minimum of 8 days. Initiation of IFN injections 6 days after birth had no effect on either liver function or mortality rate. Treatments of less than 8 days, which were begun on the day of birth, resulted in transient liver degeneration from which most mice recovered.

These studies were performed with crude IFN preparations leaving the question of the actual mediator of the side effects open to question. Subsequent studies with electrophoretically pure IFN confirmed the early studies [51]. Using electrophoretically pure IFN (6.6×10^5 units/injection), identical liver lesions and mortality rates were observed. Ultrastructural studies of the liver of IFN-treated animals showed the presence of tubular aggregates associated with granular endoplasmic reticulum of hepatocytes [47].

Moss et al. [85] and Morel-Maroger [84] also showed that mice injected early in life with IFN developed glomerulonephritis. Mice injected with IFN daily from birth for 6–8 days (5×10^4 units/injection) began to die after 38 days from glomerulonephritis. Mice sacrificed on the eighth day suffered from liver degeneration but had no kidney lesions. In the other mice, by the 35th day the liver had recovered but kidney lesions were still apparent. Immunofluorescence studies showed IgG, IgM, and C3 deposits along the glomerular basement membrane.

Again, the use of electrophoretically pure IFN confirmed that the toxic effects were induced by IFN [105]. Mice treated with pure IFN for the first eight days of life (6.6×10^5 units/injection) developed kidney lesions by the 37th day. Examination of kidneys nine days after birth showed essentially normal structures under light microscopy although the subcortical glomeruli were immature as compared with controls. Electron micrographs showed marked thickening of lamina rara interna of the basement membrane. Kidneys obtained from mice sacrificed after 37 days showed advanced disease with virtually all glomeruli sclerotic. The tubules showed diffuse atrophy of the epithelium and dilated lumens were filled with proteinaceous casts. Immunofluorescence showed granular coarse deposits of IgG, IgM, and C3 along the glomeruli basement membranes.

The effects of IFN on glomerulonephritis also have been observed in NZB mice [1, 58, 99, 100]. These mice characteristically develop spontaneous autoimmune hemolytic anemia, while F_1 hybrids between NZB × NZW (NZB/W) develop a disease similar to systemic lupus erythematosis, with symptoms including predominantly antinuclear (ANA) and anti-dsDNA antibodies as well as immune complex glomerulonephritis [74]. NZB mice given IFN three times per week for 37 weeks (2×10^5 units/injection) had an increased incidence of anti-erythrocyte antibodies. NZB/W mice given 10^6 units IFN for the same period developed glomerulonephritis 3–6 months earlier than controls. This was accompanied by an increase in renal immune complex deposits, and an earlier appearance of ANA and anti-dsDNA antibodies. No elevation in the level of serum immune complexes was observed.

Interferon has been shown to depress peripheral leukocyte counts (WBC) in mice [48]. A single injection of 1.6×10^6 units of IFN intraperitoneally resulted in a decreased WBC within 24 hours with recovery occurring by the seventh day. In vitro studies have shown that IFN inhibits the proliferation of leukocyte and erythroid progenitor cells [28, 76, 78, 87, 111, . These include inhibition of granulopoietic differentiation [111, 112] megakaryocytic progenitor differentiation [28], erythropoiesis [78, 87] and macrophage maturation [76]. In all cases stem cell inhibition was dose-dependent and reversible.

5. CONCLUSIONS AND FUTURE PROSPECTS

Interferon is a relatively non-toxic agent that exhibits potential as an antitumor agent. The mechanisms by which IFN inhibit tumor growth are not well defined. Clearly, IFN inhibits the proliferation of some tumors; however, each tumor appears to have a unique response to each IFN class and subclass. Moreover, tumors obtained from separate lesions within a single patient appear to vary in their response to the antiproliferative effects of IFN, which may complicate therapeutic approaches.

The implication that the immune response is an important mechanism in IFN-mediated antitumor activity has little supporting data. The hypothesis is based on two lines of evidence: 1) animal tumors that are not susceptible to the antiproliferative activity of IFN in vitro remain susceptible to the antitumor effects in vivo; and 2) considerable evidence demonstrates that IFN modulates various immune parameters both in vivo and in vitro but the effect of this modulation on tumor growth remains unclear. No direct evidence linking IFN-induced immune modulation with tumor therapy has been reported.

Clinical trials testing the efficacy of IFN as an antitumor agent have been reported for urologic as well as non-urologic tumors. The conclusions have always been 'IFN is a potentially active agent but...' and the 'buts' are endless. With sufficient quantities of recombinant IFN products available, long-term controlled studies are needed. It is time to determine whether recombinant IFNα or IFNβ are more than 'potentially' effective as single agents.

This issue of efficacy, however, will not be settled by these studies. As indicated in the text, distinct IFNα subclasses may mediate different biological effects which may affect therapeutic results obtained by administering single recombinant subclasses. Furthermore, preliminary evidence suggests that administration of mixtures of IFN classes produces synergistic effects and therefore, may provide a better therapeutic regimen. Finally, IFNγ has not been tested extensively in the clinic and there is evidence in animal tumor models that it is more effective as a single agent than either IFNα or IFNβ. Clearly, a considerable amount of work remains to define the role of IFN in tumor therapy.

ACKNOWLEDGEMENT

This work was supported in part by grant number CA28860 from the National Cancer Institute through the National Bladder Cancer Project.

REFERENCES

1. Adam C, Thona Y, Ronco P, Verroust P, Tovey M, Morel-Maroger L: The effect of exogenous interferon: Acceleration of autoimmune and renal diseases in (NZB/W)F$_1$ mice. Clin Exp Immunol 40:373, 1980.
2. Aguet M: High-affinity binding of ^{125}I-labeled mouse interferon to a specific cell surface receptor. Nature 284:459, 1980.

3. Aguet M, Belardelli F, Blanchard B, Marcucci F, Gresser I: High-affinity binding of ^{125}I-labeled mouse interferon to a specific cell surface receptor. IV. Mouse gamma interferon and cholera toxin do not compete for the common receptor site of alpha/beta interferon. Virology 117:541, 1982.

4. Aleman C, Khan A, Hill JM, Pardue A, Hilario R, Hill NO: Response of diffuse transitional cell carcinoma to low dose interferon. 18th Annual ASCO meeting (Abstract), 1982.

5. Ankel H, Krishnamurti C, Besançon F, Stefanos S, Falcoff E: Mouse fibroblast (type I) and immune (type II) interferons: Pronounced differences in affinity for gangliosides and in antiviral and antigrowth effects on mouse leukemia L-1210R cells. Proc Natl Acad Sci USA 77:2528, 1980.

6. Balkwill F, Moodie EM, Freedman V, Fantes KH: Human interferon inhibits the growth of established human breast tumors in the nude mouse. Int J Cancer 30:231, 1982.

7. Balkwill F, Taylor.Papdimitriore J, Fantes KH, Sebesteng A: Human lymphoblastoid interferon can inhibit the growth of human breast cancer xenographs in athymic (nude) mice. Eur J Cancer 16:569, 1980.

8. Baron S, Merigan TC, McKerlie ML: Effect of crude and purified interferons on the growth of unifected cells in culture. Proc Soc Exp Biol Med 121:50, 1966.

9. Bast RC, Bast BS: Non-specific immunostimulation as therapy for cancer. Critical review of previously reported animal studies of tumor immunotherapy with non-specific immunostimulants. Ann NY Acad Sci 277:60, 1976.

10. Belardelli F, Gresser I, Maury C, Maunoury M-T: Antitumor effects of interferon in mice injected with interferon-sensitive and interferon-resistant Friend leukemia cells. Int J Cancer 30:813, 1982.

11. Belardelli F, Gresser I, Maury C, Maunoury M-T: Antitumor effects of interferon in mice injected with interferon-sensitive and interferon-resistant Friend leukemia cells. II. Role of host mechanisms. Int J Cancer 30:821, 1982.

12. Berendt MJ, North RJ, Kerstein DP: The immunological basis of endotoxin-induced tumor regression. Requirement for T-cell mediated immunity. J Exp Med 148:1550, 1978.

13. Berendt MJ, North RJ: T cell mediated suppression of anti-tumor immunity. J Exp Med 151:69, 1980.

14. Bernstein ID, Thor DE, Zbar B, Rapp HJ: Tumor immunity: tumor suppression in vivo initiated by soluble products of specifically stimulated lymphocytes. Science 172:729, 1971.

15. Blalock JE: A small fraction of cells communicates the maximal interferon sensitivity to a population (40622). Proc Soc Exp Biol Med 162:80, 1979.

16. Blalock JE, Georgiades JA, Langford MP, Johnson HM: Purified human immune interferon has more potent anticellular activity than fibroblasts or leukocyte interferon. Cell Immunol 49:390, 1980.

17. Bocci V: Pharmacokinetic studies of interferons. Pharmac Ther 13:421-440, 1981.

18. Borden EC, Holland JF, Dao TL, Gutterman JU, Wiener L, Chang Y-C, Patel J: Leukocyte-derived interferon (alpha) in human breast carcinoma. Ann Intern Med 97:1, 1982.

19. Borden EC, Hogen TF, Voelkel JG: Comparative antiproliferative activity in vitro of natural interferons alpha and beta for diploid and transformed human cells. Cancer Res 42:4948, 1982.

20. Bradley EC, Ruscetti FW: Effect of fibroblast, lymphoid and myeloid interferons on human tumor colony formation in vitro. Cancer Res 41:244, 1981.

21. Branca AA, Baglioni C: Evidence that types I and II interferons have different receptors. Nature 294:768, 1981.

234

22. Cesario T, Tilles JG: Inactivation of human interferon by urine. J Infect Dis 127:311, 1973.
23. Christophersen IS, Jordal R, Osther K, Lindenberg J, Pedersen PH, Berg K: Interferon therapy in neoplastic disease. Acta Med Scand 204:471, 1978.
24. Czarniecki CW, Fennie CW: Potentiation of cell growth inhibitory effects with combinations of human recombinant α, β and γ interferons. Third Annual International Congress for Interferon Research (Abstract), 1982.
25. DeClercq E, Georgiades J, Edy VG, Sobis S: Effect of human and mouse interferon and of polyriboinosinic acid: polyribocytidylic acid on the growth of human fibrosarcoma and melanoma tumors in nude mice. Eur J Cancer 14:1273, 1978.
26. DeClercq E, Zhang Z-X, Huygen K: Synergism in the antitumor effects of type I and type II interferon in mice inoculated with leukemia L1210 cells. Cancer Lett 15:223, 1982.
27. Deryneck R, Leung DW, Gray PW, Goeddel DV: Human interferon γ is incoded by a single class of mRNA. Nucl Acids Res 10:3605, 1982.
28. Dukes PP, Izadi P, Ortega JA, Shore NA, Gomperts E: Inhibitory effects of interferon on mouse megakaryocytic progenitor cells in culture. Exp Hematol 8:1048, 1980.
29. Edy VG, Billiau A, DeSomer P: Comparisons of the rate of clearance of human fibroblast and leukocyte interferon from the circulatory system of rabbits. J Infect Dis 133:A18-A21, 1976.
30. Edy VG, Billiau A, DeSomer P: Non-appearance of injected fibroblast interferon in circulation. Lancet 1:451, 1978.
31. Epstein LB, Marcus SG: Review of experience with interferon and rug sensitivity testing of ovarian carcinoma in semisolid agar culture. Cancer Chemother Pharmacol 6:273, 1981.
32. Evinger M, Rubinstein M, Pestka S: Antiproliferative and antiviral activities of human leukocyte interferons. Arch Biochem Biophys 210:319, 1981.
33. Evinger M, Maeda S, Pestka S: Recombinant human leukocyte interferon produced in bacteria has antiproliferative activity. J Biol Chem 256:2113, 1981.
34. Farrar WL, Johnson HM, Farrar JJ: Regulation of the production of immune interferon and cytotoxic T lymphocytes by interleukin 2. J Immunol 126:1120, 1980.
35. Fidler I: Therapy of spontaneous metastases by intravenous injection of liposomes containing lymphokines. J Science 208:1469, 1980.
36. Fidler IJ, Sone S, Fogler WE, Barnes ZL: Eradication of spontaneous metastases and activation of alveolar macrophages by intravenous injection of liposomes containing muramyl dipeptide. Proc Natl Acad Sci USA 78:1680, 1981.
37. Fleischman WR, Kleyn KM, Baron S: Potentiation of antitumor effect of virus-induced interferon by mouse immune interferon preparations. J Natl Cancer Inst 65:963, 1980.
38. Glasgow AH, Nimberg RB, Menzoian JO, Saporoschetz I, Cooperband SR, Schmidt K, Mannick JA: Association of energy with an immunosuppressive peptide fraction in the serum of patiens with cancer. N Engl Med 291:1263, 1974.
39. Glasgow LA: Leukocytes and interferon in the host response to viral infections. II. Enhanced interferon response of leukocytes from immune animals. J Bacteriol 91:2185, 1966.
40. Golub SH, Dorey F, Hara D, Morton DL, Burk MW: Systemic administration of human leukocyte interferon to melanoma patients. I. Effects on natural killer function and cell populations. J Natl Cancer Inst 68:703, 1982.
41. Grant S, Bhalla K, Weinstein JB, Pestka S, Fisher PB: Differential effect of recombinant human leukocyte interferon on leukemic and normal myeloid progenitor cells. Biochem Biophys Res Commun 108:1048, 1982.
42. Gresser I, Bourali C: Inhibition by interferon preparations of a solid malignant tumor and pulmonary metastasis in mice. Nature (New Biol) 236:78, 1972.

43. Gresser I, Bourali C: Antitumor effects of interferon in mice. J Natl Cancer Inst 45:365, 1970.
44. Gresser I, Tovey MG: Antitumor effects of interferon. Biochim Biophys Acta 516:231, 1978.
45. Gresser I, Bourali C, Levy JP: Increased survival of mice inoculated with tumor cells and treated with interferon preparations. Proc Natl Acad Sci USA 63:51-57, 1969.
46. Gresser I, Maury C, Brouty-Boye D: On the mechanism of the antitumor effect of interferon in mice. Nature 239:167, 1972.
47. Gresser I, Maury C, Tovey M, Morel-Maroger L, Pontillion F: Progressive glomerulonephritis in mice treated with interferon preparations at birth. Nature 263:420, 1976.
48. Gresser I, Guy-Grand D, Maury C, Maunoury M-T: Interferon induced peripheral lymphadenopathy in mice. J Immunol 127:1569, 1981.
49. Gresser I, Bandu M-T, Brouty-Boye D: Interferon and cell division. IX. Interferon-resistant L1210 cells: Characteristics and origin. J Natl Cancer Inst 52:553, 1974.
50. Gresser I, DeMaeyer-Guignard J, Tovey MG, DeMaeyer E: Electrophoretically pure mouse interferon exerts multiple biological effects. Proc Natl Acad Sci USA 76:5308, 1979.
51. Gresser I, Aguet M, Morel-Maroger L, Woodrow D, Puvion-Dutilleul F, Grillon JC, Maury C: Electrophorectically pure mouse interferon inhibits growth, induces liver and kidney lesions, and kills suckling mice. Am J Pathol 102:396, 1981.
52. Gresser I, Tovey MG, Maury C, Chouroulinkov I: Lethality of interferon preparations for newborn mice. Nature 258:76, 1975.
53. Gutterman JU, Fine S, Quesada J, Horning SJ, Levine JF, Aleranian R, Bernhardt L, Kramer M, Speigel H, Colburn W, Trown P, Merigan T, Diewanowski Z: Recombinant leukocyte A interferon: Pharmacokinetics, single-dose tolerance and biologic effects in cancer patients. Ann Intern Med 96:549, 1982.
54. Gutterman JU, Rios A, Quesada JR, Rosenblum M: Partially pure human immune (gamma) interferon: A phase I pharmacological study in cancer patients. Abstract Third Annual Congress for Interferon Research, 1982.
55. Gutterman JU, Fine S, Quesada J, Horning SJ, Levine JF, Aleranian R, Bernhardt L, Kramer M, Speigel H, Colburn W, Trown P, Merigan T, Diewanowska Z: Recombinant leukocyte A interferon: pharmacokinetics, single-dose tolerance and biologic effects in cancer patients. Ann Intern Med 96:549, 1982.
56. Hanna N, Fidler IJ: Role of natural killer cells in the destruction of circulating tumor emboli. J Natl Cancer Inst 65:801, 1980.
57. Hellstrom KE, Hellstrom J: Immunologic enhancement of tumor growth. In: Mechanisms of Tumor Immunity, Green J, Cohen S, McCluskey R, (eds). New York: Wiley and Sons, Inc, p 147, 1977.
58. Heremans H, Billian A, Colombatti C, Hilgers J, DeSomer P: Interferon treatment of NZB mice: Accelerated progression of autoimmune disease. Infect Immun 21:925, 1978.
59. Hibbs JB, Chapman HA, Weinberg JB: The macrophage as an antineoplastic surveillance cell: Biologic perspectives. J Reticuloendothelial Soc 24:549, 1978.
60. Ho M: Recent advances in the study of interferon. Pharmacol Rev 34:119, 1982.
61. Horoszewicz JS, Leong SS, Ito M, Buffet RF, Karakousi C, Holyoke E, Job L, Dolen JG, Carter WA: Human fibroblast interferon in human neoplasia: Clinical and laboratory study. Cancer Treatm Rep 62:1899, 1978.
62. Ikic D, Kirhmajer V, Maricic Z, Jusic D, Krusic J, Knezevic M, Rode B, Soos E: Application of human leukocyte interferon in patients with carcinoma of the uterine cervix. Lancet 1:1027, 1981.
63. Ikic D, Maricic Z, Oresic V, Rode B, Nola P, Smudj K, Knezevic M, Jusic D: Application

236

of human leukocyte interferon in patients with urinary bladder papillomatosis, breast cancer and melanoma. Lancet 1:1022, 1981.
64. Ikic P, Singer Z, Beck M, Soos E, Sips DJ, Jusic D: Interferon treatment of uterine cervical precancerosis. J Cancer Res Clin Oncol 101:303, 1981.
65. Isaacs A, Lindenmann J: Virus interference: The interferon. Proc Royal Soc B147:258, 1957.
66. Johnson HM, Stanton JG, Baron S: Relative ability of mitogens to stimulate production of interferon by lymphoid cells and to induce suppression of the in vitro immune response (39622). Proc Soc Exp Biol Med 154:138, 1977.
67. Kadmon D, Shapiro A, Catalona WJ, Heston WDW, Oakley D, Ratliff TL: Effect of interferon gamma on the growth of the mouse bladder tumor, MBT-2, as determined by a clonogenic assay (submitted).
68. Kasai J, Leclerc JC, McVay-Boudreau L, Shen FW, Cantor H: Direct evidence that natural killer cells in non-immune spleen cell populations prevent tumor growth in vivo. J Exp Med 149:1260, 1979.
69. Kassel RL, Pascan PR, Vas A: Interferon-mediated oncolysis in spontaneous murine leukemia. J Natl Cancer Inst 48:1155, 1972.
70. Kawase I, Urdel DL, Brooks CG, Henney CS: Selective depletion of NK cell activity in vivo and its effect on the growth of NK-sensitive and NK-resistant tumor cell variants. Int J Cancer 29:567, 1982.
71. Knezevic M, Rode B, Knezevic-Krivak S, Ikic D, Maricic Z, Krusic J, Padovan I, Nola P, Brodarec I, Jusic D, Soos E: Histopathologic and histoenzymatic observations in carcinomas treated with human leukocyte interferon. Int J Clin Pharm Ther Tox 20:27, 1982.
72. Krim M: Towards tumor therapy with interferons. Part I. Interferons: production and properties. Blood 55:711, 1980.
73. Krusic J, Kirhmajer V, Knezevic M, Skic D, Maricic Z, Rode B, Jusic D, Soos E: Influence of human leukocyte interferon on squamous cell carcinoma of uterine cervix: Clinical, histological and histochemical observations. J Cancer Res Clin Oncol 101:309, 1981.
74. Lambert PH, Dixon FJ: Pathogenesis of the glomerulonephritis of NZB/W mice. J Exp Med 127:507, 1968.
75. Leandersson T, Lundgren E: Antiproliferative effect of interferon on a Burkitt's lymphoma cell line. Exp Cell Res 130:421, 1980.
76. Lee SHS, Epstein LB: Reversible inhibition by interferon of the maturation of human peripheral blood monocytes to macrophages. Cell Immunol 50:177, 1980.
77. Ludwig H, Swetly P: In vitro inhibitory effect of interferon on colony formation of myeloma stem cells. Cancer Immunol Immunother 9:139, 1980.
78. Lutton JD, Levere RD: Suppressive effects of human interferon on erythroid colony growth in disorders of erythropoiesis. J Lab Clin Med 96:328, 1980.
79. Madajewicz S, Creaven P, Ozer H, O'Malley J, Grossmayer B, Pontes E, Mittelman A, Soloman J, Ferraresi R: A phase I study of rising doses of recombinant DNAα2 interferon from E. coli. Abstract Third Annual International Congress on Interferon Research, 1982.
80. Maricic Z, Nola P, Skic C, Smudj K, Oresic V, Knezevic M, Rode B, Jusic D, Soos E: Human leukocyte interferon in therapy of patients with urinary bladder papillomatosis, breast cancer and melanoma. J Cancer Res Clin Oncol 101:317, 1981.
81. Mastrangelo MJ, Berd D, Bellet RE: Critical review of previously reported clinical trials of cancer immunotherapy with non-specific immunostimulants. Ann NY Acad Sci 277:94, 1976.
82. McPherson TA, Tan YH: Phase I pharmacotoxicology study of human fibroblast interferon in human cancers. J Natl Cancer Inst 65:75, 1980.

83. Mogensen KE, Bandu M-T, Vignaux F, Aguet M, Gresser I: Binding of ^{125}I-labeled human α interferon to human lymphoid cells. Int J Cancer 28:575, 1981.

84. Morel-Maroger L: Glomerular lesions induced by interferon. Transplant Proc 14:499, 1982.

85. Moss J, Woodrow DF, Sloper JC, Riviere Y, Grillon JC, Gresser I: Interferon as a cause of endoplasmic reticulum abnormalities within hepatocytes in newborn mice. Br J Exp Pathol 63:43, 1982.

86. Murphy GP: Current report on the interferon program at Roswell Park Memorial Institute. J Surg Oncol 17:99, 1981.

87. Ortega JA, Ma A, Shore NA, Dukes PP, Merigan TC: Suppressive effects of interferon on erythroid cell proliferation. Exp Hematol 7:145, 1979.

88. Osther K, Hill NO: Personal communication.

89. Osther K, Salford LG, Hornmark-Stenstam B, Flodgren P, Christopherson IS, Magnusson et al.: In: The Biology of the Interferon System, DeMaeyer E, Galasso G, Schellekens H (eds). Amsterdam: Elsevier/North Holland Biomedical Press, pp 415-419, 1981.

90. Pacini A, Bocci V, Muscettola M, Panlesu L, Pessina GP, Russi M: In: Interferon: Properties and Clinical Uses, Khan A, Hill NO, Dorn GL (eds). Dallas, Texas: Leland Fikes Foundation Press, pp 291-298, 1979.

91. Panniers LRV, Clemens MJ: Inhibition of cell division by interferon: changes in cell cycle characteristics and in morphology of Ehrlich ascites tumour cells in culture. J Cell Sci 48:259, 1981.

92. Paucker K, Cantell K, Henle W: Quantitative studies on viral interference in suspended L cells. III. Effect of interfering viruses and interferon on the growth rate of cells. Virology 17:324, 1962.

93. Priestman TJ, Lucken RN, Finter NB: Toxicity of inferferon. Br Med J 283:562, 1981.

94. Quesada JR, Swanson DA, Trindade A, Gutterman JU: Renal cell carcinoma: Antitumor effects of leukocyte interferon. Cancer Res 43:940, 1983.

95. Rohatiner AZS, Balkwill FR, Griffin DB, Malpas JS, Lister TA: A phase I study of human lymphoblastoid interferon administered by continuous intravenous infusion. Cancer Chemother Pharmacol 9:97, 1982.

96. Sarkar FH: Pharmacokinetic comparison of leukocyte and Escherichia coli derived human interferon type alpha. Antiviral Res 2:103-106, 1982.

97. Scorticatti CH, De La Pena NC, Bellora OA, Mariotto RA, Casabe AR, Comolli R: Systemic IFN-alpha treatment of multiple bladder papilloma grade I or II patients: Pilot study. J Interferon Res 2:339, 1982.

98. Senik A, Stefanos S, Kolb JP, Lucero M, Falcoff E: Enhancement of mouse natural killer cell activity by type II interferon. Ann Immunol (Inst Pasteur) 131C:349, 1980.

99. Sergiescu D, Cerutti I, Kahan A, Pialier D, Efthymiou E: Isoprinosine delays the early appearance of autoimmunity in (NZB/NZW)F₁ mice treated with interferon. Clin Exp Immunol 43:36, 1981.

100. Sergriescu D, Cerutti I, Efthymiore E, Kahan A, Chany C: Adverse effects of interferon treatment on the life span of NZB mice. Biomed 31:48, 1979.

101. Sherwin SA, Knost JA, Fein S, Abrams PG, Foon KA, Ochs JJ, Schoenberger C, Maluish AE, Oldham RK: A multiple-dose phase I trial of recombinant leukocyte A interferon in cancer patients. J Am Med Assoc 248:2461, 1982.

102. Smedley H, Kartrak M, Sikora K, Wheeler T: Neurological effects of recombinant human interferon. Br Med J 286:262, 1983.

103. Sonnenfeld G, Mandell AD, Merigan TC: The immunosuppressive effect of type II mouse interferon preparations on antibody production. Cell Immunol 34:193, 1977.

104. Stackpole C, Jacobson J: Escape from immune destruction. In: Handbook of Cancer Immunology, Waters H (ed). New York: Garland Publishing, Inc, p 55, 1978.

238

105. Stewart II WE: In: The Interferon System. New York, NY: Springer-Verlag, 1979.
106. Taetle R, Buick RN, McCulloch EA: Effect of interferon on colony formation in culture by blast cell progenitors in acute myeloblastic leukemia. Blood 56:549, 1980.
107. Taramelli D, Holden HT, Varesio L: In vitro induction of tumoricidal and suppressor macrophages by lymphokines: possible feedback regulation. J Immunol 126:2123, 1981.
108. Tomita Y, Cantell K, Kuwata T: Effects of human gamma interferon on cell growth, replication of virus and induction of 2′-5′-oligo-adenylate synthetase in three human lymphoblastoid cell lines and K562 cells. Int J Cancer 30:161, 1982.
109. Tsuruo T, Vida H, Tsukazoski S, Oku T, Kishida T: Different susceptibilities of cultures mouse cell lines to mouse interferon. Gann 73:42, 1982.
110. Tyring S, Klimpel GP, Fleischmann WR, Baron S: Direct cytolysis by partially-purified preparations of immune interferon. Int J Cancer 30:59, 1982.
111. Verma DS, Spitzer G, Gutterman JU, Beran M, Zander AR, McCredie KB: Human leukocyte interferon-mediated granulopoietic differentiation arrest and its abrogation by lithium carbonate. Am J Hematol 12:39, 1982.
112. Verma DS, Spitzer G, Zander AR, Gutterman JU, McCredie KB, Dicke KA, Johnston DA: Human leukocyte interferon preparation-mediated block of granulopoietic differentiation in vitro. Exp Hematol 9:63, 1981.
113. Von Hoff DD, Gutterman J, Portnoy B, Coltman CA Jr: Activity of human leukocyte interferon in a human tumor cloning system. Cancer Chemother Pharmacol 8:99, 1982.
114. Wallach D, Fellous M, Revel M: Preferential effect of gamma interferon on the synthesis of HLA antigens and their mRNAs in human cells. Nature 299:833, 1982.
115. Warren SL: Practitioner's guide to interferon. Ann Allergy 45:37, 1980.
116. Wheelock EF: Interferon-like virus inhibitor induced in human leukocytes by phytohemagglutinin. Science 169:310, 1965.
117. Zhang Z-X, DeClercq E, Heremans H, Verhaegen-Lewalle M, Content J: Antiviral and anticellular activities of human and murine type I and type II interferons in human cells monosomic, disomic and trisomic for chromosome 21. Proc Soc Exp Biol Med 170:103, 1982.

Editorial Comment

MATHILDE KRIM

That '... a considerable amount of work remains to define the role of IFN in tumor therapy' is the appropriate, immediate conclusion to be derived from an examination of the little that is known today about interferons in human cancer, including urological cancer. Having acknowledged this, it is nevertheless of interest to reflect further on the three following questions:
1. Do the properties of interferons make them a possible new modality for the treatment of urological cancer?
2. If so, what relative priority should be given to the development of therapy with interferons?
3. Do urological cancers present certain advantages as tumor systems in which to study the antitumor effects of interferons?

This Editorial Comment attempts to address these three questions, using the good general review of Drs Ratliff, Shapiro and Catalona as background information, and some additional data for the sake of either completeness or discussion.

1. ARE INTERFERONS A POSSIBLE NEW THERAPEUTIC MODALITY FOR UROLOGICAL CANCER?

As reported by the above-mentioned reviewers, all interferons have the capacity of reducing the rate of cell multiplication in vitro and in vivo although susceptibility to this effect varies greatly among cells [8]. It should be pointed out that this occurs in normal as well as in tumor cells, the effect being only better documented in the latter since tumor cells are easily propagated as continuous cell lines, or as transplantable tumors in animals. Suppression of the growth of normal cells, detectable in vitro [8, 59] and first demonstrated in vivo through the inhibition of liver regeneration in partially hepatectomized rats [26], is believed to be the cause, at least in part, of the transient leukopenia, moderate hair loss and gastrointestinal symptoms observed in patients receiving high dose interferon therapy [38, 84]. It has not been feasible to assess whether tumor cells are *relatively* more susceptible than normal cells to growth inhibition by interferons because it is difficult, if at all possible, to propagate in vitro, for valid comparisons, the true normal counterparts of established tumor cell lines. Also, what relative importance tumor cell growth inhibition has, per se – i.e. as measured in vitro – on tumor inhibition by interferons in vivo is still largely unknown, although, under certain in vitro conditions, growth-inhibited tumor cells have been shown to die, while normal cells did not [101]. Similarly, it cannot yet be assumed that the inhibition, by human interferons, of the growth of human tumor cells xenografted in the athymic 'nude' mouse is predictive of clinical response [4]. This animal has a fully active natural cytotoxicity system which may be activated by the presence of tumor cells and contribute to their suppression [73]. Interferon-induced inhibition of colony formation by tumor cells in semi-solid culture media [76, 107] has also still uncertain predictive value. Thus, it is not yet possible to assess the potential of interferons as antitumor agents in human urological cancer using cells derived from urological tumors in any of these assays. Systematic in vitro/in vivo comparative studies should be done in order to verify the predictive value and the potentially important practical use of these assay systems.

There is somewhat circuitous, but nevertheless suggestive, evidence that inhibition of tumor cell growth alone can translate into in vivo antitumor activity. Interferon-induced inhibition of cell growth is – as is the interferon-induced antiviral state of cells – generally associated with increased activity of the enzyme 2′-5′ oligo(A)synthetase [82] and an inhibition of the activity of the enzymes ornithine decarboxylase and S-adenosylmethionine decarboxylase [93]. These enzymes are required for the synthesis of polyamines which are abundant in rapidly dividing cells, particularly neoplastic cells, and are necessary for their continuous proliferation [69]. The drug α-difluoromethylornithine (DFMO) blocks irreversibly the activity of ornithine decarboxylase, the first and rate-limiting enzyme in the synthesis of polyamines [64]. DFMO inhibited the proliferation of certain cultured human cancer cells [53] and, in combination with methylglyoxal (bis)guanylhydrazone, an inhibitor of S-adenosylmethionine decarboxylase, DFMO was capable of inducing remissions in children with leukemia [85]. When murine interferon and DFMO were used in combination, they completely inhibited the growth of murine B16 melanoma cells grown either in vitro or as transplantable tumors in C57/BL mice, while either agent alone was only partially effective [94]. Thus, a drug, DFMO, inhibitory of cell growth through a biochemical pathway also used by interferons, is capable of at least partial tumor suppression in vivo, and its effect has been much enhanced by combination with interferon. Cell growth inhibition alone appears to be able to account for DFMO's in vivo antitumor effect. The same may conceivably be true for interferons.

However, growth inhibition is certainly not the only direct effect of interferons on cells and, specifically, on tumor cells. Other effects, which may also be of considerable importance, have generally received less attention. This has also been the case in the above review. These are the interferons' intriguing effects on cell membranes, cytoskeletal structures and the transformed or malignant phenotype itself: murine and human interferons have been shown to modify cell structure and behavior and, in particular, to suppress the ability, typical of tumor cells, to grow either in a multilayered and irregular fashion on solid surfaces [54], or to form colonies in semi-solid media [9–11, 14, 15, 29, 45]. These phenomena may be associated with, but appear distinct from, growth inhibition, i.e., the slowing down of the rate of cell multiplication.

When transformed murine cells were propagated as monolayers in the presence of homologous interferon, not only did they regain 'contact inhibition', but they became incapable of growing as colonies in semi-solid media, and, when inoculated into animals, they had lost their previous tumorigenicity. They behaved, in fact, very much like non-transformed cells [9–11]. Human fibroblasts and HeLa tumor cells were also altered in their phenotype by interferon treatment in vitro in such ways (increased organization of actin-containing microfilaments, decreased motility and proliferation) as to acquire a more 'normal' phenotype [97]. Interestingly, in murine cells transformed by bovine papilloma virus (BPV), phenotypic reversion induced by interferon was accompanied by a reduction in the amount of extra-chromosomal BPV DNA and the 'cure' of some cells of such DNA [104].

Interferons can have still other direct effects on tumor cells, such as could also modify the tumor–host relationship: they can enhance or inhibit the production of various classes of pharmacologically active cell products, e.g. hormones [13], prostaglandins [20, 111], plasminogen activator [78], and histamine [49]. In addition, interferon treatment in vitro has been shown to enhance the expression of Fcγ receptors [2, 28] and of HLA antigens and associated β_2 microglobulin [24, 41], all of which could facilitate immune recognition and a host response to the presence of aberrant, virus-infected or neoplastic cells. In short, interferons can have, in vitro and in vivo, many direct effects on tumor cells which could account for an interferon-induced modification of the natural course of neoplastic disease.

As has been reported in the above review, interferons also have, when administered in vivo, a spectrum of effects on the cells of the tumor-bearing host. That such activities are likely to contribute importantly to an inhibition of tumor development and progression is apparent from the in vivo suppression, by interferon, of the growth of transplantable murine lymphoma cells previously selected in vitro for complete resistance to interferon's antiviral and growth inhibitory action [1, 33, 35]. In view of this, it has been intellectually gratifying to know that, at least in vitro, interferons could stimulate the cytotoxicity of sensitized T lymphocytes [58], recruit pre-NK cells to maturity [75, 98] and enhance both NK cell killing [40, 103] and killing and phagocytosis of tumor cells by macrophages [79, 80]. Interferon type α was found to be actually produced, in vitro, by large granular lymphocytes (LGLs) (a population of peripheral blood lymphocytes which includes NK cells) when they come into contact with tumor cells [19, 103]. In what appears to be an interesting positive feedback mechanism, this IFNα in turn activates the interferon-producing cells to more effective killing. Furthermore, in the same experimental system, interferon was found to protect normal cells from indiscriminate NK cytotoxicity, thus perhaps rendering NK cytotoxicity both more efficient and more specific [102].

The discovery of the existence of host defense mechanisms against tumor cells, and of these defenses' stimulation by interferons, appeared to vindicate a widespread belief in a host response to autochtonous tumors and to offer a satisfying explanation for the host-mediated antitumor effects of exogenous interferons. A voluminous literature has accumulated over the last few years on interferons and cell-mediated cytotoxicity. Regrettably, it has been difficult to demonstrate that NK- or monocyte-macrophage activation does indeed play a role in the interferons' antitumor effect in vivo. In particular, no correlation could be found between NK cell activation, when demonstrable, and clinical response [22, 30]. It is not even generally agreed that NK cell activation always occurs, in vivo, upon interferon administration [62], or that, when it occurs, it can be effective against autologous tumor cells [106]. These questions remains to this day a subject of debate. It is possible that, depending on the dose, interferon may enhance or suppress NK cytotoxicity [55]. There have been few studies, particularly in man, on the effects of interferons on monocyte-macrophage activation, although such could be detected in the course of interferon treatment [99]. Even fewer studies have attempted to examine the effect of interferon treatment on tumor-infiltrating lymphocyte and macrophage cell populations, whose cytotoxicity is probably much more directly relevant to the fate of the tumor than that of circulating cells [108]. It is clear that much work remains to be done [87].

What conclusions can be derived today regarding *how* interferons operate as antitumor agents? It seems obvious, first of all, that they do so through a variety of complex mechanisms [31, 32]. This should not be surprising since even their better understood antiviral activity is also mediated through several intracellular biochemical pathways which either independently, or in concert, achieve the blocking of viral multiplication [82]; in addition, an interferon-induced activation of cytotoxic cells could play a role in host-mediated attack, and elimination, of virus-infected cells [77]. Nevertheless, a continuing inability to understand how treatment with interferons can achieve tumor suppression still undermines confidence in the interferons' potential as antitumor agents.

If such an understanding, and, therefore, rational use of interferons as antitumor agents are still elusive, can one derive at least some encouragement from empirical evidence, such as has been obtained so far from the administration of interferon preparations to tumor-bearing animals and humans? There can be no doubt that this is entirely justified.

Murine interferon preparations have had effects on many types of mouse tumors such as to establish unequivocally their antitumor activity [31, 32, 34]. In fact, when their efficacy is compared to that of drugs on the basis of activity per unit weight of active material, they prove to be powerful antitumor agents [36]. Similarly, in man, some impressive tumor regressions have been reported in adults given daily doses of 3 million units of interferon. Because of the very high specific activity of all interferons (10^8 to 10^9 units/mg protein), this represents only 50–500 nanograms (or $50-500 \times 10^{-6}$ mg) interferon protein per kg body weight, i.e. a much lesser amount of active substance than required for antitumor activity by any chemotherapeutic drug.

In assessing the potential of interferon therapy in human cancer, it is first of all necessary to keep in mind that clinical investigations with interferons are still at a very early stage. Phase I trials have barely been completed with natural IFNα (derived from suspensions of human leukocytes or cultured lymphoblastoid cells) and with IFNαA and α_2 (each produced by a cloned recombinant *E. coli*). These four types of preparations are now in early phase II trials in several benign and malignant diseases. They are still usually administered as single therapy, at doses that span a wide range from clearly insufficient to excessive (in the last case for being not only barely tolerable but clearly beyond the dose likely to produce optimal biologic response modification). IFNβ and γ have not as yet been systematically studied in the clinic. Except for anecdotal evidence of their also having antitumor activity in man, their relative effectiveness or their selectivity as antitumor agents cannot even be approximated. In short, today's evidence is limited to the sum total of results achieved with preparations of IFNα used as single therapy, for the most part in heavily pre-treated patients who have advanced disease. In these early phase I and II trials, a variety of mostly empirical doses and regimens of treatment were used, most of which were clearly not optimal. In this situation, it is quite misleading to compare – as has unfortunately often been done – the present efficacy of interferon treatment to that of the best established therapies. A fair comparison would be between the known efficacy of IFNα preparations and that of active drugs *at a similar stage of their development*. This was recently done by Dr Robert K. Oldham, of the Division of Cancer Treatment, NCI.* He reported that the history of chemotherapeutic agents has followed a consistent pattern. Upon emerging from successful screening in animal tumor models, i.e. when in clinical phase I trials, the most promising drugs elicited only rare, if any, partial responses (PR, i.e. >50% tumor shrinkage). It has generally been only in phase II trials, following definition of a maximum tolerable dose and of an appropriate schedule of administration, that a few PRs were observed. Combination of the new experimental drug with other active agents progressively lead to an increase in the frequency of PRs and the occurrence of some complete responses (CR, i.e. complete disappearance of all measurable disease). If, upon further refinements in the regimen of treatment and drug combinations, the rate of PRs plus CRs ('response rate') could be raised to 25% or better, then true benefit to some patients did result in the form of significant prolongation of survival and even some 'cures' (>5 year disease-free survival). The complete process required many years of work for each active compound developed, even when this could be done under conditions of no shortage of drug. Clinical investigations with interferons have, until very recently, been plagued by acute shortages of interferon preparations.

Oldham further stated that, historically, active chemotherapeutic agents have achieved a response rate of only 0 to 10% in phase I trials. Under the same trial conditions, and using the same stringent criteria of response (≥50% decrease in tumor load), IFNα has achieved a 10%, or better, rate of response. When the broadly and highly active adriamycin was used as single agent

* Presentation at an Interferon Workshop sponsored by the Office of Biologicals, Food and Drug Administration; the National Cancer Institute and the Institute for Allergy and Infectious Diseases, NIH; and the WHO Collaborating Center for Interferon Reference and Research. September 28–30, 1983, Bethesda, Maryland.

in phase II trials, it achieved a response rate of 25 to 40% and this in only some diseases. Results were poorer in others. IFNα appears to have, as does adriamycin, a broad spectrum of activity, and some selectivity. However, the overall rate of response achieved through IFNα's use as single agent in phase II trials was better than for adriamycin. It has not only been, on average, higher, but IFNα elicited less severe and moreover completely and rapidly reversible side effects.

The tumors which appear so far most responsive to IFNα treatment are, perhaps not surprisingly, benign tumors such as juvenile laryngeal papilloma and several types of warts. In them, interferon-induced regression has been the rule rather than the exception. Furthermore, complete regressions could be achieved in these diseases with very low doses of interferon given parenterally [5, 39, 68, 105], which elicited either no or inconsequential side effects. Systemic treatment of benign diseases with a significantly toxic drug such as adriamycin could not even be contemplated.

In malignant diseases, a rate of response to IFNα reaching 50–65% was reported by several investigators in various non-Hodgkin's lymphomas [25, 47, 60] and it could be even higher in certain leukemias [46], particularly chronic myelogenous leukemia [95, 96], and hairy cell leukemia [37, 71]. The overall rate of response of various solid malignant tumors has, so far, been less, although for malignant melanoma it is as good or better than that obtained with chemotherapy [17, 23, 56]. Colon and lung carcinomas appear relatively resistant to interferon treatment, as they are to chemotherapeutic drugs. Nevertheless – and of particular relevance to this Editorial Comment – there are now several reports of an encouraging rate of response to IFNα in another solid tumor, metastatic renal cell carcinoma, a disease notoriously resistant to chemo- and other therapies [63]. In very recent trials, certain IFNα preparations have induced regressions of metastatic lesions at a rate higher than can be achieved with other modalities of treatment [57, 72].

As related in the review by Ratliff et al., responses have also been obtained in small groups of patients with bladder papillomatosis and transitional cell cancer that have been treated with IFNα preparations [3, 16, 46, 50, 67, 81]. If this evidence appears at present still scant, it is because very few patients were actually so treated, rather than because response rates were low.

Minor responses seen under phase I trial conditions in a few cases of advanced (stage 4D) prostate cancer [61; Gutterman, 1983, personal communication] have so far not encouraged phase II trials. In this disease, response rate data is therefore lacking altogether.

Thus, results in urologic tumors are still few but they are clearly encouraging, given the early stage of clinical research with IFNα. It is noteworthy that many patients who had received prior treatment with other modalities could still respond to interferon treatment. This suggests that any benefits patients may derive from interferon therapy could be additional to those derived from other modalities of treatment.

In answer to our first question, it can therefore be reasonably stated that: (a) the interferons' direct and host-mediated effects on tumor cells have not been proven to cause tumor inhibition or regression but they are consistent with such activities in vivo; (b) like murine interferons, human interferons have had unquestionable tumor inhibitory activity when administered to patients with various types of benign and malignant diseases, including solid metastatic tumors; these have included major types of urologic tumors. Even at this early stage of their evaluation as antitumor agents, when used as single therapy, interferons are generally as or more effective than were some of the most active therapeutic drugs at a similar stage of their development.

For these reasons, interferons can be considered to have distinct promise as active agents with broad spectrum antitumor activity which encompasses urologic malignancies. However, to date, the interferons' optimal efficacy – in terms of rate, extent and duration of induced responses – is still uncertain for any disease, even for IFNα used as single therapy. The necessary further clinical investigations must be guided by intensive laboratory studies required to gain an understanding of the mechanisms underlying the interferons' antitumor effect, so as to ensure their future rational and maximally effective application.

2. WHAT RELATIVE PRIORITY SHOULD BE GIVEN TO THE STUDY OF INTERFERON THERAPY FOR UROLOGICAL CANCER?

The question must take into consideration tumor type and stage as well as the relative promise of other new therapeutic approaches.

Although this writer does not pretend to be able to evaluate all possible new approaches to the therapy of urological cancer, it seems to her that presently used systemic modalities of treatment – hormones and chemotherapy – have failed, so far, to have a significant impact on the natural course of advanced disease. With them, in addition to surgery and radiation, foreseeable advances will likely consist of incremental benefits derived from both earlier and more accurate diagnosis, refinements in treatment combinations, and their more aggressive and widespread use.

A search for new chemotherapeutic agents, or else other new modalities of systemic treatment, is clearly in order. Biological therapies are attractive because immunological factors seem to play a role in the occurrence and progression of all three major types of urological cancer, namely kidney, bladder and prostate [42]. In addition, though rarely, remissions have occurred spontaneously in urological cancer [27, 43, 88], and immunological approaches to treatment have, sometimes, resulted in prolongation of survival [21, 83], all of which suggests that the tumor-host relationship can sometimes be tipped by host-mediated mechanisms in favor of host survival. What has already been achieved with IFNα clearly suggests that this particular approach to biological therapy warrants being pursued.

In metastatic renal cell cancer, responses to IFNα were seen in phase I trials [47, 61] and several recent phase II trials which used preparations from different sources as single therapy and at relatively low doses, concur in reporting a response rate which may already be equal or superior to that achieved with presently available chemotherapy [57, 71, 72]. There is a distinct possibility, as is generally true with chemotherapeutic drugs, that enhanced therapeutic efficacy will be achieved not only through optimizing doses and regimens of treatment but through future combination therapies including interferons. Furthermore, since there is experimental evidence in tumor-bearing animals that the effectiveness of biological response modifiers is inversely proportional to tumor load, it is perhaps already justified to contemplate adjuvant therapy with IFNα in two thirds of the renal cancer patients who do not present with metastases and will have minimal tumor load after nephrectomy. Low doses of natural IFNα used as adjuvant therapy in human osteogenic sarcoma appear to have doubled the number of long-term (> 5 years) disease-free survivors as compared to a group of contemporary controls treated with surgery alone [91, 92].

Although, when initially seen, superficial papillomas and transitional cell carcinomas of the bladder should be curable by simple transurethral resection, accurate staging of the disease is difficult and has often lead to inappropriate therapy. Among patients who develop invasive tumors, about two thirds die of distant metastases within less than two years [86]. Partial or complete regressions of bladder papillomas have been obtained as a result of systemic [3, 16, 46, 67] or intralesional [50] treatment with natural IFNα preparations. The significance of these limited observations is strengthened by results previously obtained in controlled trials in bladder cancer which involved the use of compounds known to be inducers of interferons. The double-stranded synthetic ribonucleic acid Poly I · C is an efficient interferon inducer in vitro and in animals, including – though to a much lesser extent – in man [112]. Selected patients with bladder tumors (papillomas, carcinoma in situ, and low grade, low stage bladder tumors) were randomized to receive standard treatment with or without Poly I · C (25 μg/kg, i.v., every two weeks, for one year). All patients had been rendered grossly free of disease by trans-urethral resection and/or fulguration, procedures which were repeated when necessary in order to maintain a very low tumor load. Results gave no evidence of an effect of Poly I · C on the natural history of the disease per se, but the four year survival rate was significantly better in the group of 18 patients who had received Poly I · C than among 15 placebo-treated controls [51].

BCG has been studied extensively for the treatment of bladder cancer [83]. A recent prospective, randomized trial has confirmed earlier results in demonstrating that fulguration and intravesical BCG resulted in fewer tumors and more prolonged disease-free intervals than fulguration alone [70]. Whether Poly I · C and BCG are active agents in this disease because they are interferon inducers is not known. Whatever the case, these studies show that certain biological response modifiers can be effective when administered intravesically and this provides a sound rationale for the exploration of a similar topical use of interferons. A fully controlled trial of high dose intravesical IFNα$_2$ has recently been undertaken [Neri, 1983, personal communication]. If final results confirm the early impression of efficacy, treatment with intravesical interferon should be explored extensively since its simplicity, safety and lack of side effects would make it a highly desirable form of treatment for general application. IFNα, natural and produced by recombinant *E. coli*, is now available in virtually unlimited amounts for extensive clinical investigations.

In view of (a) an urgent need for new therapies in urological cancer, (b) the fact that experimental treatment with interferons is now possible on an adequate scale, and (c) that it is promising, at least in metastatic renal cell carcinoma, bladder papillomatosis and transitional cell cancer, the answer to our second question is that trials with interferons in these and perhaps other urological cancers appear to deserve a high priority.

3. DO UROLOGICAL CANCERS PRESENT CERTAIN ADVANTAGES AS TUMOR SYSTEMS IN WHICH TO STUDY THE ANTITUMOR EFFECTS OF INTERFERONS?

An answer to this question will be based on: (a) the availability, for in vitro research, of authenticated cell lines derived from animal and human urological cancers and/or the relative ease with which primary explants of tumors can generate viable tumor cells that can be maintained either in vitro or in vivo, such as in the athymic nude mouse; (b) the availability and relative convenience of good animal tumor models of human urological cancers; and, finally (c) the availability of patients with urological cancer and the accessibility of their lesions for objective measurement of responses to treatment.

Many established cell lines derived from animals and human urological tumors are readily available for in vitro studies. In some of them, sensitivity to growth inhibition by human interferon preparations has already been tested. Cultured cells (RT112) derived from a human transitional cell carcinoma [74] were studied for their sensitivity to natural human interferons of types α and β. Although IFNβ was some 10-fold more effective, both interferons were effective in decreasing the cells' growth rate [7]. Natural IFNβ also effectively inhibited their growth when these cells – or T24 cells derived from a similar human tumor [74] – were growing as xenografts in athymic nude mice [48]. Although, as discussed above, in vitro studies are not necessarily predictive of the in vivo responsiveness of human transitional cell carcinomas to interferons α and β, they at least suggest that cells derived from this type of tumor have no intrinsic resistance to the direct action of these interferons.

There exist some good animal models for renal cell carcinoma, transitional cell carcinoma of the bladder, and prostate cancer. A murine renal cell carcinoma which originated spontaneously in a Balb/C mouse [65] has the advantage of being transplantable and of metastasizing widely and reproducibly within a predictable period of time (28 days) when implanted beneath the renal capsule. Animals have palpable disease for 14 to 21 days, a length of time during which experimental treatment can be given and response followed. This animal model has been used for the evaluation of several chemotherapeutic agents [66] and more recently, for that of α-difluoromethylornithine (DFMO) which, like interferons, inhibits ornithine-decarboxylase. DFMO reduced tumor growth, prevented lung metastases, and increased survival [52]. This transplantable murine renal cell carcinoma could be very valuable in the study not only of the effects of interferons as single therapy but also in that of combinations of interferons with DFMO, other inhibitors of polyamine synthesis, or other chemotherapeutic drugs. Whether its slight immunogenicity will cause problems in the evaluation of biological response modifiers such as interferons, will have to be established. Immunogenicity in syngeneic hosts is not a rare occurrence among tumors transplanted for many years [44].

There exist several valuable inducible and transplantable animal tumor models for bladder cancer. Autochtonous tumors, induced in the experimental animal itself, are particularly interesting because they are better models of the human situation. The tumors are usually transitional cell carcinomas induced in rodents and several other species by injested carcinogens which have high specificity for the urothelium. These are N-butyl-N-(4-hydroxybutyl) nitrosamine (BBN), braken fern (BF) and N-[4-(5-nitro-2-furyl)-2-thiazolyl] formamide (FANFT) [12].

The carcinogenic effect of FANFT is reversible within a certain period of time, such as 6 weeks in the rat. Thereafter it is irreversible even if the carcinogenic stimulus is removed. Palpable tumors appear in the mouse after some 8 months and their incidence reaches up to 100% following 11 months of continuous carcinogen injestion [89]. The lesions induced have histologic features closely resembling those seen in humans. In both animals and man, they progress through hyperplasia, atypia, carcinoma in situ, and transitional cell tumor before becoming invasive and metastatic. They invariably kill the host. When malignant, the animal tumor cells are readily transplantable, and they rapidly form palpable, measurable lesions. Malignant cells can also be collected, separated by trypsinization, and implanted onto denuded murine urothelium. It has been speculated that 'seeding' of tumor cells occurs naturally in humans. It has been pointed out that if this is so, the curative potential of transurethral resection could be nullified, and there would be much added urgency to the development of effective topical and systemic therapies for the treatment of all patients, even those with low grade tumors [110]. The use of the animal model of bladder cancer would make it possible not only to determine the sensitivity of the murine tumors, at various stages, to various types of interferons, but to rapidly screen various doses, regimens, routes of administration and combination therapies. In particular, intravesical administration, which offers the advantage of delivering, with minimal systemic toxicity, active compounds at high concentration directly to the tumor, could be explored with interferons as has been done fruitfully with several drugs. For certain therapeutic agents, the animal model has reflected quite accurately the clinical efficacy of these drugs [89].

For cancer of the prostate, many animal and human cell lines which grow readily in the nude mouse [6], as well as several transplantable tumors in the rat species, are available [109]. It has been suggested that the treatment of nude mice with high titer anti-mouse interferon globulin permits biopsy material from human cancers of the prostate to be directly and successfully xenografted in the nude mouse and that the tumors so produced become invasive [73]. Scarcity of high titer anti-mouse interferon serum is probably responsible for the fact that this interesting observation has not been followed by concerted attempts at developing a system for the testing of therapies against individual prostate or other cancers in this animal.

Because human interferons are inactive in the animal species providing models of urological cancer, murine and rat interferons are required for studies with these models. Mouse and rat interferons can be produced on an adequate scale from cultured cells. They are available from a few commercial sources as extensively purified preparations. The murine α, β and γ interferons and the β interferon of the rat have also been cloned. The three types of these animals' interferons appear to have biological properties equivalent to those of the corresponding human interferons.

As for *human* urological tumors, they also lend themselves well to investigations with new modalities of treatment. Human metastatic renal cell carcinoma is a disease notorious for its resistance to available modalities but, for this very reason, it presents certain advantages for clinical research; because there is no accepted systemic therapy, randomization of trial patients can be to either drug or placebo, rather than to another treatment followed by patient crossover. The frequent localization of metastases to the lungs, where they are usually clearly visible on X-ray films, facilitates an objective evaluation of responses. Although the often erratic course of the natural metastatic disease creates a requirement for relatively large groups of patients per trial, approximately 2/3 of the estimated 17 000 new cases diagnosed each year in the United States alone develop metastases within a short time of primary surgical treatment [18]. There should, therefore, be no shortage of patients for meaningful trials. Furthermore, as mentioned above, the rate of response to IFNα treatment in metastatic renal cell carcinoma patients with good performance status [57, 71, 72] is close to, or has reached the 30% level of response considered to warrant attempts at adjuvant therapy [90]. This form of treatment could be readily tested and its effectiveness in this disease established within a relatively short time, given the availability of patients, and predictible, high-rate, early metastatic recurrence. A suggestion that – like its murine model – human renal cell carcinoma may be sensitive to inhibitors of polyamine synthesis has come from a clinical study trial using methyl-GAG to which a 16% rate of response was observed [100]. Although these results could not be confirmed in a phase II trial in advanced disease [113], methyl-GAG should still be considered, as well as DFMO, in the planning of future combination therapies involving interferons for the treatment of human metastatic renal adenocarcinoma.

Human bladder papillomatosis, bladder cancer in situ and metastatic bladder cancer, also lend themselves to many interesting investigations. Bladder papillomatosis is a relatively common, and frequently recurrent disease, particularly in patients who present with multiple tumors. A significant proportion of these patients eventually develop infiltrating bladder carcinoma, even among those treated with the best conventional surgical, radiation and chemotherapies.

Some of the advantageous features of bladder papillomatosis and cancer are that the different stages of the disease can be studied directly, through endoscopy. Lesions can be followed visually and photographically, and biopsy material can readily be obtained. Effects of treatment are measurable objectively, including modification of rate of recurrence which is often fairly characteristic over long periods of time for individual patients. Treatment can be administered systemically and/or topically. In the latter case this can be done by intravesical application, using high doses of drug with little risk of systemic toxicity. Finally, there being no standard effective therapy for the metastatic stage of the disease, experimental treatment can be given as single therapy in a non-adjuvant situation. The answer to our third question is, then, that in animals and man, several urological tumors are relatively convenient and most interesting systems in which to study interferons as a new modality of cancer treatment. They could help generate much information of general interest.

The authors of the preceeding review have noted that evaluations of the interferons' antitumor activity in man always conclude that interferons have 'antitumor potential, but...'. The only way to get rid of the 'buts' is to seize the present research opportunities. This writer hopes this will be done, so that, perhaps, in the not too distant future, the word 'potential' could also be replaced by the word 'activity' with regard to urological cancers.

248

REFERENCES

1. Aguet M: High-affinity binding of ^{125}I-labeled mouse interferon to a specific cell surface receptor. Nature 284:459-461, 1980.
2. Aguet M, Vignaux F, Fridman WH, Gresser I: Enhancement of Fc gamma receptor expression in interferon treated mice. Eur J Immunol 11:926-930, 1981.
3. Aleman C, Khan A, Hill JM, Pardue A, Hilario R, Hill NO: Response of diffuse transitional cell carcinoma to low dose interferon. 18th Annual ASCO Meeting (Abstract), 1982.
4. Balkwill FR, Moodie EM, Freedman V, Fantes KH: Human interferon inhibits the growth of established human breast tumors in the nude mouse. Int J Cancer 30:231-235, 1982.
5. Blanchet-Bardon C, Puissant A, Lutzner M, Orth G, Nutini MT, Guesry P: Interferon treatment of skin cancer in patients with epidermodysplasia verruciformis. The Lancet I:274, 1981.
6. Bogden AE: Characterization of animal tumors: Summary. In: Progress in clinical biological research, Vol. 37. Models for prostatic cancer, Murphy GP (ed). New York: Alan R, Liss Inc, pp 303-310, 1979.
7. Borden EC, Yamamoto N, Hogan TF, Edwards BF, Bryan GT: Interferons: Preclinical rationale for trials in human bladder carcinoma. In: Interferon. Properties, mode of action, production, clinical application, Munk K, Kirchner H (ed). Basel: Karger S, pp 42-52, 1982.
8. Brouty-Boye D: Inhibitory effects of interferon on cell multiplication. Lymphokine Rep 1:99-112, 1980.
9. Brouty-Boye D, Chang YS, Chen LB: Association of phenotypic reversion of transformed cells induced by interferon with morphological and biochemical changes in the cytoskeleton. Cancer Res 41:4174-4184, 1981.
10. Brouty-Boye D, Gresser I: Studies on the reversibility of the transformed and neoplastic phenotype. I. Progressive reversion of the phenotype of X-ray transformed C3H/10T$^{1/2}$ cells under prolonget treatment with interferon. Int J Cancer 28:165-173, 1981.
11. Brouty-Boye D, Puvion-Dutilleul F, Gresser I: Reversibility of the transformed and neoplastic phenotype. III. Long-term treatment with electrophoretically pure mouse interferon leads to the progressive reversion of the phenotype of X-ray transformed C3H/10T$^{1/2}$ cells. Experientia 38:1292-1296, 1982.
12. Bryan GT: The pathogenesis of experimental bladder cancer. Cancer Res 37:2813-2816, 1977.
13. Chany C, Mathieu D, Gregoire A: Induction of delta 3(4) ketosteroid synthesis by interferon in mouse adrenal tumor cell cultures. J Gen Virol 50:447-450, 1980.
14. Chany C, Rousset S, Bourgeade MF, Mathieu D, Gregoire A: Role of receptors and the cytoskeleton in reverse transformation and steroidogenesis induced by interferon. In: Regulatory functions of interferons, Vilcek J, Gresser I, Merigan TC (eds). Ann NY Acad Sci 350:254-265, 1980.
15. Chany C, Vignal M: Effect of prolonged interferon treatment on mouse embryonic fibroblasts transformed by murine sarcoma virus. J Gen Virol 7:203-210, 1970.
16. Christophersen IS, Jordal R, Osther K, Lindenberg J, Pedersen PH, Berg K: Interferon therapy in neoplastic disease. Acta Med Scand 204:471-476, 1978.
17. Creagan ET, Ahmann DL, Green SJ, Schutt AJ, Rubin J, Long HJ, Fein S, O'Fallon JR: Recombinant leukocyte A interferon (RO 22-8181; rIFN-αA) in disseminated malignant melanoma (DMM). ASCO Abstracts, p 58, 1983.
18. DeKernion JB, Ramning KP, Smith PB: The natural history of metastatic renal cell carcinoma: A computer analysis J Urol 120:148-152, 1978.

19. Djeu JY, Timonen T, Herberman RB: Augmentation of natural killer cell activity and induction of interferon by tumor cells and other biological response modifiers. In: Progress in cancer research and therapy. Mediation of cellular immunity in cancer by immune modifiers, Chrigos MA, Mitchell M, Mastrangelo MJ, Krim M, (eds). New York: Raven Press 19:161-166, 1981.

20. Dore-Duffy P, Perry W, Kuo HH: Interferon-mediated inhibition of prostaglandin synthesis in human mononuclear leukocytes. Cell Immunol 79:232-239, 1983.

21. Eidinger D, Morales A: BCG immunotherapy of metastatic adenocarcinoma of the kidney. Natl Cancer Inst Monogr 49:339-341, 1978.

22. Einhorn S, Ahre A, Blomgren H, Johansson B, Mellstedt H, Strander H: Interferon and natural killer cell activity in multiple myeloma. Lack of correlation between interferon-induced enhancement of natural killer activity and clinical response to human interferon-alpha. Int J Cancer 30:167-172, 1982.

23. Ernstoff MS, Reiss M, Davis CA, Rudnick SA, Kirkwood JM: Intravenous (i.v.) recombinant alpha-2 interferon (IFNα-2) in metastatic melanoma. ASCO Abstracts, p 57, 1983.

24. Fellous M, Kamoun M, Gresser I, Bono R: Enhanced expression of HLA antigens and beta 2-microglobulin on interferon-treated human lymphoid cells. Eur J Immunol 9:446-449, 1979.

25. Foon K (unpublished): Report of the National Biological Response Modifiers Program to NIH Interferon Workshop, September 28-30, 1983.

26. Frayssinet C, Gresser I, Tovey M, Lindahl P: Inhibitory effect of potent interferon preparations on the regenaration of mouse liver after partial hepatectomy. Nature 245:146-147, 1973.

27. Freed SZ, Halperin JP, Gordon M: Idiopathic regression of metastases from renal cell carcinoma. J Urol 118:538-542, 1977.

28. Fridman WH, Gresser I, Bandu M-T, Aguet M, Neauport-Santes C: Interferon enhances the expression of Fcγ receptors. J Immunol 124:2436-2441, 1980.

29. Glasgow LA, Crane JL Jr, Kern ER, Younger JS: Antitumor activity of interferon against murine osteogenic sarcoma in vitro and in vivo. Cancer Treat Rep 62:1881-1888, 1978.

30. Golub SH, D'Amore P, Rainey P: Systemic administration of human leukocyte interferon to melanoma patients. II. Cellular events associated with changes in natural killer cytotoxicity. J Natl Cancer Inst 68:711-717, 1982.

31. Gresser I: Antitumor effects of interferon. In: Cancer — A comprehensive treatise, Vol 5, Chemotherapy, Becker F (ed). New York: Plenum Press, pp 521-571, 1977.

32. Gresser I: How does interferon inhibit tumor growth? Phil Trans Roy Soc London B299:69-76, 1982.

33. Gresser I, Bandu M-T, Brouty-Boye D: Interferon and cell division. IX. Interferon-resistant L1210 cells: Characteristics and origin. J Natl Cancer Inst 52:553.559, 1974.

34. Gresser I, DeMaeyer-Guignard J, Tovey M, DeMaeyer E: Electrophoretically pure mouse interferon exerts multiple biological effects. Proc Natl Acad Sci USA 76:5308-5312, 1979.

35. Gresser I, Maury C, Brouty-Boye D: On the mechanism of the antitumor effect of interferon in mice. Nature 239:167-168, 1972.

36. Gresser I, Maury C, Tovey M: Interferon and murine leukemia. VII. Therapeutic effect of interferon preparations after diagnosis of lymphoma in AKR mice. Int J Cancer 17:647-653, 1976.

37. Gutterman JU (unpublished): Hairy cell leukemia. Report to NIH Interferon Workshop, September 28-30, 1983.

38. Gutterman JU, Fine S, Quesada J, Horning SJ, Levine JF, Alexanian R, Bernhardt L,

Kramer M, Speigel H, Colburn W, Trown P, Merigan T, Djewanowska Z: Recombinant leukocyte A interferon: Pharmacokinetics, single-dose tolerance and biologic effects in cancer patients. Ann Intern Med 96:549, 1982.

39. Haglund S, Lundquist PG, Cantell K, Strander H: Interferon therapy in juvenile laryngeal papillomatosis. Arch Oto Laryngol 107:327-332, 1981.

40. Herberman RB, Ortaldo JR, Riccardi C, Timonen T, Schmidt A, Maluish A, Djeu J: Interferon and NK cells. In: Interferons. UCLA Symposia on Molecular and Cellular Biology, Merigan TC, Friedman RM (eds). New York: Academic Press, pp 287-294, 1982.

41. Heron I, Hokland M, Berg K: Enhanced expression of β2-microglobulin and HLA antigens on human lymphoid cells by interferon. Proc Natl Acad Sci USA 75:6215-6219, 1978.

42. Hersch EM, Wallace S, Johnson DE, Bracken RB: Immunological studies in human urological cancer. In: Cancer of the genitourinary tract, Johnson DE, Samuels ML, (eds). New York: Raven Press, pp 47-56, 1979.

43. Hewitt CB: Renal cell carcinoma: A clinical challenge. In: Renal Neoplasia, Stanton King J Jr, (ed). Boston: Little Brown and Company, pp 3-12, 1967.

44. Hewitt HB: Animal tumor models and their relevance to human tumor immunology. J Biol Resp Mod 1:107-119, 1982.

45. Hicks NJ, Morris AG, Burke DC: Partial reversion of the transformed phenotype of murine sarcoma virus-transformed cells in the presence of interferon: A possible mechanism for the anti-tumor effect of interferon. J Cell Sci 49:225-236, 1981.

46. Hill NO, Pardue A, Khan A, Aleman C, Dorn G, Hill JM: Phase I human leukocyte interferon trials in cancer and leukemia. J Clin Hematol Oncol 11:23-35, 1981.

47. Horning S (unpublished): Lymphomas. Report to NIH Interferon Workshop, September 28-30, 1983.

48. Horoszewicz J, Leong SS, Ito M, Buffet RF, Karakousi SC, Holyoke E, Job L, Dolen JG, Carter WA: Human fibroblast interferon in human neoplasia. Cancer Treatm Rep 62:1899-1906, 1978.

49. Ida S, Hooks JJ, Siraganian RP, Notkins AL: Enhancement of IgE-mediated histamine release from human basophils by viruses: Role of interferon. J Exp Med 145:892-906, 1977.

50. Ikic D, Maricic Z, Oresic V, Rode B, Nola P, Smudj K, Knezevic M, Jusic D: Application of human leukocyte interferon in patients with urinary bladder papillomatosis, breast cancer and melanoma. Lancet 1:1022-1024, 1981.

51. Kemeny N, Yagoda A, Wang Y, Field K, Wrobleski H, Whitmore W: Randomized trial of standard therapy with or without Poly I:C in patients with superficial bladder cancer. Cancer 48:2154-2157, 1981.

52. Kingsworth AN, McCann PP, Diekema KA, Ross JS, Malt RA: Effects of α-difluoromethylornithine on the growth of experimental Wilms' tumor and renal adenocarcinoma. Cancer Res 43:4031-4034, 1983.

53. Kingsworth AN, Russell WE, McCann PP, Diekema KA, Malt RA: Effects of α-difluoromethylornithine and 5-fluorouracil on the proliferation of a human colon adenocarcinoma cell line. Cancer Res 43:4035-4038, 1983.

54. Knigth E: Interferon: Effect on the saturation density to which mouse cells will grow in vitro. J Cell Biol 56:846-849, 1973.

55. Koren HS, Brandt CP, Tso CY, Laszlo J: Modulation of natural killing activity by lymphoblastoid interferon in cancer patients. J Biol Resp Modif 2:151-165, 1983.

56. Krown SE, Burk M, Kirkwood JM, Kerr D, Nordlund JJ, Morton DL, Oettgen HF: Human leukocyte interferon (HuLeIF) in malignant melanoma (MM): Preliminary report of the American Cancer Society clinical trials. Proc Am Assoc Cancer Res 22:158, 1981.

57. Krown SE, Einzig AI, Abramson JD, Oettgen HF: Treatment of advanced renal cell cancer (RCC) with recombinant leukocyte A interferon (rINF-αA). ASCO Abstracts, p 58, 1983.

58. Lindahl P, Leary P, Gresser I: Enhancement by interferon of the specific cytotoxicity of sensitized lymphocytes. Proc Natl Acad Sci USA 69:721-725, 1972.

59. Lindahl-Magnusson P, Leary P, Gresser I: Interferon and cell division. VI. Inhibitory effect of interferon on the multiplication of mouse embryo and mouse kidney cells in primary cultures. Proc Soc Exp Biol Med 138:1044-1050, 1971.

60. Louie AC, Gallaguer JG, Sikora K, Levy R, Rosenberg SA, Merigan TC: Follow-up observations on the effect of human leukocyte interferon in non-Hodgkin's lymphoma. Blood 58:712-717, 1981.

61. Madajewicz S, Creavan P, Ozer H, O'Malley J, Grossmeyer E, Pontes E, Mittelman J, Soloman J, Ferraresi R: A phase I study of rising doses of recombinant DNA α2 interferon from E.coli. Abstract Third Annual International Congress on Interferon Research, Miami, November 8-10, 1982.

62. Maluish A, Ortaldo JR, Conlon JC, Sherwin SA, Leavitt R, Strong DM, Weirnik P, Oldham RK, Herberman RB: Depression of natural killer cytotoxicity after in vivo administration of recombinant leukocyte interferon. J Immunol 131:503-507, 1983.

63. McDonald MW: Current therapy for renal cell carcinoma. J Urol 127:211-217, 1982.

64. Metcalf BW, Bey P, Danzin C, Jung MJ, Casara P, Veveri JP: Catalytic irreversible inhibition of mammalian ornithine decarboxylase by substrate and product analogs. J Am Chem Soc 100:2551-2552, 1978.

65. Murphy GP, Hrushesky WL: A murine renal cell carcinoma. J Natl Cancer Inst 50:1013-1021, 1973.

66. Murphy GP, Williams GP: Testing of chemotherapeutic agents in murine renal cell adenocarcinoma. Res Commun Chem Pathol Pharmacol 9:265-277, 1974.

67. Osther K, Salford LG, Hornmark-Stenstam B, Flodgren P, Christopherson I, Magnusson K and the Southern Sweden Neuro-Oncology Group: Local versus systemic human leukocyte interferon treatment. In: The Biology of the Interferon System, DeMaeyer E, Galasso G, Schellekens H (eds). Amsterdam: Elsevier/North Holland Biomedical Press, pp 415-419, 1981.

68. Pazin GJ, Ho M, Haverkos HW, Armstrong JA, Breinig MC, Wechsler HL, Arvin A, Merigan T, Cantell K: Effects of interferon-alpha on human warts. J Interferon Res 2:235-243, 1982.

69. Pegg AE, McCann PP: Polyamine metabolism and function: A brief review. Am J Physiol 243:C212-C221, 1982.

70. Pinsky C, Camacho D, Kerr H, Herr N, Geller N, Whitmore W, Oettgen H: Treatment of superficial bladder cancer with intravesical BCG. ASCO Abstracts, #C-223, p 57, 1983.

71. Quesada JR, Ruben J, Manning JT, Hersh E, Gutterman JU: Alpha Interferon for induction of remission in hairy cell leukemia. N Eng J Med 310:15-18, 1984.

72. Quesada JR, Swanson DA, Trindade A, Gutterman JU: Renal cell carcinoma: Antitumor effects of leukocyte interferon. Cancer Res 43:940-947, 1983.

73. Reid LM, Minato N, Gresser I, Holland J, Kadish A, Bloom BR: Influence of anti-mouse interferon serum on the growth and metastasis of tumor cells persistently infected with virus and of human prostatic tumors in athymic nude mice. Proc Natl Acad Sci USA 78:1171-1176, 1981.

74. Rigby CC, Franks LM: A human tissue culture cell line from a transitional cell tumor of the urinary bladder. Growth, chromosome pattern, and ultrastructure. Br J Cancer 24:746-754, 1970.

75. Saksela E, Timonen T, Cantell K: Human natural killer cell activity is augmented by interferon via recruitment of 'Pre-NK' cells. Scand J Immunol 10:257-266, 1979.

76. Salmon SE, Duric BGM, Young L, Lin RM, Trown PW, Stebbing N: Effects of cloned human leukocyte interferons in the human tumor stem cell assay. J Clin Oncol 3:217-224, 1983.

77. Schellekens H, Weimar W, Cantell K, Stitz L: Antiviral effect of interferon in vivo may be mediated by the host. Nature 278:742, 1979.

78. Schroder EW, Chou IN, Jaken S, Black P: Interferon inhibits the release of plasminogen activator from SV 3T3 cells. Nature 276:828-829, 1978.

79. Schultz RM: Macrophage activation by interferon. In: Lymphokine Reports, Pick E (ed). New York: Academic Press, 1:63-97, 1980.

80. Schultz RM, Chirigos MA: Similarities among factors that render macrophages tumoricidal in lymphokine and interferon preparations. Cancer Res 38:1003-1007, 1978.

81. Scorticatti CH, De La Pena NC, Bellora OA, Mariotto RA, Casabe AR, Comolli R: Systemic IFN-alpha treatment of multiple bladder papilloma grade I or II patients: Pilot study. J Interferon Res 2:339-343, 1982.

82. Sen GC: Mechanism of interferon action: Progress towards its understanding. In: Prog Nucl Acid Res and Mol Biol, Cohn W (ed). New York: Academic Press 27:105-156, 1982.

83. Shapiro A, Kadmon D, Catalona WJ, Ratliff TL: Immunotherapy of superficial bladder cancer. J Urol 128:891-894, 1983.

84. Sherwin SA, Knost JA, Fein S, Abrams PG, Foon KA, Ochs JJ, Schoenberger C, Maluish AE, Oldham RK: A multiple-dose phase I trial of recombinant leukocyte A interferon in cancer patients. J Am Med Assoc 248:2461, 1982.

85. Siimes M, Seppanen P, Alhonen-Hongisto L, Janne J: Synergistic action of two polyamine antimetabolites leads to a rapid therapeutic response in childhood leukemia. Int J Cancer 28:567-570, 1981.

86. Skinner DG: Current perspectives in the management of high-grade invasive bladder cancer. Cancer 45:1866-1874, 1980.

87. Smalley RV, Oldham RK: Interferon as a biological response modifying agent in clinical trials. J Biol Resp Mod 2:401-408, 1983.

88. Smith JA, Herr HW: Spontaneous regression of pulmonary metastases from transitional cell carcinoma. Cancer 46:1499-1515, 1980.

89. Soloway MS: Intravesical and systemic chemotherapy of murine bladder cancer. Cancer Res 37:2918-2929, 1977.

90. Soloway MS: CIS-diaminedichloroplatinum II in advanced urothelial cancer. J Urol 120:716, 1978.

91. Strander H: Interferons: Anti-neoplastic drugs? Blut 35:277-288, 1977.

92. Strander H (unpublished): Osteosarcoma. NIH Interferon Workshop, September 28–30, 1983.

93. Streevalsan T, Taylor-Papadimitriou J, Rozengurt E: Selective inhibition by interferon of serum-stimulated biochemical events in 3T3 cells. Biochem Biophys Res Commun 87:679-685, 1979.

94. Sunkara P, Prakash NJ, Mayer GD, Sjoerdsma A: Tumor suppression with a combination of α-difluoromethylornithine and interferon. Science 219:851-853, 1983.

95. Talpaz M, McCredie KB, Keating MJ, Gutterman JU: Clinical investigation of leukocyte interferon (HuIFN-α) in chronic myelogenous leukemia. Am Soc Hematology Meeting Abstracts, 1983.

96. Talpaz M, McCredie KB, Mavligit G, Gutterman JU: Leukocyte interferon: Control of myeloid proliferation in chronic myelogenous leukemia. Blood 62:689-692 1983.

97. Tamm I, Wang E, Landsberger FR, Pfeffer L: Interferon modulates cell structure and function. In: UCLA Symposia on Molecular and Cellular Biology. Interferons, Merigan TC, Friedman RM (eds). New York: Academic Press 25:159-179, 1982.

98. Targan S, Dorey F: Interferon activation of 'pre-spontaneous killer' (pre-SK) cells and alteration of kinetics of lysis of both 'pre-SK' and active SK cells. J Immunol 124:2157-2161, 1980.

99. Territo M, Sarna G, Figlin R: Effect of in vivo administration of interferon on human monocyte function. J Biol Resp Mod 2:450-457, 1983.

100. Todd RF III, Garnick MB, Canellos GY, Richie JP, Gittes RF, Mayer RJ, Skarin AT: Phase I-II trial of methyl-GAG in the treatment of patients with metastatic renal adenocarcinoma. Cancer Treatm Rep 65:17, 1981.

101. Tovey MG, Brouty-Boye D: The use of the chemostat to study the relationship between cell growth rate, viability and the effect of interferon on L1210 cells. Exp Cell Res 118:383-388, 1979.

102. Trinchieri G, Granato D, Perussia B: Interferon-induced resistance of fibroblastst to cytolysis mediated by natural killer cells. Specificity and mechanism. J Immunol 126:335-340, 1981.

103. Trinchieri G, Santoli D, Dee RR, Knowles BB: Antiviral activity induced by culturing lymphocytes with tumor-derived or virus-transformed cells. Identification of the antiviral activity as interferon and characterization of the human effector lymphocyte subpopulation. J Exp Med 147:1299-1313, 1978.

104. Turek LP, Byrne JC, Lowy DR, Dvoretsky I, Friedman RM, Howley PM: Interferon induces morphologic reversion with elimination of extra-chromosomal viral genomes in bovine papillomavirus-transformed mouse cells. Proc Natl Acad Sci USA 79:7914-7918, 1982.

105. Uyeno K, Ohtsu A: Interferon treatment of viral warts and some skin diseases. In: Proc Conf on Clinical Potentials of Interferons in Viral Diseases and Malignant Tumors, Tokyo, Japan, December 2-4, 1980, (Abstracts, pp 32-33), 1980.

106. Vanky F, Argov SA, Einhorn S, Klein E: Role of alloantigens in natural killing. J Exp Med 151:1151-1165, 1980.

107. Von Hoff DD, Gutterman J, Portnoy B, Coltman CA Jr: Activity of human leukocyte interferon in a human tumor cloning system. Cancer Chemother Pharmacol 8:99-103, 1982.

108. Vose BV, Vanky E, Argou S, Klein E: Natural cytotoxicity in man: Activity of lymph node and tumor infiltrating lymphocytes. Eur J Immunol 7:753, 1977.

109. Webber MM: In vitro models for prostatic cancer: Summary. In: Progress in Clinical Biological Research, Vol. 37. Models for Prostatic Cancer, Murphy GP (ed). New York: Alan R, Liss Inc, pp 133-147, 1979.

110. Weldon TE, Soloway MS: Susceptibility of urothelium to neoplastic cellular implantation. Urology 5:824-827, 1975.

111. Yaron M, Yaron I, Gurari-Rotman D, Revel M, Lindner HR, Zor V: Stimulation of prostaglandin E producing cultured fibroblasts by poly(I) poly(C) and human interferon. Nature 267:457, 1977.

112. Young CW: Interferon induction in cancer. Med Clin North Am 55:721-728, 1971.

113. Zeffren J, Yagoda A, Watson RC, Natale RB, Blumenreich MS, Chapman R, Howard J: Phase II trial of methyl-GAG in advanced renal cancer. Cancer Treatm Rep 65:525, 1981.

10. Surgical Management of Post-Chemotherapy Residual Testis Tumor

RANDALL G. ROWLAND

1. INTRODUCTION

In considering the management of residual testis cancer after chemotherapy, one needs to review the previous modes of therapy of advanced testis cancer as well as review the changes in chemotherapy and staging procedures which have allowed the mode of therapy to evolve to its current day form increasing survival from 5–10% a decade ago to greater than 80% at this time. Each of these aspects will be considered in turn followed by current recommendations for workup of the patient and for evaluation of the patient after completion of chemotherapy. Also the preoperative preparations will be discussed along with intraoperative surgical considerations and postoperative management. The results of this combined treatment regimen will be considered as well as the complications of the treatment. Finally, an overall flow sheet of the management of patients with disseminated testis cancer will be presented. This flow sheet emphasizes the indications for surgery and its interrelationship with chemotherapy for advanced seminoma as well as non-seminomatous germ cell testis tumors.

2. EARLY APPROACH TO DISSEMINATED TESTIS CANCER

Prior to the development of a highly effective combination chemotherapy, surgical excision of the bulk of tumor followed by chemotherapy or radiation therapy was the primary mode of treatment in advanced testis cancer. Even though this approach represented a significant advance in survival of the previous 5–10% rate for advanced non-seminomatous germ cell testis cancer reported in the previous decade, the surgery followed by chemotherapy approach yielded results considerably below those currently available. In 1976 Merrin [1] reported 11 patients who underwent primary

T. L. Ratliff and W. J. Catalona (eds), Urologic Oncology. ISBN 0-89838-628-4.
© *1984. Martinus Nijhoff Publishers, Boston. Printed in the Netherlands.*

cytoreductive surgery followed by postoperative chemotherapy with a 6 drug regimen. He initially reported 8 patients with a complete response. Follow-up on the initial report however was 8.2 months. The long-term survival of these patients was quoted as 43% [2]. In reality the issue at hand seemed to be the development of effective cell cycle-specific agents which could be administered in full therapeutic doses in the patient that had not been rendered immunologically suppressed by massive disease or by an extensive surgical procedure. A similar experience was noted in a small number of patients at Indiana University. All four patients treated with primary surgical cytoreduction suffered significant postoperative morbidity and complications. Three patients relapsed [3]. The subsequent development of effective combination chemotherapy made it possible to switch the sequence of events in the treatment of disseminated disease. Einhorn and Donohue [4] reported the use of adjunctive surgery after using cytoreductive chemotherapy as primary therapy. Also Merrin and his associates who had previously championed the approach of surgery first followed by chemotherapy suggested from their data that the opposite approach was more satisfactory [5]. Before proceeding further one needs to review the advances in chemotherapy which made possible the switch from cytoreductive surgery to cytoreductive chemotherapy as the primary mode of treatment in disseminated testis cancer.

3. ADVANCES IN CHEMOTHERAPY

Considering matters in a chronological order, one of the first major advances in chemotherapy for disseminated testis cancer occurred in 1960 in which Li [6] reported the use of combination actinomycin D, chlorambucil, and methotrexate. Encouraging single agent data was also reported on vinblastine [7], mithramycin [8], and bleomycin [9]. In all of these reports the total response rate was in the 50%–70% range. It should be noted that one of the significant advances was a 10–20% durable complete remission rate with these agents. One other significant single agent study, although it had a small number of patients, was reported by Watt in 1967 [10]. In this report he noted a 40% complete response rate of disseminated testis cancer to single agent methotrexate. He did have prolonged survivorship in this group.

The next significant advance in the treatment of disseminated testis cancer was made by Samuels and his associates. They noted that the combination of vinblastine and bleomycin produced a complete response rate of 33% in 51 patients which was higher than would be predicted by the single agent data [11]. There were other reports of various protocols which gave similar results using the combination of velban and bleomycin with the addition of actinomycin D [12, 13]. The next significant advance came with the use of cis-platinum. This agent was noted by Rosenberg and his associates to cause a significant inhibition of bacterial replication [14]. It also was shown to be active in a phase I study in testicular carcinoma [15]. These reports led to the institution of a combination of vinblastine, bleomycin and platinum beginning in August of 1974 at Indiana University. Fifty patients with advanced germ cell testis cancer were treated between 1974 and 1976 with the three drug protocol [16]. Thirty-three of forty-seven evaluable patients (70%) achieved a complete clinical remission with this combination of drugs. Of the remaining 14 patients, an additional five patients were rendered disease-free by the surgical resection of residual tumor. Of the 70% who had achieved a clinical remission only 10% experienced a subsequent relapse.

Although this therapeutic regimen was extremely effective four of fifty patients died in complete remission. Two of the deaths were attributable to the chemotherapy. One was a case of gram-negative sepsis and the other from bleomycin-induced pulmonary fibrosis. The other two deaths were attributable to pre-existing conditions. Since that time, however, 78 additional patients have been treated with platinum, vinblastine, bleomycin with or without adriamycin and there have been no additional drug-induced mortalities in these additional patients [17].

Although there was a relatively low mortality rate there was a significant rate of granulocytopenic fevers (38%) and sepsis (15%) with this treatment regimen. In order to try to reduce the toxicity of the chemotherapy a three arm study was undertaken at Indiana University and the Southeastern Cancer Study Group. In this study one group received the standard 0.4 mg/kg of vinblastine with each course of treatment. The second group received a reduced dose of vinblastine 0.3 mg/kg every three weeks. The third group received 0.2 mg/kg of vinblastine and 50 mg/m^2 of doxorubicin every three weeks. Patients in each group received platinum 20 mg/m^2 each of five days every three weeks along with bleomycin 30 units intravenously weekly for 12 weeks. There was no significant difference in the rate of complete remission, the percentage of patients further rendered free of disease with surgery, or the partial remission rate. Also there was no significant difference in the relapse rate. There was a significant decrease however in the toxicity of the regimen in terms of granulocytopenic fevers and documented sepsis. The group that received the lower dose of vinblastine without adriamycin had the lowest rate of granulocytopenic fever (15%) and had no documented sepsis in a total of 27 patients. Due to the lower toxicity rate in the 0.3 mg/kg group, the regimen containing the higher dose of vinblastine was abandoned.

The question of maintenance therapy was also examined. Initially patients received vinblastine 0.3 mg/kg monthly for 20 months. A randomized study was set up to examine the efficacy of maintenance vinblastine therapy after the initial 12 weeks induction course of chemotherapy. One hundred and thirteen patients have been evaluated in this protocol. There is no significant difference in the relapse rate in the maintenance group (9%) versus the group with no maintenance (7%) and the disease-free status at the current time was not significantly different [18].

As a result of the above-mentioned studies the current treatment regimen for advanced abdominal testis cancer (stage B_3) or patients with metastatic disease in the chest (stage C) consists of four courses of platinum (20 mg/m^2 per day × 5 days every three weeks), vinblastine (0.3 mg/kg every 3 weeks), and bleomycin (30 units every week for a total of 12 weeks).

The response to such a treatment regimen can best be expressed as a summation of the results from the various treatment groups which have been shown to be statistically equivalent. The overall complete response rate in 125 patients treated with platinum, vinblastine, bleomycin with or without adriamycin was 69%. Table 1 shows the distribution of these patients by type of therapy administered. The results are related to the extent of disease present initially. For this purpose minimal pulmonary disease is defined as less than 6 pulmonary metastases per lung with none

Table 1. Number of patients treated by type of therapy [a].

Therapy	No. of patients
PVB (0.4 mg/kg)	73
PVB (0.3 mg/kg)	27
PVB + A	25

[a] Data extracted from report by Einhorn and Williams [17].

Table 2. Results of chemotherapy (PVB ± A) by extent of disease [a].

Extent of disease	No. of patients	No. of CR
Minimal pulmonary disease	24	21 (88%)
Advanced pulmonary disease	29	16 (55%)
Minimal abdominal + pulmonary disease	22	21 (95%)
Advanced abdominal disease	39	18 (46%)
Elevated markers only	7	7 (100%)
Miscellaneous	4	3 (75%)
	125	86 (69%)

[a] Data extracted from report by Einhorn and Williams [17].

being greater than 2 cm in diameter. Advanced pulmonary disease is defined as masses greater than 2 cm in diameter and/or greater than 6 pulmonary metastases per lung. Advanced abdominal disease was defined as a palpable abdominal mass or the presence of hepatic metastases. Table 2 shows the combined results of the various chemotherapeutic regimen by extent of disease. The overall complete remission rate seems to be inversely related to the amount of disease present as illustrated by a 100% complete remission rate in 7 patients with elevated markers only versus a 46% complete remission rate in 39 patients that had advanced abdominal disease. Recently Vugrin, Whitmore, and Golbey reported similar results (68% complete remission) using a VAB-6 protocol [19].

4. ADVANCES IN DIAGNOSIS AND STAGING

In addition to advances in chemotherapy, one needs to review the progress that has been made in the techniques of diagnosis and staging. The use of high resolution whole lung tomograms (WLT) and abdominal computed axial tomographic (CAT) scans have permitted a much greater degree of accuracy in detecting small to moderate amounts of retroperitoneal and chest disease than previously possible with conventional chest X-rays, intravenous pyelograms (IVP), and lymphangiograms.

At Indiana University, WLT is more accurate than chest CAT scans in detecting small pulmonary metastases. This may not be true in all institutions based upon the particular skills of the radiologists and the type of equipment that is available.

Both ultrasound and CAT scans have been used extensively to evaluate the retroperitoneum. Ultrasound has the advantage of not exposing the patient to ionizing radiation. It is, however, limited by bony structures and bowel gas. CAT scans, on the other hand, are not limited by gas or bone. The resolution is now in the range of 1–1.5 cm. Occasionally, difficulty will be encountered in a particularly thin patient in terms of loss of definitions of natural tissue planes between structures based on a lack of body fat. In this instance, ultrasound can be very helpful in defining structures more clearly.

There are several series reported in the literature on the accuracy of ultrasound and CAT scans in detecting retroperitoneal tumor [20–22]. As one might imagine, if the amount of disease increases, the accuracy of the techniques also increases. In stage B_1 disease, the pick up rate is low (1 of 12) as would be expected since this is microscopic or very low volume disease [22]. In stage B_2 disease, the rate of detection increases to 67%. In stage B_3, virtually all patients have scans which are interpreted as positive. The

Table 3. CAT scan in staging testis cancer.

Series	No. of patients	True (+)	True (−)	False (+)	False (−)	Sensi-tivity	Speci-ficity
Williams [20]	32	14	14	3	1	93%	82%
Richie [21]	30	13	9	1	7	65%	90%
Rowland [22]	63	16	27	5	15	50%	84%
	125	43	50	9	23	66%	85%

sensitivity and specificity of CAT scans of the abdomen from a combined series of 125 patients is shown in Table 3.

In terms of patients with disseminated testis cancer, detecting the presence of chest metastases and evaluating the extent of disease in the chest and abdomen are the most important factors in determining the plan of therapy and predicting the response to therapy.

Whole lung tomograms, CAT scans and ultrasound scans of the abdomen are crucial to the evaluation of the patient's response to primary chemotherapy. This again plays a critical role in determining the patient's subsequent treatment, if any.

Serum markers, alpha-fetoprotein (AFP), human chorionic gonadotropin (HCG) and occasionally lactate dehydrogenase (LDH) are very valuable in detecting the original disease, evaluating the extent of disease and the response to therapy, and detecting early relapse.

AFP has a molecular weight of approximately 70,000. It has been shown to be present in the yolk sac cell. Its half-life is approximately 5 days [23]. About 70% of all patients with embryonal cell carcinoma or teratocarcinoma will have elevated serum levels [24].

Human chorionic gonadotropin has a molecular weight of approximately 38,000 and has an alpha and a beta subunit. The beta subunit is similar to those of LH, FSH and TSH. The half-life of the beta chain is approximately 45 minutes [25]. Despite the development of very specific antibodies against the beta subunit (B-HCG), there can be significant crossover with LH. The syncytiotrophoblasts in testis tumors have been shown to contain B-HCG. Approximately 60% of non-seminomatous testis tumors will produce elevated serum levels of B-HCG. Reports of elevated B-HCG levels for seminoma vary from 5–10% of cases.

LDH is occasionally elevated with massive disease or with liver metastases. In dealing with patients with disseminated disease and elevated markers initially, persistence of elevated markers identifies those patients who have active cancer after chemotherapy. These patients are excluded from surgery (vide infra). However, it should be noted that a return of markers to normal does not rule out the persistence of active cancer since 10% [24] to

20% (vide infra) will have active tumor in a residual mass after chemotherapy.

5. INDICATIONS FOR POST-CHEMOTHERAPY SURGICAL MANAGEMENT OF RESIDUAL DISEASE

There are two separate groups of patients in the scheme of management in disseminated testis cancer which come to surgery. The first set of patients are those who had a partial remission with primary chemotherapy. The second set are those who had a complete remission after primary chemotherapy but who relapsed and then only achieved a partial remission with salvage chemotherapy treatment.

Let us consider the first group of patients that undergo a partial remission after primary combination chemotherapy. If a patient does not completely normalize his findings on an abdominal CAT scan or occasionally on a abdominal ultrasound scan, he is considered a candidate for radical retroperitoneal lymph node dissection. If the residual mass is high in the abdomen and extends into the retrocrural area or apparently involves the diaphragm with or without extension into the chest, a combined abdominal and thoracic approach is indicated. This has to be planned on an individual basis and may require either a thoracoabdominal incision or a median sternotomy in combination with a midline abdominal incision. When patients have residual unilateral chest disease, either parenchymal or mediastinal, this can usually be approached with a thoracotomy incision by itself assuming that the abdomen has completely normalized or was not abnormal to begin with. In this group of patients if there are residual abdominal findings as well, a thoracoabdominal incision is frequently performed and both the chest and the abdominal disease are addressed. If a patient has bilateral parenchymal or mediastinal masses and the abdomen has normalized or was never abnormal, then the patient is approached through a median sternotomy or if the disease is in the posterior mediastinum the patient may be approached through two separate thorocotomy incisions. If, on the other hand, there is disease in the thorax as well as the abdomen and both chest cavities need to be entered, the incision of choice is a median sternotomy in combination with a midline abdominal incision.

If in any of these patients there is a persistently elevated serum alpha-fetoprotein or serum B-HCG, they are not considered candidates for surgical resection. Experience has shown that they are unlikely to benefit from surgery at this point. The patients therefore advance to salvage chemotherapy measures.

The second group of patients that are candidates for surgical management

Table 4. Indications for surgery after chemotherapy.

Finding	RPLND	Thoracotomy	Mediansternotomy
Residual abdominal mass on CAT or ultrasound	+		
Retrocrural mass on CAT	+	+/0	+/0
Unilateral parenchymal mass on WLT		+	
Unilateral mediastinal mass on WLT		+	
Bilateral parenchymal or mediastinal masses			+
Elevated serum AFP	0	0	0
Elevated serum B-HCG	0	0	0

of residual disease are those patients with a complete clinical remission initially with primary chemotherapy that have relapsed and have gone on to have only a partial remission with salvage chemotherapy. The same criteria are used in this group as were outlined above for the patient undergoing partial resection with chemotherapy. Again it should be emphasized that if the patients have positive alpha-fetoprotein or B-HCG after the salvage chemotherapy they would be candidates for further chemotherapy rather than surgical treatment. The indications for surgery are summarized in Table 4.

6. PREOPERATIVE EVALUATION

Normally the patient undergoes re-evaluation at the beginning of the fourth course of chemotherapy. This evaluation includes whole lung tomograms and abdominal CAT scan. Also a set of serum markers are drawn at this time. Assuming that the whole lung tomograms and abdominal CAT scan show evidence of only a partial objective response to the chemotherapy by virtue of a decrease in size or number of the metastases, the patient is treated with the fourth course of chemotherapy and admitted for surgical exploration in 4–6 weeks.

At the time of admission for surgical exploration, the patient undergoes a repeat whole lung tomogram and abdominal CAT scan. In the case where patients have stage C disease the size of the chest metastases is compared to the previous CAT scans. If there is complete disappearance of the chest disease the patient can be spared a thoracic exploration. On the other hand if there is persistence of disease in the chest the appropriate thoracic exploration and excision of masses can be planned.

An abdominal CAT scan is obtained and, again, it is compared to the earlier studies. If there is still residual disease present the patient would be a candidate for radical retroperitoneal lymph node dissection. Occasionally there will be complete clearing of the metastatic disease as assessed by whole lung tomograms and abdominal CAT scan between the interval of the last studies and the one obtained as part of the preoperative evaluation. In this case the patient does not undergo surgical exploration assuming that the serum AFP and B-HCG remain negative.

In addition to the above-mentioned studies, abdominal ultrasound scans are obtained on occasion. In a previous report it has been noted that abdominal ultrasound rarely adds information that is not gained by abdominal CAT scan [22]. However on occasion particularly in the extremely thin patient where the tissue planes are obscured by lack of fat on the abdominal CAT scan the ultrasound can be helpful. In addition to the above-mentioned staging evaluation, the patient has routine preoperative lab work performed as outlined in Table 5. These studies are used to monitor the patient for persistence of myelosuppression, abnormal liver enzymes and evidence of abnormal renal function. Also an electrocardiogram is obtained. This is of significance particularly in those patients who have had exposure to doxorubicin.

Table 5. Post-chemotherapy preoperative evaluation.

CBC, platelet count, prothrombin time, partial thromboplastin time
SMA_{12}, serum B-HCG, AFP
Whole lung tomograms
Abdominal computerized axial tomograms $\pm$ abdominal ultrasound scan
Spirometry, diffusion capacity, arterial blood gases on room air
Electrocardiogram

A thorough evaluation of the patient's pulmonary functions is also performed. Arterial blood gases are obtained on room air. It is not uncommon after having had chemotherapy including bleomycin to have a patient with an arterial P_AO_2 in the 70–80 Torr range. Since bleomycin is known to cause pulmonary fibrosis with a restrictive component as well as a diffusion defect, we pay particular attention to diffusion capacity, forced vital capacity, and forced excretory volume (FEV_1). A mild diffusion defect or mild restrictive disease has not caused significant difficutlies.

7. PREOPERATIVE PREPARATION

After obtaining the preoperative evaluation studies as outlined above, if the patient's hemoglobin is less than 10 grams/dl he undergoes a preoperative transfusion. Beginning 24–48 hours before the time of surgery the patient undergoes a mechanical bowel preparation. This normally consists of clear liquid diet along with a 12 ounce bottle of citrate of magnesia as a cathartic. In the afternoon of the preoperative day an intravenous line is started and the patient is kept moderately hydrated with dextrose and half normal saline at a rate of 100 ml/hr. Also if a patient appears to be volume depleted, 500 ml of 5% plasma protein can be given as a portion of the fluids. This will also help minimize the crystaloids given and maximize the colloids in order to try to maintain a normal or slightly elevated intravascular osmotic pressure.

The patient is also instructed in the techniques of pulmonary exercises preoperatively. Blow bottles or suction devices along with incentive spirometry seem to be used more effectively on the patient's part if he has exposure to them preoperatively when he is not experiencing surgical pain.

8. OPERATIVE SET-UP AND MONITORING

In order to help control the patient's temperature during the procedure a warming blanket is placed on the operating table prior to the arrival of the patient. The patient customarily arrives in the operating room with a peripheral venous line in place. After the routine monitoring devices for blood pressure and cardiogram are established, anesthesia is induced. After the patient had been anesthetized, a central venous line and an arterial line are placed. A large caliber sump type nasogastric tube is placed as well as an esophageal temperature probe. A Foley catheter is placed and is led to straight drainage. If a retroperitoneal lymph node dissection is the only procedure that is planned or if it is planned in conjunction with a median sternotomy then the patient is left in the supine position. If a thoracotomy is to be performed first as a separate procedure the patient is placed in the appropriate flank position. If, on the other hand, a thoracoabdominal incision is planned, the ipsilateral arm is placed on an ether screen to support it at the level of the shoulders and the patient's shoulders are sightly torqued.

If a thoracotomy is to be performed as the initial surgical procedure this is completed by the thoracic surgery service and the patient is returned to the supine position. He is reprepped and draped and a retroperitoneal lymph node dissection is initiated. If a combined thoracoabdominal incision or median sternotomy and midline abdominal incision is planned, normally the thoracic surgery service initiates the case and completes the chest portion of the dissection. At this point the chest incision is left open and is covered with a sterile towel. The midline abdominal incision is then opened and the retroperitoneal lymph node dissection is carried out. The details of the technique will be considered below. Once the abdominal portion is completed both the abdominal and chest wound are closed simultaneously.

9. TECHNICAL CONSIDERATION OF RETROPERITONEAL LYMPH NODE DISSECTION

A previous report by Donohue [26] has thoroughly described the technique of full bilateral retroperitoneal lymph node dissection with extension into the suprahilar zones. As described in that article the dissection is started in the suprahilar zone and then is continued more inferiorly removing the aortocaval lymph node packages.

In cases where a fairly extensive amount of tumor is still present in the aortocaval area it is frequently advantageous to begin the dissection in this area. In the original description the concept of splitting the adventitia overlying the great vessels and rolling the tissue laterally off the vessels is described. This is also applied in the post-chemotherapy retroperitoneal lymph node dissection; however, at times it is advantageous to excise tumor masses if they are fairly bulky in extent in order to facilitate better surgical exposure for the remaining portions of the dissection.

It must be emphasized that a full bilateral dissection including suprahilar zones is indicated in the post-chemotherapy node dissection. The need for this has been pointed out in a previous report on the distribution of metastatic tumor in lymph nodes after chemotherapy [27]. Even though gross disease may be visible in one particular zone, it has been noted that there is a significant incidence of microscopic disease in other zones of the dissection. It is also impossible to distinguish visually between necrotic changes, teratoma and carcinoma. As a result, a complete dissection within the confines of the standard node dissection must be carried out in order to insure accurate assessment of the disease status of the retroperitoneum. After the dissection has been completed the abdominal wound is usually closed with a single layer of interrupted inverted figure of 8 sutures of #0 or #1 nonabsorbable or monofilament synthetic absorbable sutures. If the patient has had particularly massive disease it is also common to use abdominal retention sutures.

10. POSTOPERATIVE CARE

Customarily for the first 24 hours postoperatively the patient goes to a surgical intensive care unit. The central venous and arterial pressure monitoring can be continued in this setting. During the first 24 to 48 hours, 5% plasma protein is usually administered at a rate of 250–500 ml every 8 hours. This is used as a portion of the patient's total intravenous intake which usually runs in the range of 125 ml/hr. The use of the plasma protein again helps to maintain the colloid osmotic pressure and minimize problems with overhydration. After the initial 24–28 hr period, assuming that the patient has remained stable, the Foley catheter, central venous line, and arterial line are removed and the patient is returned to a normal surgical nursing unit. From this point on, postoperative care does not differ significantly from that of the patient who has undergone a routine radical retroperitoneal lymph node dissection with the one exception that extra emphasis is placed on respiratory care. The usual postoperative period of hospitalization is 8–10 days.

11. RESULTS OF SURGERY

A total of 123 patients who had partial remissions after primary or salvage chemotherapy and have undergone surgery have been reported [27–30]. In reviewing the results, the location of residual mass(es), chest and/or retroperitoneum, and the type of previous therapy must be considered.

Table 6 shows the histologic findings by the location of residual masses. Patients had RPLND alone, thoracotomy alone, or combined chest and retroperitoneal procedures. The patients in the RPLND only group were composed of those who had partial remissions after primary chemotherapy or who had relapsed after complete remission from primary chemotherapy and had a partial response to salvage chemotherapy. Overall, there was roughly a 1/3–1/3–1/3 division among the findings of fibrotic–cystic–necrotic tissue, teratoma (mature or immature), and carcinoma as previous-

Table 6. Histologic findings in surgery after chemotherapy.

Group	No. of patients	Fibrotic–cystic–necrotic tissue	Teratoma	Carcinoma
RPLND only [27, 28]	51 [a]	16 (31.5%)	16 (31.5%)	19 (37%)
Thoracotomy only [29, 30]	48	14 (30%)	17 (35%)	17 (35%)
RPLND + thoracotomy [30]	24 [b]	4 (17%)	13 (54%)	7 (29%)
	123	34 (28%)	46 (37%)	43 (35%)

[a] These patients represent partial remissions after primary chemotherapy and relapses after complete remission who went on to have partial remissions with salvage chemotherapy.
[b] In 17 patients the pathology in the chest and retroperitoneum agreed and in 7 they differed.

ly reported [28]. Patients having combined chest and retroperitoneal procedures had a higher percentage of teratoma (54%) than those patients with either chest or retroperitoneal surgery alone. In 17 of 24 patients having combined procedures, the pathologic findings in the chest and retroperitoneum were in agreement while in 7 patients there was a difference between the two regions [30].

A review of updated results at Indiana University which is the subject of a future report considers the differences in results of patients having RPLND after primary chemotherapy with those having RPLND after salvage chemotherapy. A portion of this data was reported earlier by Donohue as a single group [28]. Table 7 shows the approximate results in the updated series on 125+ patients having post-chemotherapy RPLND. Instead of an equal distribution between the three types of histologic findings, carcinoma is found in approximately 20% of patients having RPLND after primary chemotherapy versus approximately 50% after salvage chemotherapy. There was a corresponding drop in necrotic tissue in the salvage chemotherapy group. The incidence of teratoma was unchanged in the two groups.

Table 7. Histologic findings in RPLND specimens after partial response to chemotherapy.

Type of treatment	Fibrotic–cystic–necrotic tissue	Teratoma	Carcinoma
Primary chemotherapy	40%	40%	20%
Salvage chemotherapy	10%	40%	50%

It must be emphasized that all of these patients had partial remissions after chemotherapy. Any patient having a complete remission was observed and surgery was not performed. After primary chemotherapy of those patients achieving a complete clinical remission (70% of those originally treated), only 10% experienced a relapse. This corresponds very well with the findings of Richie who noted a 10% incidence of residual cancer in patients having a RPLND after a complete remission with primary chemotherapy [31]. Our findings and those of Richie contrast with those of Bracken et al. [32] who report residual carcinoma in 5 of 22 (23%) and teratoma in an additional 3 (14%). This discrepancy however can probably be explained by differences in staging techniques. The authors acknowledge that had CAT scans been available, only 2 of the 22 (9%) would have been classified as complete remissions and as having residual carcinoma. These findings would then correlate with the other data including the report of Vugrin et al. [19], which noted a 12% relapse rate after VAB-6 treatment complete clinical remissions.

12. COMPLICATIONS OF SURGERY

There have been two major reports of complications in patients undergoing retroperitoneal lymph node dissection for testis cancer [3, 33]. Both of these series reported complications for low stage diseases as well as high stage disease. In high stage disease the vast majority of the patients who were operated had undergone previous chemotherapy and were analogous to the types of patients that are being discussed in this report.

Donohue's group reported a series of 235 patients that had undergone radical retroperitoneal lymph node dissection. Forty-nine of these patients underwent retroperitoneal node dissection for advanced disease. Of these 49, 45 received previous chemotherapy. In the 49 patients the total complication rate was 26% and the death rate was 2%. This contrasts with an overall complication rate of 14% and a death rate of 0.5% in patients who were operated on for lesser stage disease. Skinner's group reported a series of 149 patients. Fifty-two patients in this group were operated on for advanced disease. The complication rate was 23% with a death rate of 4%. Again, this is contrasted to a complication rate of 7% and no deaths for patients undergoing node dissection for low stage disease. These data are shown in Table 8.

Table 8. Complications of surgery.

	Stages A, B_1, B_2			Stages B_3-C		
Series	No. of patients	Total complications	Deaths	No. of patients	Total complications	Deaths
Donohue and Rowland [3]	186	27 (14%)	1 (0.5%)	49	13 (26%)	1 (2%)
Skinner et al. [33]	97	7 (7%)	0	52	12 (23%)	2 (4%)

In Mandelbaum's report of 48 patients having thoracotomy or median sternotomy alone and of 24 patients having combined chest and retroperitoneal procedures, there were no operative deaths and minimal complications as evidenced by a 10–14 day postoperative period of hospitalization in the latter group [30].

Special attention must be paid to the potential complications generated by the patients' exposure to prior chemotherapy. Each agent should be considered separately. Platinum's primary toxicity is renal. Based upon improved techniques of administering platinum with adequate hydration the incidence of renal failure is minimal at the time of administration of the agent. However, one needs to guard against dehydration during the operative period and if a patient encounters an episode of sepsis the use of aminoglycosides must be avoided if at all possible due to enhanced sensitivity of the kidneys to these agents after exposure to platinum chemotherapy.

Exposure to bleomycin can cause some compromise of pulmonary function. This is most frequently seen as a mild restrictive component and also as a decrease in diffusion capacity of the lungs. In practical terms this makes it difficult for the patient to respond to overhydration and it may cause serious problems with pulmonary hypertension and increased interstitial edema with a subsequent increase in the diffusion defect causing hypoxia [34]. In order to help prevent complications as a result of the pulmonary changes careful monitoring during the intraoperative and postoperative periods is required to guard against overhydration. Also, efforts are made to maintain a normal or even slightly increased colloid osmotic pressure.

Vinblastine causes myelosuppression at the time of administration however usually the patients have recovered from this aspect by the time that they come to surgery. Other than monitoring for the return of the patient's white count and platelet count this usually presents no significant problem.

Overall the complication rate of the patients undergoing retroperitoneal lymph node dissection and/or thoracotomy for advanced disease after administration of chemotherapy is approximately twice that of patients undergoing surgery as their primary mode of treatment. However, when compared to the potential benefit gained in terms of assessing need for additional treatment, the benefits far outweigh the complications. It should be noted that the vast majority of complications encountered prolong the hospital stay by a few days and infrequently cause long-term problems. A death rate in the range of 1–2% is acceptably low considering the extent of the surgery and the complicating factors induced by the previous exposure to chemotherapy.

13. POSTOPERATIVE FOLLOW-UP OF THE SURGICALLY TREATED PATIENT

Routinely the patient is seen for his first postoperative visit approximately 3–4 weeks after discharge from the hospital. At that time he undergoes a physical examination looking for evidence of recurrent abdominal tumor or evidence of inguinal, axillary or cervical adenopathy. In addition routine chest X-ray is obtained along with serum B-HCG and AFP. For the remainder of the first postoperative year the patient is asked to get monthly chest X-rays and serum markers. He is routinely seen by his primary physician on an every other month basis for physical examination, again paying particular attention for evidence of recurrent abdominal or nodal disease. He is

Table 9. Routine follow-up of the postsurgical patient.

Follow-up	First year	Second year	Subsequent years
Chest X-rays	monthly	every other month	semi-yearly or yearly
Serum markers AFP, B-HCG	monthly	every other month	semi-yearly or yearly
Physical exam by primary physician	every other month	every 3–4 months	semi-yearly or yearly
Physical exam at medical center	every 3–4 months	every 6 months	yearly
CAT, ultrasound, WLT	as needed	as needed	as needed

also seen at the medical center by the urologist and the medical oncologist approximately 3–4 times in the first year. During the second year of follow-up the chest X-rays and serum markers are obtained on an every other month basis. The physical examinations are also decreased to every 3–4 months. The patient is seen by the urologist and the medical oncologist at the medical center approximately every 4–6 months during the second year. After that time, the likelihood of relapse is low and we suggest follow-up on an every 6–12 month basis again with physical examination, chest X-ray and serum markers.

During the entire period of follow-up if there is any questions about an abnormal abdominal finding we do not hesitate to obtain additional CAT scans or ultrasound examinations of the abdomen. After surgical dissection with the use of metalic surgical clips there is frequently a considerable amount of distortion induced in the CAT scan. In this situation abdominal ultrasound scans have been of added benefit in terms of improving our diagnostic accuracy. Also if there is any question on the chest X-rays additional CAT scans of the chest or whole lung tomograms are obtained. Table 9 summarizes the recommended follow-up scheme.

14. OVERVIEW OF THE ROLE OF SURGERY IN MANAGING DISSEMINATED TESTIS CANCER

Advances in chemotherapy, namely the development of effective combination therapy such as cis-platinum, vinblastine, and bleomycin have made it possible to change the role of surgery for disseminated seminoma and non-seminomatous testis cancer from that of a primary cytoreductive treatment prior to chemotherapy which had a limited capacity to kill tumor to that of an adjuvant treatment after a significant response from chemotherapy. Surgical resection of residual mass(es) in the chest and retroperitoneum after chemotherapy actually serves both diagnostic and therapeutic purposes. On one hand, resection of teratoma is therapeutic in most and resection of carcinoma is therapeutic in many. On the other hand, the knowledge of the presence or absence of active carcinoma allows the planning of the appropriate additional therapy. In the case where only scar or teratoma is present, observation can be used. If active cancer is demonstrated, additional courses of induction chemotherapy can be used if a complete resection of tumor was felt to have been achieved or the patient can progress to salvage chemotherapy if a complete resection was not possible.

Figure 1 illustrates the concepts discussed in this review. The relative frequency of the various responses to chemotherapy and surgical findings are indicated. Several points need to be emphasized. After four courses of primary induction chemotherapy (PVB), those patients with no demonstrable disease by WLT, abdominal CAT scan, physical exam, or serum AFP or B-HCG are not operated. Approximately 10% of that group or 7% of the original population which presented with disseminated disease will relapse. The vast majority of these patients (80%) will achieve complete remission status with salvage chemotherapy. Those who achieve only a partial remission from salvage chemotherapy (20%) will have a high rate of persistent

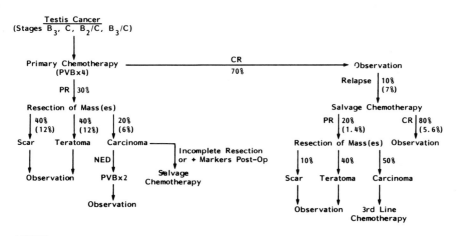

TREATMENT SCHEME FOR DISSEMINATED TESTIS CANCER
AT INDIANA UNIVERSITY

LEGEND
( ) = percentage of original population
CR = complete clinical remission
PR = partial clinical remission
NED = no evidence of disease

carcinoma (50%) at surgery. These patients are then advanced to third-line chemotherapy and as of this time have very limited success.

If a patient has persistently positive AFP and/or B-HCG after primary chemotherapy, they are advanced to salvage chemotherapy without surgery since surgery has not proven to be helpful in this setting. In most patients there is a one log reduction in the markers for each course of chemotherapy. Therefore, the patient with elevated markers after four courses of primary therapy is felt to have persistent disease which is refractory to the induction agents.

Even though exposure to chemotherapy increases the risk of operative mortality and morbidity, the benefits to the patient in terms of therapy and planning for future treatments far outweigh the 1–2% mortality of the combined treatment mode. Advances in staging techniques and the sensitivity of the markers has allowed increased accuracy in determining which patients should be subjected to surgery after chemotherapy. Perhaps in the future, new or more sensitive markers, radionuclide scans, or nuclear magnetic resonance scans will afford such a high level of confidence in evaluating patient responses to chemotherapy that surgical exploration and resection can be limited to those patients who have teratoma or carcinoma and those with only scar or necrotic tissue can be spared.

At the current time, it must be emphasized that resection of residual mass(es) after primary or salvage chemotherapy is indicated. An aggressive approach should be taken in both the chest and the abdomen. Not infrequently, at exploration more masses are found in the chest than are appreciated during the workup. In the retroperitoneum a thorough bilateral dissection including the suprahilar zones should be performed due to the heterogeneity of the tissue. Complete resection helps assure accurate assessment of the disease status of the retroperitoneum.

Although the results described in this report are being achieved in many centers using similar aggressive combined modes of therapy, one should not forget that the key to success in the treatment of these patients with disseminated germ cell testis cancer seems to lie in compulsive follow-up for a minimum of two years. This type of approach integrating chemotherapy and surgery has yielded cure rates in disseminated seminoma and non-seminomatous germ cell testis cancer in excess of 80%.

REFERENCES

1. Merrin C, Takita H, Weber R, Wajsman Z, Baumgartner G, Murphy GP: Combination radical surgery and multiple sequential chemotherapy for the treatment of advanced carcinoma of the testis (stage III). Cancer 37:2029, 1976.
2. Donohue JP: Surgical management of testis cancer. In: Testicular Tumors: Management and Treatment, Einhorn LH (ed). New York: Masson Publishing USA Inc, pp 29–46, 1980.

3. Donohue JP, Rowland RG: Complications of retroperitoneal lymph node dissection. J Urol 125:338-340, 1981.

4. Einhorn LH, Donohue JP: Chemotherapy for disseminated testicular cancer. Urol Clin North Am 4(3):407-426, 1977.

5. Merrin C, Bleckley S, Takita H: Multimodal treatment of advanced testicular tumor with reductive surgery and multisequential chemotherapy with cis-platinum, bleomycin, vinblastine, vincristine and actinomycin D. J Urol 120:73-76, 1978.

6. Li MC, Whitmore WF, Golbey R, Grabstald H: Effects of combined drug therapy on metastatic cancer of the testis. JAMA 174:145-153, 1960.

7. Samuels ML, Howe CD: Vinblastine in the management of testicular cancer. Cancer 25:1009-1017, 1970.

8. Kennedy BJ: Mithramycin therapy in advanced testicular neoplasms. Cancer 26:755-766, 1970.

9. Blum RH, Carter S, Agre K: A clinical review of bleomycin – a new antineoplastic agent. Cancer 31:903-914, 1973.

10. Wyatt JK, McAninch LH: A chemotherapeutic approach to advanced testicular carcinoma. Can J Surg 10:421-426, 1967.

11. Samuels ML, Lanzotti VJ, Holoye PY, Boyle LE, Smith TL, Johnson DE: Combination chemotherapy in germinal cell tumors. Cancer Treat Rev 3:185-204, 1976.

12. Wittes RE, Yagoda A, Silvay O, Magill GB, Whitmore W, Krakoff IH, Golbey RB: Chemotherapy of germ cell tumors of the testis. Cancer 37:637-645, 1976.

13. Cvitkovic E, Cheng E, Whitmore WF Jr et al.: Germ cell tumors. Chemotherapy update. Proc Am Assoc Cancer Res 18:324, 1977.

14. Rosenberg B, VanCamp L, Krigas T: Inhibition of cell division in E. coli by electrolysis products from a platinum electrode. Nature 205:678-699, 1965.

15. Highby DJ, Wallace HJ, Albert DJ, Holland JF: Diaminodichloroplatinum: a phase I study showing responses in testicular and other tumors. Cancer 33:1219-1225, 1974.

16. Einhorn LH, Donohue JP: Cis-diamminedichloroplatinum, vinblastine and bleomycin chemotherapy in disseminated testicular cancer. Ann Intern Med 87:293-298, 1977.

17. Einhorn LH, Williams SD: The management of disseminated testicular cancer. In: Testicular Tumors: Management and Treatment, Einhorn LH (ed). New York: Masson Publishing USA Inc, pp 117-149, 1980.

18. Einhorn LH: Testicular cancer. In: Medical Oncology, Schein P, Calabres P (eds). New York City: MacMillan (in press).

19. Vugrin D, Whitmore WF Jr, Golbey RB: Vinblastine, actinomycin D, bleomycin, cyclophosphamide and cis-platinum combination chemotherapy in metastatic testis cancer – a 1-year program. J Urol 128:1205-1208, 1982.

20. Williams RD, Feinberg SB, Knight LC, Fraley EE: Abdominal staging of testicular tumors using ultrasonography and computed tomography. J Urol 123:872-875, 1980.

21. Richie JP, Garnick MB, Finberg H: Computerized tomography: how accurate for abdominal staging of testis tumors? J Urol 127:715-717, 1982.

22. Rowland RG, Weisman D, Williams SD, Einhorn LH, Klatte EC, Donohue JP: Accuracy of preoperative staging in stages A and B non-seminomatous germ cell testis tumors. J Urol 127:718-720, 1982.

23. Gitlin D, Boesman M: Serum alpha-fetoprotein, albumin, and gammaglobulin in the human conceptus. J Clin Invest 45:1826-1838, 1966.

24. Lange PH, McIntire KR, Waldman TA: Tumor markers in testicular tumor: current status and future prospects. In: Testicular Tumors: Management and Treatment, Einhorn LH (ed). New York: Masson Publishing USA Inc, pp 69-81, 1980.

25. Javadpour N: The National Cancer Institute's experience with testicular cancer. J Urol 120:651-659, 1978.

274

26. Donohue JP: Retroperitoneal lymphadenectomy: the anterior approach including bilateral supra-hilar dissection. Urol Clin North Am 4(3):509-521, 1977.
27. Donohue JP, Roth LM, Zachary JM, Rowland RG, Einhorn LH, Williams SG: Cytoreductive surgery for metastatic testis cancer: tissue analysis of retroperitoneal masses after chemotherapy. J Urol 127:1111-1114, 1982.
28. Donohue JP, Einhorn LH, Williams SD: Cytoreductive surgery for metastatic testis cancer: considerations of timing and extent. J Urol 123:876-880, 1980.
29. Mandelbaum I, Williams SD, Einhorn LH: Aggressive surgical management of testicular carcinoma metastatic to lungs and mediastinum. Ann Thor Surg 30:224-229, 1980.
30. Mandelbaum I, Yaw PB, Einhorn LH, Williams SD, Rowland RG, Donohue JP: The importance of one-stage median sternotomy and retroperitoneal node dissection in disseminated testicular cancer. Presented at Soc of Thoracic Surgeons, San Francisco, January 1983. Ann Surg 36:524-528, 1983.
31. Richie JP: Personal communication.
32. Bracken RB, Johnson DE, Frazier OH, Logothetis CJ, Trindade A, Samuels ML: The role of surgery following chemotherapy in stage III germ cell neoplasms. J Urol 129:39-43, 1983.
33. Skinner DG, Melamed A, Lieskovsky G: Complications of thoracoabdominal retroperitoneal lymph node dissection. J Urol 127:1107-1110, 1982.
34. Rowland RG, Moorthy SS, Donohue JP: Anesthetic considerations for post-chemotherapy radical retroperitoneal lymph node dissection. Presented North Central Section American Urological Association, Marco Island, Florida, October 1982.

Editorial Comment

MICHAEL A. S. JEWETT

Doctors Comisarow and Grabstald initially reported the efficacy of secondary surgery for residual retroperitoneal metastatic testicular tumor [1]. It is now well established that this type of surgery is feasible with low morbidity rates and virtually no mortality. Patients regularly survive disease-free after excision of residual active tumor which was apparently drug-resistant although further chemotherapy is usually administered.

The current issues include the indications and timing of the procedure. The principles apply to all sites of residual testis tumor. Most candidates are now seen after initial chemotherapy which was given as part of a planned protocol for extensive disease. Initial surgery in the face of large tumor burden is no longer practiced [2]. As Doctor Rowland indicated the majority of patients coming to this type of surgery have only achieved a partial response to this induction chemotherapy. It is frequently possible to predict the patients who will ultimately require surgery. Few large abdominal masses will completely disappear on chemotherapy alone. Early experience revealed a tendency to prolong induction chemotheapy if residual tumor remained with poorer survival. It is important to operate as soon as possible after the usual induction drug protocol has been completed, if regression is seen, and before tumor regrowth. A sufficient interval must be allowed for the recovery of any neutropenia or thrombocytopenia and a reassessment of renal and pulmonary function.

Although it is generally agreed that persisting elevation of markers after chemotherapy is a bad prognostic sign, there are a few surviving patients in various series who were marker-positive preoperatively. Two of six such patients in our early experience have survived free of disease for more than 5 years. With the occasional patient failing salvage chemotherapy protocols and with persistently elevated markers, it is difficult to decide against surgery when it appears to be the last available modality. However if a decision is made to proceed, the retroperitoneal and intra-abdominal disease is often more extensive than appreciated and in fact may be unresectable. In general, therefore, a policy of further chemotherapy in the face of elevated markers is correct. This particularly applies to central nervous system disease.

Most centers choose not to explore patients who have achieved a complete response on chemotherapy. Despite some limitations, current techniques of imaging and available markers rarely understage in this setting. If all evidence of retroperitoneal disease has disappeared after chemotherapy, the incidence of microscopic or small volume disease is less than 10%. The same must be assumed for pulmonary disease as most patients presenting with pulmonary metastases alone and who achieve a complete response remain disease-free.

Perioperative issues include familiarizing the Anesthetic Service with this type of patient. Peripheral venous access is frequently poor after extensive chemotherapy and the potential complications from pretreatment must be known. Bleomycin has been discussed by Doctor

Rowland. In addition we maintain patients on 30% oxygen because of the suggestions that a potential for oxygen toxicity exists in addition to the generally recognized intolerance to large extracellular volumes [3]. This precludes the use of blood substitutes in the occasional patient who will not accept transfusion. A Cell-Saver may be used in these cases if significant blood loss is anticipated.

The operative approach is determined by the site(s) of the tumor as described. The operating surgeon should be comfortable planning the appropriate incisions to include operating within the thorax. It is wise to recruit one or two thoracic surgical colleagues to focus expertise. Similarly vascular complications are frequently encountered. We have patched or replaced the abdominal aorta on three occasions and sacrificed what remained of the inferior vena cava on one occasion. Unilateral nephrectomy was performed in continuity with excision of the abdominal mass on three occasions to avoid cutting through what appeared to be active tumor. A renal artery has been reconstructed in one additional case. Doctors Donohue and Rowland have emphasized the importance of thorough and meticulous lymphadenectomy. Although residual retroperitoneal disease is usually macroscopic localized to visible and palpable masses, microscopic nodal and extranodal tumor can occur. This is usually when the macroscopic disease contains active tumor. A lumpectomy-type procedure would therefore be inadequate therapy alone [4].

The histology of the excised tumor mass will reveal one or more components including active carcinoma (usually embryonal carcinoma but frequently also immature elements of almost sarcomatous appearance), necrosis/fibrosis only and/or teratoma. The proportions of each pattern in any one series will vary according to local indications and timing of surgery in relation to pretreatment, pathological criteria, the number of sections taken by the pathologist, the completeness of surgery, and the accuracy of preoperative screening for extra-abdominal metastases which might preclude surgery. In our first 30 patients who underwent a retroperitoneal procedure with or without pulmonary resection, 12 (40%) had carcinoma. 5/5 are free of disease more than 12 months after surgery. Fibrosis/necrosis was present in 11 (37%) patients and all 8 followed more than 1 year are disease-free. Teratoma was found in 7 (23%) patients. Despite reports that the finding of teratoma generally confers a good prognosis, only 3 survived disease-free at 12 months. The finding of teratoma must not induce complacency during follow-up and prophylactic chemotherapy might still be considered depending on local experience. Finally, it is not uncommon to have a discrepancy between the histology of the pulmonary and retroperitoneal metastatic disease. The practical implication of this observation is that both areas must be explored and fully assessed. At present no means exist to distinguish the different histologies preoperatively. Even if no direct therapeutic benefit arises from excision of necrotic tumor, further chemotherapy may be avoided.

The indications and timing will continue to be refined with more accurate imaging and new markers although these prospects do not appear to be immediately on the horizon. The techniques can now be standardized and perioperative management is satisfactory in major centers.

There are few areas in oncology that require such fine tuning by a closely knit team of experienced medical and surgical oncologists. Not only should experience be concentrated in a few centers to improve understanding but the rate of complete excision and survival improves with experience. Doctor Rowland has thoroughly and thoughtfully reviewed a complex subject. His very large personal experience at Indiana University will be apparent to any reader who has treated similar patients.

REFERENCES

1. Comisarow RH, Grabstald H: Re-exploration for retroperitoneal lymph node metastases from testis tumor. J Urol 115:569–571, 1976.

2. Javadpour N, Ozols RF, Anderson T, Barlock AB, Wesley R, Young RC: A randomized trial of cytoreductive surgery followed by chemotherapy versus chemotherapy alone in bulky stage III testicular cancer with poor prognostic features. Cancer 50:2004–2010, 1982.
3. Goldiner PL, Schweizer O: The hazards of anesthesia and surgery in bleomycin-treated patients. Semin Oncol 6:121–124, 1979.
4. Hendry WF, Goldstraw JE, Husband JE, Barrett A, McElwain TJ, Peckham MJ: Elective delyaed excision of bulky para-aortic lymph node metastases in advanced non-seminoma germ cell tumours of testis. J Urol 53:648–653, 1981.

11. Prognostic Value of HLA in Genitourinary Tumors

ARTHUR I. SAGALOWSKY

1. INTRODUCTION

Before one may properly interpret available data on associations of the HLA system with genitourinary tumors, one first must understand the basic structure and function of HLA and the possible mechanisms linking it with disease.

Every vertebrate species studied thus far has a major histocompatibility complex (MHC) [1]. In man this entire region is called HLA for 'human leukocyte antigens' and is located on the short arm of chromosome 6. These HLA antigens consist of two polypeptide chains, a variable heavy glycoprotein moiety and a constant light chain, with molecular weights of 44 000 and 16 000 daltons, determined on chromosomes 6 and 15, respectively [2]. HLA-A, B, and C locus antigens are detected serologically, while those at the D locus are defined by mixed lymphocyte culture (MLC). HLA antigens are present on cell membranes, leukocytes, T and B lymphocytes, platelets and all nucleated cells which have been tested.

The HLA system is highly polymorphic and the list of identified alleles continues to grow. By 1981 more than thirty-five million HLA phenotypes were theoretically possible although only a small fraction of these have been observed. While HLA extreme polymorphism is exemplified by the difficulty in overcoming rejection in organ transplantation, its fundamental purpose remains obscure. The prevailing belief is that HLA capacity allows broad protection and preservation of the organism's concept of self against somatic mutation and invasion by pathogens [3, 4]. Several human studies suggest HLA heterozygosity is advantageous. Macurova and associates studied 19 HLA specificities in 83 patients, 350 and 100 controls, ages greater than 80, 40–80, and less than 20 years, respectively [5]. There was an increase in HL-AW10 (corrected p, pc 0.02) and generalized greater number of specificities among the healthy octagenarians. Bender and associates

T. L. Ratliff and W. J. Catalona (eds), Urologic Oncology. ISBN 0-89838-628-4.
© *1984. Martinus Nijhoff Publishers, Boston. Printed in the Netherlands.*

found increased numbers of antigens in healthy patients over 70 years of age compared to children less than 12 [6]. Gerkins and associates typed for 25 HLA specificities in 4 patient groups: (a) 126 healthy non-Jewish caucasians over age 75: (b) 66 solid tumor patients diagnosed over age 75; (c) 148 healthy controls less than 36 years old; (d) 72 patients with onset of cancer at less than 36 years [7]. Healthy elderly patients had a slight increase in frequency of HL-A1 and A8 and the highest number of identified antigens (2 first or second locus antigens, or all 4 antigens in 86 and 72%, respectively).

HLA haplotypes are inherited by Mendelian transmission. However, recombination from gene crossover during meiosis occurs in 1% of divisions and the offspring haplotypes differ from either parent's in these cases [2]. Certain genes on a chromosome tend to segregate together by the process of linkage. Linkage disequilibrium refers to the non-random association of antigens in a population. Possible reasons for this phenomenon include selective advantage, lack of random distribution of recent haplotypes, and new genes or haplotypes introduced by population migration (founder effect) [8].

At least six possible mechanisms of HLA association with disease have been proposed. The first concept is genetic determination of generalized immune responsiveness. Immune response (Ir) genes which determine the specific recognition of antigens exist in the mouse H2 region which is analogous to HLA in man [1, 9]. Ia antigens located at the mouse D locus may be the result of Ir genes and may play the central role in mediating the overall immune response (humoral and cellular). Indirect evidence also exists for human Ir genes and Ia-like antigens, perhaps at the site determining the MLC reaction (D locus) [2]. An essential question is whether or not Ia (murine) or Ia-like (human) antigens are the product of Ir genes, and whether or not the locus for this genetic information is the same as that defining the MLC response. Dausset cautions that one must allow for the possibility that immunologic reaction to cancer is weak even though the weight of extensive current experimentation and opinion is to the contrary [10]. If a limited role of the immune system in cancer proves correct it could explain the difficulty thus far in associating HLA with specific tumors. HLA association with generalized immune responsiveness is but one possible mechanism linking HLA and cancer.

The second mechanism is HLA-directed tumor susceptibility [11]. In 1967 Lilly and associates demonstrated that a gene(s) in the H2 locus is the major determinant of murine susceptibility to Gross leukemia virus. This was the first association of histocompatibility with naturally occurring or environmentally induced neoplasia [12]. The findings of increased HLA-B antigens in patients with Hodgkin's disease and subsequently in breast cancer were among the first associations of HLA with human disease [13, 15]. Lynch and associates described a family with a significantly increased frequency of the HL-A2, A12 haplotype, and vertically transmitted increased frequency of colon and endometrial tumors which occurred multiply and ten to fifteen years earlier than in the general population. This is one example of the 'cancer family syndrome' and genetic susceptibility [16]. Predisposition to cancer may be a direct effect of single or multiple HLA antigens. Identification of multiple, related susceptibility antigens is difficult because these antigens segregate as a single locus in families. Histocompatibility antigens also may be indirectly associated with cancer thru linkage disequilibrium with a non-HLA tumor-related antigen [10, 17, 18]. Recessive HLA susceptibility genes in linkage disequilibrium with an HLA tumor marker are revealed by the occurrence of tumor more often in patients who are homozygous for the marker than chance allows. Finally, a tumor susceptibility gene may be linked to the HLA complex without linkage disequilibrium. In this case no specific HLA antigen is identifiable. Such a linkage is only revealed by rare cases of the same tumor developing in several family members.

Third, HLA antigens may confer resistance to development or progression of malignancy [10, 14, 17]. Resistance antigens are more prevalent in long-term disease survivors than in the total population with the disease, or in the healthy controls. Prospective and retrospecitve studies must be compared to identify resistance antigens with confidence. Retrospective studies of long-term survivors alone omit the early fatalities which may include the majority of patients for malignant diseases. Antigens associated with long-term survival reveal more about disease resistance than incidence or susceptibility. Examples of antigens associated with increased survival are HLA-B8 in breast cancer, HLA-AW19 and HLA-B5 in lung cancer, and HLA-A2 and A9 in acute lymphocytic leukemia [14, 19]. Conversely HLA-AW19 and B5 and HLA-BW40 are associated with a poor prognosis in Hodgkin's disease and acute lymphocytic leukemia, respectively [14, 19]. Theoretical explanations of how genes confer resistance include: decreased pathogen replication in target cells; higher tolerance for chemotherapy and radiotherapy; stronger non-specific immune response; and higher spontaneous regression rate [10]. In most studies subject patient number is less than controls and the frequency of the study antigen in controls is less than 50%. Under these circumstances it is more difficult to demonstrate a statistically significant negative association (i.e., resistance) than a positive one (i.e., susceptibility). This mathematical fact of life emphasizes the need for maximum subject numbers rather than for limiting use of controls. For all these reasons genetic susceptibility is studied more often than resistance.

Fourth, HLA antigens may serve as cell membrane receptors or hormonal ligands for pathogens [17, 21]. Fifth, cross-reactivity between pathogenic and MHC antigens may cause tolerance and failure of the host immune surveillance system in recognizing the foreign antigen. Sixth, HLA antigens may be markers for other genes which cause disease states by mediating deficiency of specific normal proteins such as complement [21].

Several practical points regarding HLA study design should be made. Antigen frequency varies greatly among differing racial, ethnic, and religious groups [2, 22]. The impact of ethnic influences is well illustrated in the accompanying Table 1 adapted from a study by Takasugi and associates [22], which shows marked variation in HLA antigen frequencies in cancer patients, caucasian controls, and controls with Jewish or Mexican names. Within a given race the genetic pool may not yet be at equilibrium (e.g., American caucasians and American blacks) and this may bias results. On the other hand highly inbred populations may suggest spurious genetic associations with disease. Environmental exposure may be a stronger influence on the disease under study and mask a weaker genetic role [14, 17]. Therefore, the need for matching patient and control populations as closely as possible is obvious. Accurate typing sera may be difficult to obtain due to cytotoxic autoantibodies to non-HLA determinants.

Genetic studies of disease are essentially of two types [10, 20]. First, population studies which compare antigen frequencies in patients and matched controls are the easiest to perform. This type of study shows statistical associations which are not necessarily genetically linked or directly related to causing the disease. Second, family studies of two or more affected members may be performed. Statistical genetic linkage with a disease is easier to prove in family studies than in large population trials. However, family studies are more difficult to conduct for a variety of reasons. Subject numbers are far more limited than in populations studies. Instances of family-related neoplasia are few. Family studies may be biased by incomplete penetrance of disease, variable age at disease onset, and incomplete availability of genetic information on other family members. Statistical significance should be distinguished from strength of association. Significance values (p) should be corrected (pc) by multiplying for the number of antigens tested. Strength of association is defined as a cross-product or incidence ratio yielding the relative risk of developing a given disease when a given antigen is present versus the risk when the antigen is absent. Relative risk greater than unity or less than one indicates susceptibility or resistance respectively. Study size of both subjects and controls determines whether or not the strength of association parallels statistical significance.

Table 1. Frequencies of HLA specificities among ethnically different normal controls and patients with bladder and prostate cancer. [b] The frequencies are compared to the total normals by χ^2 tests.

	No. tested	HL-A						W				HL-A					W							
		1	2	3	9	10	11	28	32	29	30	5	7	8	12	13	5	22	27	14	15	17	18	10
Laboratory normals	47	23	53	19	28	6	15	13	9	2	15	2	23	11	30	6	30	6	4	0	15	11	6	21
Parous women	204	25	48	16	26	8	12	16	6	6	16	13	21	16	25	5	22	9	8	7	10	8	9	14
Other donors	300	29	47	26	21	13	8	11	9	8	9	13	25	23	22	6	21	3	10	10	5	6	10	14
Volunteer blood donors	228	30	47	25	19	10	15	8	8	8	6	11	26	23	25	2	21	5	7	7	7	10	8	10
Kidney donors	127	20	51	33	18	16	13	11	7	7	9	7	29	21	24	2	26	5	7	6	9	6	6	19
Total normals	906	27	48	24	21	11	12	12	8	7	10	11	25	21	24	4	22	5	8	7	8	8	9	14
Jewish names (normals)	103	19	43	19	31	20	9	9	6	8	9	9	22	11	23	6	21	2	13	17	3	11	12	12
Mexican names (normals)	277	15	47	15	28	12	15	21	4	5	18	18	10	9	17	4	34	4	7	9	6	5	13	13
Bladder	139	22	45	26	22	14	12	11	6	6	10	10	27	15	24	8	13 [a]	6	9	12	7	9	10	9
Prostate	214	21	51	20	19	14	14	14	5	8	13	10	24	14	24	6	24	6	12	9	11	9	12	10

[a] Frequencies with $0.002 < p < 0.05$.

[b] Adapted from Takasugi M, Terasaki PI, Henderson B, Mickey MR, Menck H, Thompson RW: HL-A Antigens in solid tumors. Cancer Res 33:648–650, 1973 [22].

2. SPECIFIC HLA RELATIONSHIPS WITH GENITOURINARY TUMORS

2.1 *Kidney*

2.1.1 *Renal cell carcinoma.* Valleteau and associates described a family with renal cell carcinoma in four of seven siblings [23]. All seven siblings shared the HLA-A2, A12 haplotype. The three unaffected siblings should be closely followed but a direct cause and effect relationship of the haplotype and renal cancer in this family is not established. HLA-A2, A12 is the second most common caucasian A locus haplotype.

Braun and associates found renal cell carcinoma in two successive generations in each of three unrelated caucasian families [24]. The frequency of HLA-W17 was increased in patients with tumor compared to unaffected family members (5/6 or 83% versus 10/13 or 77%) and compared to the incidence in 485 controls (83% versus 10%, $p = 0.0011$, $pc = 0.066$). The control frequency of HLA-W17 in this study is similar to that previously reported in a larger series of 906 controls (8%). The authors subsequently identified a fourth family with renal cell carcinoma in two brothers with HLA-W17. HLA-W17 was not identified in any of 13 random cases of renal cell carcinoma in this study. Thus, HLA-W17 may only be a marker for renal cancer in the affected families. HLA-W31 was present in two of the four families and HLA-W32 was present in one family.

Pilepich and associates identified two brothers with renal cell carcinoma and the HLA-A2BW21 haplotype [25]. HLA-BW21 cross-reacts with BW17 and therefore this family may carry the same association as the families described in the preceding study. A sister of these two patients, as well as a son carry the HLA-A2BW21 haplotype and are being followed for development of renal cancer.

Kuntz and associates tested for 28 HLA-A and B antigens in 44 unrelated caucasian patients with renal cell carcinoma and 300 healthy matched controls [26]. HLA-AW30/31 frequency was significantly increased in patients (25% versus 7%, $p = 0.00025$, $pc = 0.007$). Thus, an association of HLA-W31/32 with renal cancer has been shown in both population and family studies. Increases in HLA-B8 (25% versus 13%) and absence of HLA-B17 (0% versus 9%) among patients were not significant.

Terasaki and associates found a statistically increased frequency of the HLA-A1, B8 haplotype ($p < 0.05$) in renal cell carcinoma in a collected review of histocompatibility data in 32 diseases [27]. These authors subsequently reported an increased frequency of HLA-AW29 in renal cell carcinoma [28].

2.1.2 *Wilms' tumor.* Majsky and associates studied 23 HLA specificities in 46 patients with Wilms' tumor and 301 healthy controls [29]. The frequencies of HLA-A1 (46% versus 28%, $p = 0.024$, $pc = 0.552$) and HLA-A9 (37% versus 19%, $p = 0.006$, $pc = 0.138$) were significantly increased in patients with Wilms' tumor. However the statistical significance is lost after correcting the p value.

Evers and associates tested for 27 HLA specificities in 30 patients with Wilms' tumor and 800 ethnically matched controls [30]. The patients all had non-familial, unilateral tumors and there was an equal number of males and females. There was one occurrence each of aniridia and a chromosomal abnormality (13q−), factors which have previously been linked with Wilms' tumor. The frequencies of HLA-BW21 (17% versus 6%, $p = 0.01$) and HLA-BW40 (27% versus 11%, $p = 0.0046$) were increased in the patient group. However, the results are not significant after p value correction. The authors point out that the high familial association of Wilms' tumor (38%) and the improved survival with current therapy will allow vertical transmission studies on the genetics of WIlms' tumor similar to previous work with retinoblastoma.

Finally, Ryder, Andersen and Svejgaard included in the third report of the HLA and disease registry the unpublished observation by Beming and associates that no association of specific HLA-A or B antigens was found in forty-six Wilms' tumor patients [31].

2.2 Neuroblastoma

Majsky and associates studied 23 HLA specificities in 20 patients aged one to twenty-four years and in 301 healthy controls [32]. Patient survival ranged from one to twenty-three years and there were only nine survivors beyond five years. The frequencies of HLA-B13 (25% versus 9%, $pc = 0.69$) and HLA-B21 (15% versus 5%) were slightly increased among patients compared to controls.

2.3 Bladder

The immunologic response to transitional cell carcinoma of the bladder has been studied extensively. Catalona has provided a comprehensive review of this work [33]. Generalized and specific host immunologic reactivity against tumor-associated cell surface antigens exist in the form of serologic and leukocyte cytotoxicity. Further, immune responsiveness declines as disease progresses and correlates with prognosis.

In an early study Takasugi and associates tested for 23 HLA specificities in 139 American patients with bladder cancer and in 906 healthy controls (Table 1) [34]. HL-W5 (BW35) frequency was insignificantly decreased in patients with bladder tumors. This result must be interpreted with caution as W5 serotyping was difficult when this study was performed and indeed

W5 showed the greatest extremes in variation of any of the 23 antigens tested.

In another American study, Terasaki and associates reported a statistically increased frequency of both HLA-A2 and BW21 in 217 caucasian bladder cancer patients compared to controls ($pc < 0.05$) [27]. However, in a subsequent study including 264 bladder tumor patients, these authors found no tumor-associated HLA-A or B antigens [28].

The Japanese study by Obata and associates is particularly important from several standpoints [35]. Bladder cancer is rare in Japan and accounted for only 2 078 reported deaths per year in 1978. The authors believe epidemiologic studies on bladder cancer mortality in Japan and elsewhere suggest there are populations at high genetic risk for bladder tumor. They tested for 38 HLA-A and B antigens in 84 patients and in 95 healthy controls. Patients with bladder tumors had increased frequency of HLA-B12 (26.7% versus 15.8%, $p > 0.05$) and decreases of HLA-A10 (12.8% versus 29.8%, $p = 0.01$, $pc > 0.05$) and HLA-B7 (4.7% versus 10.5%, $p > 0.05$) compared to controls (Tables 2 and 3). The frequency of HLA-BW35 in patients with bladder tumors also was decreased slightly as in the earlier report by Takasugi and associates. Two members of one family who shared the HLA-AW19 and HLA-B40 specificities developed bladder tumors. However, other unaffectd family members also shared these antigens and the question of direct or indirect genetic tumor susceptibility remains. One potentially important factor influencing results in this study

Table 2. HLA-A: phenotype and gene frequencies in bladder cancer [a].

Antigen	Bladder cancer ($N = 86$)			Contorls ($N = 95$)		
	PF%	GF%	SE%	PF%	GF%	SE%
A1	3.5	1.8	1.0	1.1	0.6	0.5
A2	37.2	20.8	3.2	46.3	26.7	3.5
A3	0.0	0.0	0.0	0.0	0.0	0.0
A9	62.8	39.6	4.2	48.4	28.2	3.6
A10	12.8	6.6	1.9	29.8	16.0	2.8
A11	16.3	8.5	2.2	15.8	8.2	2.0
A28	0.0	0.0	0.0	0.0	0.0	0.0
A29	0.0	0.0	0.0	0.0	0.0	0.0
AW19	18.6	9.8	2.3	27.4	14.8	2.7
AW34	0.0	0.0	0.0	0.0	0.0	0.0
AW36	0.0	0.0	0.0	0.0	0.0	0.0
AW43	0.0	0.0	0.0	0.0	0.0	0.0
Blank	48.6	28.4	3.8	31.6	17.3	2.9

[a] From Obata K, Ohno Y, Murase T, Aoki K, Tsugi K: Bladder cancer and HLA antigens. Nagoya J Med Sci 43:65–70, 1981 [35].

Table 3. HLA-B: phenotype and gene frequencies in bladder cancer [a].

Antigen	Bladder cancer ($N = 86$)			Controls ($N = 95$)		
	PF%	GF%	SE%	PF%	GF%	SE%
B5	33.7	18.6	3.1	34.7	19.2	3.0
B7	4.7	2.4	1.2	10.5	5.4	1.7
B12	26.7	14.4	2.8	15.8	8.2	2.0
B13	3.5	1.8	1.0	1.1	0.6	0.5
B15	14.0	7.3	2.0	21.1	11.2	2.3
BW16	4.7	2.4	1.2	8.4	4.3	1.5
B17	1.2	0.6	0.6	0.0	0.0	0.0
BW22	27.9	15.1	2.8	18.9	9.5	2.2
BW35	12.8	6.6	1.9	17.8	9.3	2.2
B37	3.5	1.8	1.0	1.1	0.6	0.5
B40	36.0	20.0	3.2	47.4	27.5	3.5
Blank	31.4	17.2	3.0	23.2	12.4	2.5

[a] From Obata K, Ohno Y, Murase T, Aoki K, Tsugi K: Bladder cancer and HLA antigens. Nagoya J Med Sci 43:65–70, 1981 [35].

must be noted. The patients with bladder tumors and the controls came from different regions of Japan (Nagoya and Kanto districts, respectively). Although the Japanese population is fairly homogeneous, regional genetic variation has been demonstrated.

Braf and associates compared the frequency of 27 HLA-A and B specificities in 44 Israeli patients with bladder tumors and in 400 ethnically matched controls [36]. The majority of patients had low stage tumors (9, 27, 2, 4, 2 patients with stage 0, A, B, C, D, respectively). No statistically significant HLA associations with tumor were found (Table 4). Similarly, there were no differences in antigen frequencies when each stage of disease was compared to controls or other stages of disease.

Arce and colleagues tested for 25 HLA specificities in 40 Cuban patients with bladder tumor and in 109 controls [37]. The patients had a statistically significant increase of HLA-A9 (40% versus 16%, $p = 0.002$, $pc = 0.05$) (Table 5).

2.4 Prostate

Ng anc co-workers performed detailed serologic and immunochemical analyses of two human prostate cancer cell lines, DU-145 and H494 [38]. Both tumor lines expressed HLA-A and B antigens, beta 2 microglobulin, and other tumor-associated glycoproteins. In addition, H494 cells expressed Ia-like antigens which were serologically recognized by monoclonal antibodies to cultured B cells. Expression of Ia-like activity by prostate cancer cells in vivo remains to be demonstrated.

Table 4. Comparison of HLA-A and HLA-B loci alleles between 44 patients with transitional cell carcinoma of the bladder and 400 normal matched controls [a].

HLA antigens	Carcinoma patients No. (%)	Control No. (%)
A1	8 (18)	135 (31)
A2	14 (32)	129 (29)
A3	10 (23)	81 (18)
A9	14 (32)	115 (26)
A10	8 (18)	110 (25)
A11	1 (2)	51 (12)
A28	7 (16)	39 (9)
A29	5 (11)	40 (9)
Aw19	14 (32)	101 (23)
Blank	7 (16)	82 (19)
B5	8 (18)	67 (15)
B7	5 (11)	43 (10)
B8	4 (9)	32 (7)
B12	6 (14)	76 (17)
B13	6 (14)	40 (9)
Bw14	7 (16)	71 (16)
Bw15	3 (7)	26 (6)
Bw16	9 (20)	89 (20)
Bw17	3 (7)	55 (13)
Bw18	6 (14)	34 (8)
Bw21	2 (4)	40 (9)
Bw22	3 (7)	21 (5)
Bw35	13 (30)	141 (32)
Bw37	1 (2)	9 (2)
Bw40	6 (14)	35 (8)
Bw27	2 (4)	24 (5)
Blank	4 (9)	74 (17)

χ^2 for the total distribution 0.05. None of the comparisons of individual antigens was significant by the χ^2 test.
[a] From Braf ZF, Gazit E, Many M: HLA-A and B antigens in transitional cell carcinoma of the bladder. J Urol 122:465–466, 1979 [36].

Takasugi and associates reported no significant differences in 23 HLA antigen frequencies between 214 patients with prostate cancer and 906 healthy controls (Table 1) [22]. In a second study Terasaki and co-workers reported prostate cancer was associated with increased HLA-A28 and BW22 and decreased HLA-A1 and B8 frequencies [28].

Barry and associates studied the frequency of 32 HLA-A and B antigens in 100 caucasian men with prostate cancer and 169 matched caucasian controls (Table 6) [39]. The relative risk for developing prostate cancer was greater than 2 for HLA-A11 and A29 and was less than 0.2 for HLA-AW23,

Table 5. Frequencies of 25 HLA-A specificities among 109 normal Cuban controls and 40 bladder cancer patients [a].

Antigen HL-A	Normal population 109 controls		Bladder cancer 40 patients		χ_2 with Yates correction
	Positive cases	Phenotypic frequency	Positive cases	Phenotypic frequency	
Locus A					
HLA-A1	14	0.12	6	0.15	0.004 NS
HLA-A2	46	0.42	20	0.50	0.440 NS
HLA-A3	18	0.16	7	0.18	0.010 NS
HLA-A9	16	0.14	16	0.40	9.677 $p<0.002$
HLA-A10	12	0.11	3	0.08	0.106 NS
HLA-A11	15	0.13	4	0.10	0.111 NS
HLA-A28	9	0.08	1	0.03	0.764 NS
HLA-A29	20	0.18	4	0.10	0.951 NS
HLA-AW30	5	0.04	1	0.03	0.10 NS
HLA-AW33	15	0.13	3	0.08	0.568 NS
Locus B					
HLA-B5	17	0.14	7	0.18	0.001 NS
HLA-B7	19	0.17	7	0.18	0.055 NS
HLA-B8	9	0.08	5	0.13	0.222 NS
HLA-B12	27	0.24	8	0.20	0.154 NS
HLA-B13	6	0.55	0	0.00	1.090 NS
HLA-BW15	6	0.05	4	0.10	0.365 NS
HLA-BW16	5	0.04	1	0.03	0.010 NS
HLA-BW17	13	0.11	4	0.10	0.001 NS
HLA-B18	11	0.10	4	0.10	0.084 NS
HLA-BW21	6	0.05	5	0.13	1.198 NS
HLA-BW22	5	0.04	1	0.03	0.010 NS
HLA-B27	6	0.05	4	0.10	0.365 NS
HLA-BW35	31	0.29	15	0.38	0.739 NS
HLA-BW37	5	0.04	1	0.03	0.010 NS
HLA-BW40	7	0.06	8	0.20	4.550 NS

[a] From Arce S, Lopez R, Almaguer M, Ballester JM, Filgueiras E, Ustariz C, Perez S, Hernandez E: HL-A antigens and transitional-cell carcinoma of the bladder. Materia Medica Polona 10:98–100, 1978 [37].

BW21, BW22. However, none of the differences in antigen frequency were statistically significant after *p* value correction.

Finally, the study by Feingold and associates is included for completeness [40]. HLA antigen frequencies were studied in patients with a variety of tumors, including prostate cancer, from 26 different populations around the world. The authors report a negative association between HLA-B12 and prostate cancer. Analysis of the data is very difficult because antigen-related

Table 6. Frequency of human leukocyte A and B antigens in 100 white patients with adenocarcinoma of the prostate and 169 controls [a].

Antigen	% Positive	
	Patients	Controls
A1	27	36
A2	47	53
A3	25	27
A9	3	2
Aw23	1	6
Aw24	19	14
A10	1	2
A25	6	3
A26	6	3
A11	22	12
A28	6	8
A29	11	5
Aw30	2	6
Aw31	4	7
Aw32	8	4
Aw33	1	1
B5	10	15
B7	26	24
B8	25	25
B12	25	29
B13	4	3
B14	2	5
B15	11	15
Bw16	3	5
B17	8	8
B18	8	7
Bw21	1	5
Bw22	1	8
B27	11	6
Bw35	16	17
B37	0	2
B40	19	19

[a] From Barry JM, Goldstein A, Hubbard M: Human leukocyte A and B antigens in patients with prostatic adenocarcinoma. J Urol 124:847–848, 1980 [39].

susceptibility was estimated from disease frequency calculations based on disease mortality rates. Prostate cancer has a highly variable natural history and occurs predominantly in an elderly population at high risk for death from unrelated disease. Due to this circumstance prostatic cancer-related mortality rate may reveal more about genetic resistance to progression than about susceptibility.

2.5 *Testis*

Germ cell testicular tumors offer a unique opportunity to study genetic factors which mediate cellular differentiation. The incidence of testicular neoplasm varies greatly in different populations (2 per 100 000 European and North American caucasians and very rare in American and African blacks and Japanese) and suggests a genetic role in susceptibility. Immature or embryonic antigens are expressed on animal and human teratocarcinoma cell lines. Perhaps tumor production of the relatively specific biochemical tumor markers alfa-fetoprotein and beta subunit human chorionic gonadotropin is directed by these antigens [21].

Two separate teams of investigators simultaneously presented evidence for the expression of F9 antigen on human embryonal carcinoma cell lines. F9 antigen is present on murine embryonal carcinoma cells and on murine embryonic tissues, spermatozoa, and male germinal epithelium, but not on adult somatic tissues or tumor differentiated to teratoma. Murine embryonal carcinoma cells lack adult H2 antigens. Thus, F9 antigen may be associated with embryonic differentiation. Hogan and colleagues isolated a human teratocarcinoma cell line (SuSa) which expresses F9 antigen [41]. Holden and associates identified F9 antigen in pulmonary metastases from two other human testicular teratocarcinomas (Tera 1 and Tera 2) [42]. It is of interest that these authors found high levels of F9 antigen and alkaline phosphatase in Tera 2 cells and low levels of both substances in Tera 1 cells. These findings suggest that cells from Tera 1 are more differentiated than those from Tera 2. The authors propose that failure of human T cell recognition of teratocarcinoma cells in regional lymph nodes and ineffective immunologic response against the tumor may be due to the primitive genetic and biochemical expression of these cells.

Avner and co-workers found a greater genetic variability in studies of 5 human teratoma cell lines (SuSa, Tera 1, Tera 2, Huttke, PA 1). Several cells expressed both F9 and HLA antigens. Other cells expressed F9 antigen and beta 2 microglobulin but not HLA antigens. Finally, other cells expressed HLA specificities but lacked beta 2 microglobulin [43]. HLA-DR antigens were not identified in any of the five cell lines.

Andrews and associates demonstrated variable HLA-A, B, and C antigens and beta 2 microglobulin in 8 human teratocarcinoma cell lines (833KE, 1156QE, 2102Ep, 1218E, Tera 1, Tera 2, Susa, MG) [44]. Distinct subpopulations of cells which were predictably associated with the presence or absence of specific antigens were not found.

Carr and associates studied the frequency of twenty HLA antigens in twenty patients with testicular tumors and correlated antigen specificities with the risk for developing metastatic disease [45]. The frequency of HLA-AW24 was similar in patients and in the general North American caucasian

292

population (25% versus 16%). However, five of nine patients with metastases carried HLA-AW24. The difference in HLA-AW24 frequency in patients with metastases compared to that in controls (55.6% versus 16%, $p = 0.0075$) is significant. However the corrected p value in this small series is not significant. The finding of metastases in all the patients with HLA-AW24 may indicate a tendency to progression or lack of resistance in these patients and may be associated with worse prognosis. Investigation in larger numbers of patients is indicated.

Majsky and associates studied 23 HLA specificities in 62 testis tumor patients (40 seminoma, 10 embryonal, 5 teratocarcinoma, 7 mixed) and 301 healthy controls [46]. Patients with seminoma had increased frequency of HLA-BW35 (27.5% versus 14.3%, $p > 0.025$, pc not significant). Increased frequencies of HLA-A3, A10, B14, B40 and decreased frequencies of HLA-A2 and B15 were not significant. Patients with non-seminomatous tumors had increased frequency of HLA-A10 (36.4% versus 15.3%, $p < 0.025$, pc not significant) and lesser increases of HLA-B18, B40 and BW21, and decreases of HLA-B8 and B17. Five year survival in the non-seminomatous group was higher in patients with HLA-A2, A9, A10, AW19, B5, B12, B13, BW21. However, none of these associations was statistically significant.

The work by DeWolf and associates on HLA typing in testis tumor patients is particularly important because it includes D locus specificities [21]. The authors tested for 52 HLA-A, B and C antigens and for 9 HLA-D antigens (DW1-7, 10, 11) in 61 patients (30 seminoma, 27 em-

Table 7. Frequency of HLA-D determinants in patients with testicular teratocarcinoma and controls [a].

Determinant	Normal controls (%)	Patients with teratocarcinoma (%)	p value
Dw1	19/150 (13)	7/26 (27)	NS
Dw2	19/150 (13)	3/26 (12)	NS
Dw3	21/150 (14)	6/26 (23)	NS
Dw4	12/150 (8)	2/26 (8)	NS
Dw5	7/100 (7)	1/26 (4)	NS
Dw6	0/50 (0)	1/26 (4)	NS
Dw7	14/150 (9)	12/26 (46)	0.01
Dw10	5/150 (3)	0/26 (0)	NS
Dw11	18/150 (12)	0/26 (0)	NS
Single blank	69/168 (41)	8/26 (31)	NS
Double blank	30/168 (18)	6/26 (23)	NS

[a] Adapted from DeWolf WC, Lange PH, Einasson ME, Yunis EJ: HLA and testicular cancer. Nature 277:216–217, 1979 [21].

bryonal, 26 teratocarcinoma, 7 choriocarcinoma). HLA-A and B, C, and D antigens were also tested in 561, 171, and 150 matched controls, respectively. The frequency of HLA-DW7 was significantly increased in teratocarcinoma patients compared to controls (46% versus 9%, $p < 0.01$) (Table 7). The findings of increased HLA-DW7 frequency in patients with seminoma or embryonal carcinoma (29% each) and absence of this antigen in the 7 patients with choriocarcinoma, were all statistically insignificant compared to controls. The relative risk for developing teratocarcinoma in subjects with HLA-DW7 was 8.32. Thus, HLA DW7 may represent a tumor susceptibility antigen. If substantiated in larger series, this finding would support the existence of oncogenes within the MHC (DW7 as the direct cause) or cross-reactivity of HLA antigens with pathogens (DW7 as the indirect cause). The authors further speculate on the existence of a human MHC-associated region which controls embryonic differentiation and other male reproductive capacities similar to the T/t complex linked to H-2 in the mouse.

At least eighteen cases of familial testicular tumors have been reported. Thirteen tumors occurred in twin or non-twin brothers. Lapes and associates reported the fifth case of testis tumors in father and son pairs [47]. HLA typing in these cases has not been reported and would be of great interest.

3. SUMMARY AND CONCLUSIONS

The structure of the HLA system within the human major histocompatibility complex (MHC) as it is currently understood has been presented. The six following proposed mechanisms for the HLA association with disease have been discussed: 1) generalized immune responsiveness through Ir genes and Ir directed Ia-like antigens controlling the net immune response; 2) tumor susceptibility; 3) tumor resistance; 4) HLA atigens as cell membrane receptors for pathogens; 5) cross-reactivity between HLA antigens and pathogens resulting in failure of host immune surveillance and tolerance to disease; 6) HLA as a marker for other genes which are associated with disease states.

Extreme polymorphism of HLA along with racial, religious and ethnic variations in gene frequencies, and the multifactorial etiology of malignancy all make careful study design of paramount importance in investigations of HLA and cancer. The available data on HLA prognosis in genitourinary tumors has been presented in detail. Suggestions of HLA association with kidney, bladder, prostate and testicular tumors exist. However, in general these associations have been weak and resemble the findings in most other studies of HLA and malignancy. In contrast, associations of HLA and certain non-malignant diseases have been strong.

Why should this be? One must recall Dausset's caveat that perhaps immunologic response to cancer is limited. Failing this explanation what other alternatives exist? Most investigations have pursued only HLA-A and B specificities. Studies of other loci, especially D and DR, may be more rewarding. Tumor susceptibility may be linked with several genes or even an entire complex on the sixth chromosome and be more difficult to identify than single genes associated with non-malignant diseases. Non-malignant disease-related antigens may be located closer to HLA loci than are tumor-related antigens. Genetic tumor associations may be related to resistance more than susceptibility. We have seen that resistance is more difficult to demonstrate than susceptibility. Finally, neoplasia may be an older process phylogenetically than non-malignant diseases and tumor susceptibility genes may be closer to equilibrium with HLA.

Finally, the impression remains that as the pieces of the puzzle are sorted out more clearly a definite association of genetic influences on neoplasia will be appreciated. Subpopulations at high risk for tumor occurrence will be followed more closely. Likewise patients who are likely to have progressive disease will be followed more often and perhaps treated more aggressively. Last but not least, study of the genetic associations with testicular tumors may provide an increased understanding of cellular differentiation and the basic functions of the immune system.

REFERENCES

1. Dausset J, Svejgaard A: Introduction. In: HLA and Disease, Dausset J, Svejgaard A (eds). Copenhagen: Munksgaard, pp 9-10, 1977.
2. Payne R: The HLA complex: Genetics and implications in the immune response. In: HLA and Disease, Dausset J, Svejgaard A (eds). Copenhagen: Munksgaard, pp 20-31, 1977.
3. Dausset J: Les systèmes d'histocompatibilité et la susceptibilité au cancer. Presse Méd 76:1397-1400, 1968.
4. Bodmer WF: Evolutionary significance of the HLA system. Nature 237:139-145, 1972.
5. Macurova H, Ivanyi P, Sajdlova H, Trojan J: HLA antigens in aged persons. Tissue Antigens 6:269-271, 1975.
6. Bender K, Riiter G, Mayerova A, Hiller C. Studies on the Heterozygosity at the HL-A gene loci in young and old individuals. International Symposium on HL-A Reagents, Ragsmey RH, Sprack JV (eds). Basel: Karger, pp 287-290, 1973.
7. Gerkins VR, Ting A, Menck HT, Casagrande JT, Terasaki PI, Pike MC, Henderson BE: HLA heterozygosity as a genetic marker of long-term survival. J Natl Cancer Inst 52(6):1909-1911, 1974.
8. Schaller JG, Hansen JA: HLA relationships to disease. Hospital Practice 16(5):41-49, 1981.
9. McDevitt HD, Benacerraf B: Genetic control of specific immune responses. Adv Immunol 11:31-74, 1970.

10. Dausset J: HLA and association with malignancy: a critical review. In: HLA and Malignancy, Murphy GP, Cohen E, Fitzpatrick JE, Pressman D (eds). New York, NY: Alan R Liss Inc, pp 131-144, 1977.

11. Mittal KK: Possible mechanisms for association of HLA antigens and disease. In: HLA and Malignancy, Murphy GP, Cohen E, Fitzpatrick JE, Pressman D (eds). New York, NY: Alan R Liss Inc, pp 39-51, 1977.

12. Lilly F, Boyse EA, Old LJ: Genetic basis of susceptibility to viral leukaemogenesis. Lancet ii:1207-1209, 1964.

13. Amiel JL: Study of the leukocyte phenotypes in Hodgkin's disease. Histocompatibility testing. Copenhagen: Munksgaard, p 79, 1967.

14. Simons MJ, Amiel JL: HLA and malignant disease. In: HLA and Disease, Dausset J, Svejgaard A (eds). Copenhagen: Munksgaard, pp 212-232, 1977.

15. Falk J, Osoba D: The HLA system and survival in malignant disease: Hodgkin's disease and the carcinoma of the breast. In: HLA and Malignancy, Murphy GP (ed). New York: Alan R Liss Inc, pp 205-216, 1977.

16. Lynch HT, Thomas RJ, Terasaki PI, Ting A, Guirgis HA, Kaplan AR, Chaperon E, Magee H, Lynch J, Kraft C: HL-A in cancer 'Family N'. Cancer 36:1315-1320, 1975.

17. Dick HM: HLA and disease: Introductory review. Brit Med Bull 34:271-274, 1978.

18. Thomson G, Bodmer W: The genetic analysis of HLA and disease association. In: HLA and Disease, Dausset J, Svejgaard A (eds). Copenhagen: Munksgaard, pp 84-93, 1977.

19. Cohen E, Singal DP, Khurana K, Gregory SG, Cox C, Sinks L, Henderson E, Fitzpatrick JE, Highby D: HLA-A9 and survival in acute lymphocytic leukemia and myelocytic leukemia. In: HLA and Malignancy, Murphy GP (ed). New York NY: Allan R Liss Inc, pp 65-70, 1977.

20. Svejgaard A, Ryder L: Associations between HLA and disease. In: HLA and Disease, Dausset J, Svejgaard A (eds). Copenhagen: Munksgaard, pp 46-71, 1977.

21. DeWolf WC, Lange PH, Einasson ME, Yunis EJ: HLA and testicular cancer. Nature 277:216-217, 1979.

22. Takasugi M, Terasaki PI, Henderson B, Mickey MR, Menck H, Thompson RW: HL-A antigens in solid tumors. Cancer Res 33:648-650, 1973.

23. Valleteau M, Ganansia R, Hors J, Letexier A, Moria M: Cancer du rein familial et système HLA. Nouv Presse Méd 3:1539-1542, 1974.

24. Braun WE, Strimlan CV, Negron AG, Straffon RA, Sachary AA, Bartee SL, Grecek DR: The association of W17 with familial renal cell carcinoma. Tissue Antigens 6:101-104, 1975.

25. Pilepich MV, Berkman EM, Goodchild NT: HLA typing in familial renal carcinoma. Tissue Antigens 11:487-488, 1978.

26. Kuntz BME, Schmidt GD, Scholz S, Albert ED: HLA-antigens and hypernephroma. Tissue Antigens 12:407-408, 1978.

27. Terasaki PI, Mickey MR: HL-A haplotypes of 32 diseases. Transplant Rev 22:105-119, 1975.

28. Terasaki PI, Perdue ST, Mickey MR: HLA frequencies in cancer. A second study. In: Genetics of Human Cancer, Mulvihill JJ, Miller RW, Fraumeni JF (eds). New York: Raven Press, pp 321-328, 1977.

29. Majsky A, Abrahamova J, Koutecky J: Wilms' tumor and HLA antigens. Tissue Antigens 11:74, 1978.

30. Evers KG, Gutjahr P, Zachiedrich S, Haase W, Knoop U: Lack of association between HLA specificities and Wilms' tumor. Eur J Pediatr 136:47-49, 1981.

31. Ryder LP, Andersen E, Svejgaard A (eds): HLA and Disease Registry: Third Report. Copenhagen: Munksgaard, 1979.

32. Majsky A, Abrahamova J, Koutecky J: HLA antigens and neuroblastoma. Tissue Antigens 12:156, 1978.

33. Catalona WJ: Commentary on the immunobiology of bladder cancer. J Urol 118:2-6, 1977.

34. Takasugi M, Terasaki PI, Henderson B, Mickey MR, Menck H, Thompson RW: HL-A antigens in solid tumors. Cancer Res 33:648-650, 1973.

35. Obata K, Ohno Y, Murase T, Aoki K, Tsugi K: Bladder cancer and HLA antigens. Nagoya J Med Sci 43:65-70, 1981.

36. Braf JF, Gazit E, Many M: HLA-A and B antigens in transitional cell carcinoma of the bladder. J Urol 122:465-466, 1979.

37. Arce S, Lopez R, Almaguer M, Ballester JM, Filgueiras E, Ustariz C, Perez S, Hernandez E: HL-A antigens and transitional-cell carcinoma of the bladder. Materia Medica Polona 10:98-100, 1978.

38. Ng A, Pellegrino MA, Imai K, Ferrone S: HLA-A, B antigens, Ia-like antigens, and tumor associated antigens on prostate carcinoma cell lines: serologic and immunochemical analysis with monoclonal antibodies. J Immunol 127:443-447, 1981.

39. Barry JM, Goldstein A, Hubbard M: Human leukocyte A and B antigens in patients with prostatic adenocarcinoma. J Urol 124:847-848, 1980.

40. Feingold N, Degos L, Feingold J: HLA in populations: An approach for genetical suscep-tibility to cancer. J Immunogen 6:29-35, 1979.

41. Hogan B, Fellous M, Avner P, Jacob F: Isolation of a human teratoma cell line which expresses F9 antigen. Nature 270:515-518, 1977.

42. Holden S, Bernard O, Artzt K, Whitmore WF Jr, Bennett D: Human and mouse embryonal carcinoma cells in culture share an embryonic antigen (F9). Nature 270:518-520, 1977.

43. Avner P, Bono R, Berger R, Fellous M: Characterization of human teratoma cell lines for their in vitro developmental properties and expression of embryonic and major histocom-patibility locus-associated antigens. J Immunogen 8:151-162, 1981.

44. Andrews PW, Bronson DL, Wiles MV, Goodfellow PN: The expression of MHC antigens by human teratocarcinoma derived cell lines. Tissue Antigens 17:493-500, 1981.

45. Carr BI, Bach FH: Possible association between HLA-AW24 and metastatic testicular germ cell tumors. Lancet ii:1346-1347, 1979.

46. Majsky A, Abrahamova J, Korinkova P, Bek V: HLA system and testicular germinative tumors. Oncology 36:228-231, 1979.

47. Lapes M, Iozzi L, Ziegenfus WD, Antoniades K, Vivacqua R: Familial testicular cancer in a father (bilateral seminoma-embryonal cell carcinoma) and son (teratocarcinoma). Cancer 39:2317-2320, 1977.

Editorial Comment

MARILYN S. POLLACK

1. INTRODUCTION: THE ROLE OF CLASS II HLA MARKERS IN HLA-DISEASE STUDIES

As noted in the previous chapter by A. Sagalowsky, traditional studies of HLA-A, B antigen associations with human cancers of any kind and with genitourinary tumors in particular have not yielded any striking conclusions. It had been supposed for many years, on the basis of Lilly's original study of H-2-linked susceptibility to leukemia in mice [1], that HLA-linked susceptibility (and resistance) factors *must* also exist for human cancers. Their failure to be clearly identified in most cases has been attributed to the outbred nature of most human populations studied, to the multiple subtypes of cancers that are usually combined for data analyses, and to the possibility that different risk factors associated with disease onsets that may occur at different ages have been overlooked in previous studies.

The rapid advancement that has recently occurred in relation to the serological, functional and biochemical identification of human class II histocompatibility system molecules of the DR, DS (MB) and SB series [e.g. 2–7] has, however, now suggested that HLA associations of various forms of cancer with antigens of one or more of these series might be identified. The expectation that this would occur is based on the evidence that these particular determinants are likely, by analogy with mouse data [8] to be more closely related to actual 'immune response' genes. In fact, with the notable exception of HLA-B27-associated diseases, and a few other cases (e.g., the psoriasis/Cw6 association) [9], in which direct involvement of particular HLA-A, B, or C locus antigens is likely, most HLA-associated diseases (which have a significant immune component) have now been determined to have closer statistical associations with particular (DR) class II antigens than with the more traditionally studied HLA-B antigens [9–11]. Examples of these higher associations with class II determinants are shown in Table 1, which also includes evidence for an association in at least one case, celiac disease, with an MB (DC) type of class II determinant [11, 12].

2. CLASS II HLA ASSOCIATIONS WITH NON-GENITOURINARY MALIGNANCIES

Since serological and functional typing for class II antigens is relatively new, only a few forms of cancer have been clearly studied to date with respect to such possible associations. A summary of some of these associations for cancers other than genitourinary tumors is shown in Table 2. It is clear from this table that several different forms of cancer, notably both classical

Table 1. Examples of diseases in which class II HLA antigens show greater associations than do the traditional class I (HLA-B) HLA antigens.

Disease	HLA antigen	No. of studies	No. of patients (%)	No. of controls (%)	Relative risk[a]	Source of data
Multiple sclerosis	B7	17	2698 (12–46%)	14409 (14–31%)	1.75	Ryder et al. [9] (p 30)
	DR2	4	159 (40–70%)	544 (18–29%)	4.80	
Juvenile (insulin-dependent) diabetes	B8	18	1785 (19–60%)	13349 (2–29%)	2.56	Ryder et al. [9] (p 25)
	DR3	3	199 (36–59%)	376 (11–24%)	5.69	
	B15	17	1769 (4–50%)	13175 (2–26%)	2.05	Ryder et al. [9] (p 25)
	DR4	2	76 (32–58%)	216 (16–28%)	2.81	
Rheumatoid arthritis	B27	12	12971 (4–49%)	8458 (5–14%)	1.77	Ryder et al. [9] (p 41)
	DR4	1	53 (70%)	68 (28%)	5.8	
Celiac disease	B8	1	33 (73%)	400 (17%)	13.02	Betuel et al. [11]
	DR3	1	22 (64%)	100 (21%)	8.78	
	DR7	1	22 (55%)	100 (20%)	4.80	
	DR3 and/or DR7[b]	1	22 (86%)[b]	100 (37%)	10.78	

[a] Where relative risk information was not provided, these figures were calculated according to the formula described by Ryder et al. [9].

Note: All data included in this table are statistically significant.

[b] Since both DR3 and DR7 are highly associated with the same MB (DS) molecule, MB2 (Duquesnoy et al. [12], it is possible that MB2 is the primary disease risk gene in this case.

Table 2. Examples of studies of DR antigen frequencies in patients with non-genitourinary cancers.

Type of cancer	Population studied	Relevant antigens	Frequency in patients	Frequency in appropriate controls	Relative risk[a]	Source of data[a]
Classical Kaposi's sarcoma (older pts)	New York (mostly Italian & Ashkenazi)	DR3	2/19 (11%)	94/588 (16%)	0.62	Pollack et al. [13]
		DR5	12/19 (63%)	211/588 (36%)	3.06	
AIDS Kaposi's sarcoma (young pts)	New York (Italian & Ashkenazi)	DR3	1/19 (5%)	94/588 (16%)	0.29	Pollack et al. [13]
		DR5	12/19 (63%)	211/588 (36%)	3.06	
	New York (other caucasians (Northern Europe))	DR3	3/26 (12%)	38/176 (22%)	0.47	
		DR2	16/26 (62%)	44/176 (25%)	5.24	
Mycosis fungoides	New York (caucasians)	DR5	17/32 (56%)	36/176 (20%)	4.41	Safai et al. [14]
Chronic lymphocytic leukemia	New York (caucasians)	DR5	18/29 (62%)	6/28 (21%)	6.0	Winchester et al. [15]
		IVD12 (MB3)	27/29 (93%)	14/28 (50%)	13.5	

Table 2. (continued).

Type of cancer	Population studied	Relevant antigens	Frequency in patients	Frequency in appropriate controls	Relative risk[a]	Source of data
Hairy cell leukemia	New York (caucasians)	DR3 DR5 IVD12 (MB3)	0/14 (0%) 4/14 (29%) 12/14 (86%)	7/28 (25%) 6/28 (21%) 14/28 (50%)	0.02 1.05 6.00	Winchesteret al. [15]
Basal cell carcinoma	New York (Irish)	DR3	4/12 (33%)	10/23 (43%)	0.65	Myskowskit al. [16] (and unpublished data)
Hodgkin's disease	Caucasians (20–25 different studies)	B8 B18	(11–35%)[b] (3–39%)[b]	(12–33%)[b] (2–16%)[b]	1.23 1.30	Ryder et al. [9]

[a] Where relative risk information was not provided, these figures were calculated according to the formulas described by Ryder et al. [9]. Note that relative risks less than 1.00 indicate a negative association (resistance factor).
[b] Ranges of % obtained in the different studies. Note that increases in B8 and B18 were found only in retrospective studies and suggest that they (and DR3) are markers for survival or resistance to the disease.

and Acquired Immunodeficiency Syndrome (AIDS)-associated Kaposi's sarcoma [13], mycosis fungoides [14], CLL [15], and hairy cell leukemia [15], have been found in population studies to have significant positive associations with the specific HLA-DR antigens DR2 and, especially, DR5. It is of interest that in the case of Kaposi's sarcoma, different associations exist in different ethnic subpopulations of patients [13] (Table 1) and that in the case of CLL and hairy cell leukemia, it appears that there may be an even more significant association with the MB (DC) class II locus antigen MB3 than with DR5.

It is also evident from these studies that the specific HLA-DR antigen DR3 is negatively associated with malignancy in Kaposi's sarcoma [13], hairy cell leukemia [15], and basal cell carcinoma [16]. In one additional case, Hodgkin's disease, a negative assocition with DR3 can be inferred from the data relating to B8 and B18 and the known strong positive linkage dise-quilibrium of B8 and B18 with DR3 [17]. These data are particularly interesting because *increases* in the antigens B8 and B18 are actually found, but these are found only in *retrospective* studies and *not* in prospective studies [18]. The implication has been that B8 and B18 (and therefore *DR3* (see above)) are actually *increased* in the longer surviving patients because they offer a benefit in relation to survival (or resistance) to the cancer.

During the course of our study of patients with AIDS-associated Kaposi's sarcoma (Table 2), we also performed HLA typing tests for a group of 45 male homosexual patients with unex-plained lymphadenopathy who were being evaluated as possible AIDS patients at the Hemato-logy-Oncology Division of New York Hospital-Cornell University Medical Center Clinic, and 91 similar patients with lymphadenopathy who were evaluated at the Sloan-Kettering Depart-ment of Infectious Diseases. A total of 6 of the patients in these two groups who were observed for at least 2 months developed AIDS with Kaposi's sarcoma while another group of 6 of these patients developed AIDS with one or more opportunistic infection (without Kaposi's sarcoma) (overall incidence of AIDS development = 12/136 = 9% (unpublished data)). The distribution of DR antigen frequencies among these patients indicated that 3 of 6 of the patients who devel-oped opportunistic infections had HLA-DR3. In contrast, five of the six patients who developed Kaposi's sarcoma had HLA-DR5 while the sixth patient had HLA-DR2 without HLA-DR5. Two of the patients with HLA-DR5 also had HLA-DR2, and none of the six had HLA-DR3. These and the previous results suggest that HLA-DR5 and/or DR2 may be associated with susceptibility while HLA-DR3 may be associated with resistance to the Kaposi's sarcoma clin-ical manifestation among patients who are afflicted with the (as yet unknown) primary etiolog-ical agent for AIDS.

Since other diseases associated with the HLA-DR antigen HLA-DR3 are largely in the cate-gory of autoimmune diseases [e.g., Ref. 19–21 and Table 1], the association of HLA-DR3 with resistance to cancer, at least for the cases of Kaposi's sarcoma and basal cell carcinoma (Table 2) suggests that the 'hyperreactivity' of the HLA-DR3 haplotype may confer resistance to malig-nancy in general. The prognostic utility of monitoring additional potential AIDS patients with lymphadenopathy according to their HLA-DR types is currently being evaluated.

The significant increase of HLA-DR5 in Kaposi's sarcoma and mycosis fungoides patients found in our group's own studies (Table 2) is also an important observation, especially in view of the fact that these patients were tested relatively early in the course of their diseases. The increase in DR5 is, therefore, likely to represent an increase in susceptibility rather than selective resistance (survival).

Some of the other non-malignant HLA disease associations with DR5 that have been describ-ed to date, include scleroderma [22], and the earliest onset form of juvenile rheumatoid arthri-tis [23]. In both of these diseases, immunologic alterations play an important role in the patho-genesis of the disease. It is possible that similar (DR5-associated) immunologic alterations may play a role in the etiology of Kaposi's sarcoma and/or mycosis fungoides or any of the DR5-associated genitourinary malignancies (see below). It is also interesting to note in this connection

302

Table 3. Examples of studies of DR antigen frequencies in patients with genitourinary cancers.

Type of cancer	Population studied	Relevant antigens	Frequency in patients	Frequency in appropriate controls	Relative risk	Source of data
Renal cell carcinoma	Caucasians	DR5	14/26 (54%)	25/124 (20%)	4.62	DeWolfe et al. [28]
Testicular cancer (non-seminomatous)						
metastatic	Austrian caucasians	DR5	(42%)	(23%)	+ [a]	Aiginger et al. [29]
Non-metastatic	Austrian caucasians	DR2	(59%)	(22%)	+ [a]	
Testicular cancer						
pure seminoma	New York caucasians	DR2	5/13 (38%)	44/176 (25%)	1.88	Pollack et al. [30]
		DR5	7/13 (54%)	36/176 (20%)	4.54	
		DR3	0/13 (0%)	38/176 (22%)	0.02	
Non-seminomatous	New York caucasians	DR3	12/92 (13%)	38/176 (22%)	0.55	
Prostate cancer	Caucasians	B8	39/299 (13%)	818/3896 (21%)	0.56	Terasaki et al. [31]

[a] Not enough data were provided in this (abstract) reference for calculation of the relative risk. It is evident, however, that it would be positive in each of these cases.

that DR5 is well recognized to be a serologically complex antigen with at least 4 partially defined subtypes [24–27]. Analysis of the patterns of the reactivities of Kaposi's sarcoma patients in comparison with the reactivity patterns of cells from DR5-positive healthy controls should indicate whether patients with this disease may selectively express a unique subtype of DR5, in possible linkage disequilibrium with unique immune response factors.

3. CLASS II HLA ANTIGEN ASSOCIATIONS WITH GENITOURINARY MALIGNANCIES

As in the case of other malignant diseases, relatively few studies have as yet been performed in relation to associations of particular DR or other class II HLA antigens with particular genitourinary malignancies. Resulsts from a few of the studies that have been published to date are summarized in Table 3. These results indicate that DR5 is associated with renal cell carcinoma although only one patient population has yet been studied. The authors of that study [28] have speculated that spontaneous remission occurs occasionally in this malignancy and that (HLA-associated) immune response factors may play some role in its etiology.

It is also interesting to note that DR5 or DR2, the same two antigens associated with Kaposi's sarcoma, were found to be increased in one recent study among non-seminomatous testicular carcinoma patients with metastatic disease or non-metastatic disease, respectively [29]. In our own study, in which no attempt was made to distinguish patients according to their status of disease progression, no deviations were noted in the frequencies of DR antigens in the *total* group of patients with non-seminomatous disease but an increase in both the antigens DR2 and DR5 were found among the testicular carcinoma patients with pure seminoma [30] (Table 3).

In addition, in our own study of testicular carcinoma the antigen DR3 was found to be significantly decreased among *both* seminoma and non-seminomatous patients [30], as it is for some of the other malignancies studied (see above). A significant decrease in the antigen B8 was found in two different studies of patients with prostate cancer [31], which suggests (because of linkage disequilibrium, as noted above) that DR3 would also be decreased in this form of malignancy.

These preliminary results for genitourinary malignancies thus follow similar patterns for recent studies of other malignancies, namely a general trend towards increases in the antigens DR5 and DR2, and a decrease in DR3. It is also evident that additional studies will be able to further subdivide patients according to their specific ethnic origin, their exact disease subcategory and their responses to treatment, and that these studies will also be able to analyze the roles of other class II determinants. We can thus look forward to the possibility that the immunogenetic components that affect susceptibility and resistance to these and other forms of human malignancy will be more clearly understood in the near future and that their possible prognostic utility may be clearly established.

ACKNOWLEDGEMENTS

Original reserach included in these comments was supported in part by NIH grants CA-22507, CA-08748 and CA-34995. The author also wishes to thank Drs Bijan Safai, Patricia Myskowski, Craig Metroka, Jonathan Gold, William Hennesey and Davor Vugrin, Memorial Hospital, New York, New York, for referring most of the Kaposi's sarcoma, AIDS, basal cell carcinoma, and testicular carcinoma patients studied in relation to the locally generated data included in this report, and to acknowledge the expert technical assistance of Cynthia Callaway.

304

REFERENCES

1. Lilly F, Boyse EA, Old LJ: Genetic basis of susceptibility to viral leukaemogenesis. Lancet ii:1207-1209, 1964.
2. Goyert S, Shively JE, Silver J: Biochemical characterization of a second family of human Ia molecules, HLA-DS, equivalent to murine I-A subregion molecules. J Exp Med 156:550-566, 1982.
3. Zeevi A, Scheffel C, Anne K, Bass G, Marrari M, Duquesnoy RJ: Association of PLT specificity of alloreactive lymphocyte clones with HLA-DR, MB, and MT determinants. Immunogenetics 16:209-218, 1982.
4. Shaw S, Pollack MS, Payne SM, Johnson AH: HLA linked B-cell antigens of a new segregant series defined by secondary allogeneic proliferative and cytotoxic responses. Hum Immunol 1:177-186, 1980.
5. Pawelec G, Shaw S, Wernet P: Analysis of the HLA-linked SB gene system with cloned and uncloned alloreactive T-cell lines. Immunogenetics 15:187, 1982.
6. Shaw S, DeMars R, Schlossman SF, Smith PL, Lampson LA, Nadler LM: Serologic identification of the human secondary B cell antigens. Correlation between function, genetics and structure. J Exp Med 156:731-743, 1982.
7. Shackelford DA, Lampson LA, Strominger JL: Separation of three class II antigens from a homozygous human B cell line. J Immunol 130:289, 1983.
8. Uhr JW, Capara JD, Vitteta ES et al.: Organization of the immune response genes. Science 206:292-297, 1979.
9. Ryder LP, Andersen E, Svejgaard A (eds): HLA and Disease Registry: Third Report. Copenhagen: Munksgaard, 1979.
10. Tiwari JL, Terasaki PI: HLA-DR and disease associations. In: The Lymphocyte, Sell K, Miller WV (eds). New York: Alan R Liss, pp 151-163, 1981.
11. Betuel H, Gebuhrer L, Descos L et al.: Adult celiac disease associated with -HLA-DRw3 and -DRw7. Tissue Antigens 15:231-238, 1980.
12. Duquesnoy R, Marrari M, Vieira J: Definition of MB and MT by 8th International Histocompatibility Workshop B cell alloantiserum clusters. In: Histocompatibility Testing 1980, Terasaki PI, (ed). Los Angeles: UCLA, pp 861-863, 1980.
13. Pollack MS, Safai B, Dupont B: HLA-DR5 and DR2 are susceptibility factors for acquired immunodeficiency syndrome with Kaposi's sarcoma in different ethnic subpopulations. Disease Markers: 135-139, 1983.
14. Safai B, Myskowski PL, Dupont B, Pollack MS: Association of HLA-DR5 with mycosis fungoides. J Invest Dermatol 80: 395-397, 1983.
15. Winchester R, Toguchi T, Szer I, Burmester G, Galbo PL, Cuttner J, Capra JD, Nunez-Roldan A: Association of susceptibility to certain hematopoietic malignancies with the presence of Ia allodeterminants distinct from the DR series. Utility of monoclonal antibody reagents. Immunol Rev 70:155-166, 1983.
16. Myskowski PL, Pollack MS, Schor ES, Dupont B, Safai B: HLA associations in basal cell carcinoma. Clin Res 31:590A, 1983.
17. Baur MP, Danilovs JA: Reference tables of two and three locus haplotype frequencies for HLA-A,B,C,DR,Bf, and GLO. In: Histocompatibility Testing 1980, Terasaki PI (ed). Los Angeles: UCLA, pp 994-1210, 1980.
18. Hors J, Dausset J: HLA and susceptibility to Hodgkin's disease. Immunol Rev 70:167-191, 1983.
19. Batchelor JR, Morris PJ (eds): HLA and Disease. In: Histocompatibility Testing 1977, Nodmer WF, Batchelor JR, Bodmer JG, Festenstein H, Morris PJ (eds). pp 205-258, 1977.

20. Svejgaard A, Platz P, Ryder LP: Insulin-dependent diabetes mellitus. In: Histocompatibility Testing 1980, Terasaki PI (ed). Los Angeles: UCLA, pp 638-656, 1980.
21. Dawkins R: Myasthenia gravis. In: Histocompatibility Testing 1980, Terasaki PI (ed). Los Angeles: UCLA, pp 662-667, 1980.
22. Gladman DD, Keystone EC, Baron M, Lee P, Cane D, Mervert H: Increased frequency of HLA-DR5 in scleroderma. Arthritis Rhem 24:854-856, 1981.
23. Suciu-Foca N, Godfrey M, Jacobs J, Khan R, Rohowsky C, Foca-Rodi A, Woodward K, Hardy M: Increased frequency of DRw5 in Pauci-articular JRA. In: Histocompatibility Testing 1980, Terasaki PI (ed). Los Angeles: UCLA, p 953, 1980.
24. Wakisaki A, Nakai Y, Kano T, Aizawa M, Moriuchi J, Itakura K: Complexity of DRw5 in Japanese. In: Histocompatibility Testing 1980, Terasaki PI (ed). Los Angeles: UCLA, p 806, 1980.
25. Curtoni ES, Borelli I, Cornaglia M, Olivetti E: Complexity of DRw5. In: Histocompatibility Testing 1980, Terasaki PI (ed). Los Angeles: UCLA, p 805, 1980.
26. Engelfreit C, de Lange G, Hilterman T, van den Berg-Loonen E: DR5. In: Histocompatibility Testing 1980, Terasaki PI (ed). Los Angeles: UCLA, pp 518-521, 1980.
27. Mizrachi Y, Orgad S, Jonash A, Avigad S, Yaron M, Gazit E: DRw5 heterogeneity in the Jewish population. In: Histocompatibility Testing 1980, Terasaki PI (ed). Los Angeles: UCLA, p 807, 1980.
28. DeWolf WC, Lange PH, Shepard R, Martin-Alosco S, Yunis EJ: Association of HLA and renal cell carcinoma. Human Immunol 1:41-44, 1981.
29. Aiginger P, Schwarz HP, Kumits R, Kuhbock J, Schemper M, Mayr WR, Karrer K: HLA-A,B,C and DR antigens and testicular cancer: a prospective study. Proc Am Assoc Cancer Res (Abstracts), p 190, 1983.
30. Pollack MS, Vugrin D, Hennessy W, Herr HW, Dupont B, Whitmore WF: HLA antigens in patients with germ cell cancer of the testis. Cancer Res 42:2470-2473, 1982.
31. Terasaki PI, Perdue ST, Mickey MR: HLA frequencies in cancer. A second study. In: Genetics of Human Cancer, Mulvihill JJ, Miller RW, Fraumeni JF Jr (eds). New York: Raven Press, pp 321-328, 1977.

12. Luteinizing Hormone Releasing Hormone Analog Agonists in the Treatment of Advanced Prostatic Cancer

JOHN TRACHTENBERG

1. INTRODUCTION

The treatment of advanced prostatic cancer is based upon the belief that this tumor is initially androgen dependent [1]. Therapeutic modalities therefore attempt to lower the level of circulating androgens. The two major clinical methods of achieving this aim are bilateral orchiectomy and the administration of pharmacologic doses of estrogens. While both techniques are effective in diminishing the level of circulating androgens and in inducing a remission in the majority of patients they both are associated with distinct clinical problems [2].

Bilateral orchiectomy is a surgical procedure that often must be performed in the elderly and infirm. In these patients there can be significant morbidity and mortality. Furthermore many men object to castration on psychological grounds.

Estrogens when administered in adequate doses will lower serum androgens to the castrate level. This therapy has therefore been labeled a 'medical castration'. It thus theoretically should provide all the benefits of castration while avoiding the surgical procedure. Proponents of its use also believe that estrogen therapy has a direct cytotoxic effect on prostatic cancer cells. Inspite of these beliefs clinical experience has not proven estrogen therapy superior to orchiectomy.

The decline in serum androgens after the initial administration of estrogens is both time and dose dependent. At the usual dose of 3 mg of diethylstilbestrol per day serum androgens do not decline to the castrate level until approximately 14 days. At lower doses the rate of decline is slower and the extent of decline is variable. At higher doses unpleasant side effects become clinically problematic. The long-term use of estrogens are associated with a variety of both major and minor side effects. Estrogens are by their nature feminizing but more important is their deleterious effect on the cardiovas-

T. L. Ratliff and W. J. Catalona (eds), Urologic Oncology. ISBN 0-89838-628-4.
© *1984. Martinus Nijhoff Publishers, Boston. Printed in the Netherlands.*

cular system. Several trials have demonstrated a markedly increased incidence of fluid retention, hypertension, and ischaemic heart disease. Furthermore there is a real increase in morbidity and mortality due to an increase in thromboembolic phenomena [3]. These side effects must be tolerated in light of increasing evidence that hormonal therapy is only palliative in nature and does not in fact increase survival [2].

Recently, several new compounds and treatment strategies have challenged the use of estrogens as the agent of choice in the medical treatment of advanced prostatic cancer. These treatments propose to offer the benefits of castration pharmacologically without the side effects of estrogens and to possibly increase survival.

2. LUTEINIZING HORMONE RELEASING HORMONE ANALOGS

In 1971 Schally and co-workers successfully isolated, described, and synthesized the molecular structure of native luteinizing hormone releasing hormone (Pyroglu-His-Trp-Ser-Gly-Leu-Arg-Pro-Gly-NH$_2$) [4]. It is felt that the 'active center' of this molecule lies at amino acid positions two and three with important conformational sites at positions one, six, and ten. Schally and others subsequently synthesized a series of potent analog agonists of this molecule that possessed the unique property of releasing manyfold more luteinizing hormone than the native molecule. Common to many of these analogs is a substitution of glycine by D-amino acids (e.g. leucine, t-butyl serine, tryptophan, or alanine) in the sixth position of the decapeptide chain and removal of the tenth amino acid-amide group. These changes are felt to significantly increase the affinity and binding characteristics of the molecule to its receptor sites in the pituitary.

While these agents cause an abrupt increase in LH release and subsequent sex steroid release in both males and females after acute administration, paradoxically during chronic administration sex steroid levels fall to the castrate levels [5, 6]. Th exact mechanism for this action is not completely clear but probably results from alterations in the central feedback control of LH release, desensitization of the gonad to LH by reduction in gonadal LH receptor sites, and direct gonadal steroid enzyme inhibition [7].

In a variety of male animals and men these agents have been consistently demonstrated to reduce serum testosterone, impair spermatogenesis, decrease the size and weight of the testes and cause an involution of androgen-dependent tissues [5–8]. Because these agents have no estrogenic action they were immediately seized upon as possible replacements for estrogens in the medical treatment of prostatic cancer. It was hoped they would provide the 'anti-androgenic' effects of estrogens with none of estrogens' side effects.

Were this so, not only could patients be spared the feminizing effects of estrogens but also they might avoid the cardiovascular toxicity of estrogens and perhaps thus realize a survival benefit.

In a variety of trials using various analogs these agents have proven to be both safe and effective in reducing serum testosterone and in the induction and maintenance of remissions in patients with prostatic cancer [7, 9, 10]. These agents have been administered either subcutaneously in daily injections or by nasal insufflation. With both methods patient acceptance and compliance have been good. At present several large-scale long-term trials are underway to compare the relative benefits of LHRH analogs and estrogen therapy or orchiectomy in the hormonal treatment of advanced prostatic cancer. We have been involved in a 200 patient trial of the daily injection of 1 mg of a six-leucine LHRH analog (leuprolide, TAP Pharmaceuticals, North Chicago, Illinois) vs 3 mg of DES taken orally in patients with stage D_2 metastatic prostatic cancer [11]. In our center eleven patients were randomized to receive DES and twelve leuprolide. The pretreatment clinical characteristics of these two groups were identical. Both agents caused a decline in serum testosterone to the castrate range by one month of treatment and the subsequent induction of objective and subjective improvement in all patients. The leuprolide group was however, marked by a 30% increase in serum testosterone at one week of treatment because of its initial agonist effect. This was accompanied by a transient increase in bone or flank pain in 40% of patients with completely resolved by two weeks of treatment. Several strategies are now in effect to blunt this initial 'flare' period by the temporary initial use of anti-androgens or estrogens. At one year of follow-up of the entire trial, both groups have similar survival characteristics but the leuprolide group is associated with significantly fewer complications. The long-term side effects noted with leuprolide are remarkably few. They include recurrent flushing, occasional local irritation at the site of injection, and impotence. By contrast the DES group had a significant incidence of pedal edema, deep vein thromboses, myocardial infarctions, strokes, as well as gynecomastia and impotence. Thus early evidence suggests that leuprolide is as effective in inducing and maintaining a remission as estrogens but has fewer complications than estrogens. LHRH analogs may be superior to estrogens in the medical hormonal therapy of prostatic cancer.

Another approach to the use of these agents has been taken by Labrie and co-workers who have married the ability of a specific LHRH analog (buserelin, Hoechst AG, FDR) to reduce testicular steroidogenesis with an anti-androgen which blunts the initial flare effect of the analog as well as blocking residual adrenal androgen action [12]. This combination is thus said to produce total androgen ablation and the combined blockade of testicular and adrenal androgens to confer a survival advantage over the elimination of only testicular androgens in the hormonal treatment of patients with advanced prostatic cancer. Whether this 'combined' therapy is superior to single agent therapy remains to be determined.

It appears clear that in the near future new agents will become available that will provide the benefits of estrogens in the hormonal management of prostatic cancer with little of their side effects. Whether these agents are superior to estrogen therapy or orchiectomy in the treatment of advanced prostatic cancer remains to be seen.

REFERENCES

1. Huggins C, Hodges CV: Studies of prostatic cancer. I. The effect of castration, estrogen, and androgen injections on serum phosphatases in metastatic carcinoma of the prostate. Cancer Res 1:293, 1941.
2. Walsh PC: Physiological basis for hormonal therapy in carcinoma of the prostate. In: The Prostate. Urol clin North Am. Philadelphia: Saunders WB, p 125, 1975.
3. Glashorn RW, Robinson MRG: Cardiovascular complications in the treatment of prostatic cancer. Br J Urol 53:624, 1981.
4. Matsuo H, Baba Y, Nair RMG, Arimura A, Schally AV: Structure of the porcine LH and FSH releasing hormone. I. The proposed amino acid sequence. Biochem Biophys Res Commun 43:1334, 1971.
5. Sandow J, Von Rechenberg W, Jerzabek G, Engelbart K, Kuhl H, Fraser H: Hypothalamic pituitary testicular function in rats after supraphysiological doses of a highly active LRH analogue (Buserelin). Acta Endocrinol 94:489, 1980.
6. Trachtenberg J: Effect of chronic administration of potent luteinizing hormone releasing hormone analog on the rat prostate. J Urol 128:1097, 1982.
7. Tolis G, Mehta A, Kinch R, Comaru-Schally AM, Schally AV: Suppression of sex steroids by an LH-RH analogue in man. Clinical Res 28:676, 1980.
8. Linde R, Doelle GC, Alexander N, Kirchner F, Vale W, Rivier J, Rabin D: Reversible inhibition of testicular steroidogenesis and spermatogenesis by a potent gonadotropin-releasing hormone agonist in norman men. N Engl J Med 305:663, 1981.
9. Tolis G, Ackman D, Stellos A, Mehta A, Labrie F, Fazekas ATA, Comaru-Schally AM, Schally AV: Tumor growth inhibition in patients with prostatic cancer treated with luteinizing hormone releasing hormone agonists. Proc Natl Acad Sci USA 79:1658, 1982.
10. Trachtenberg J: The use of a potent luteinizing hormone releasing hormone analog agonist in the treatment of advanced prostatic cancer. J Urol (in press).
11. Trachtenberg J: A comparison of DES and a potent luteinizing hormone releasing hormone analog in the treatment of advanced prostatic cancer. In: Proceeding of the Annual Meeting of the American Urological Association. Abstract 34, 1983.
12. Labrie F, Dupont A, Belanger A, Cusan L, Lacourciere Y, Monfette G, Laberge JG, Emond JP, Husson JM: New hormonal therapy in prostatic carcinoma: Combined treatment with an LHRH agonist and an antiandrogen. Clin Invest Med 5:267, 1982.

Editorial Comment

JOSEPH A. SMITH, JR.

1. INTRODUCTION

The potential usefulness of luteinizing hormone releasing hormone analogs in the treatment of prostatic cancer is dependent upon the observed reduction in circulating levels of androgens which occurs with chronic administration of these agents. The partial androgen dependence of most prostatic adenocarcinomas has been recognized since the pioneering work of Huggins and Hodges in 1941 [1]. They were able to demonstrate that suppression of serum testosterone levels to the castrate range resulted in clinical improvement and objective regression of tumor in the majority of patients with prostatic cancer. Over 40 years later, hormonal manipulation with testosterone suppression continues to be the most effective initial treatment for patients with metastatic carcinoma of the prostate. However, as discussed by Dr Trachtenberg, there are limitations in existing endocrine treatments, primarily orchiectomy and oral estrogens.

Bilateral orchiectomy is a simple and safe surgical procedure which rapidly reduces circulating levels of serum testosterone and effects a prompt clinical response and objective disease regression in most patients with prostatic cancer. Even in elderly and chronically ill patients, the procedure can be performed easily under local anesthesia with relatively little morbidity. However, the potential adverse psychological impact of castration limits its appeal in some patients.

Oral administration of adequate doses of diethylstilbestrol reliably suppresses testosterone to castrate levels by an inhibition of pituitary gonadotropin release. However, doses of 1 mg per day may incompletely suppress testosterone [2]. In addition, higher doses are associated with an increased incidence of cardiovascular and thromboembolic complications which, in some groups, have had an adverse impact on patient survival [3]. Painful gynecomastia occurs frequently with chronic DES administration and is only partially prevented by pretreatment breast irradiation [4]. Salt and water retention and nausea and vomiting are also associated with estrogen therapy in some patients. Recognition of these limitations of orchiectomy and DES have prompted continued investigations of alternative forms of endocrine therapy and stimulated clinical trials investigating LHRH analogs as treatment of prostatic cancer.

2. MECHANISM OF ACTION

Naturally occurring luteinizing hormone releasing hormone (LHRH) causes the release of the gonadotropins luteinizing hormone (LH) and follicle stimulating hormone (FSH) from the pituitary gland. Chronic administratin of LHRH analogs has been shown to produce atrophy of reproductive organs in male rodents by suppressing testosterone production [5]. Initial investigations emphasized the fact that relatively small doses of these agonists inhibited testosterone production with virtually no systemic toxicity [6]. Leuprolide is the generic name for a potent LHRH analog developed by Abbott Laboratories/TAP Pharmaceuticals. The compound was synthesized by substitution of the D-isomer of leucine for glycine at the 6th position of naturally occurring GnRH and the 10th amino acid was replaced by an ethylamide moiety attached to the carboxyl group of proline at position 9. The short-hand notation for this compound is: (D-Leu 6, des-Gly-NH₂ 10, Pro-ethylamide 9) – GnHR.

It is important to recognize that compounds such as leuprolide are LHRH agonists, not antaqonists. However, chronic administration of these agents has the paradoxical effect of suppression of pituitary gonadotropins and, consequently, testosterone. Although the mechanism behind this action is uncertain, administration of these agents causes an initial stimulation of pituitary gonadotropin release and a rise in circulating androgen levels. Thirty patients at the University of Utah Medical Center with metastatic carcinoma of the prostate and no previous endocrine therapy have been treated with leuprolide. In the first week of treatment, there was an increase in the serum FSH and LH over basal pre-treatment levels. By day 4, FSH levels had decreased to significantly below baseline and reached a nadir of suppression at 10 weeks. Although plasma levels of FSH gradually increased and achieved a higher plateau between 25 and 97 weeks, they have remained significantly suppressed below baseline for periods of follow-up as long as two years.

Testosterone and dihydrotestosterone levels followed a pattern similar to that of the gonadotropins. Serum testosterone levels increased from a mean of 360 ng/ml to 668 ng/ml at day 4. By day 8, testosterone had decreased to levels similar to the pre-treatment status and at week 6 had been markedly suppressed to mean levels of 15.67 ng/ml. Profound suppression of testosterone has continued for as long as two years.

3. CLINICAL EFFECTS

The clinical response in patients with metastatic carcinoma of the prostate is predictable based upon these endocrine changes. Table 1 outlines the objective responses seen in patients at the University of Utah who have undergone treatment with leuprolide. The response criteria were identical to those defined previously by the National Prostatic Cancer Project [7]. Thirty patients had received no previous endocrine treatment. Of these, 14 had objective evidence of a partial response at the three month evaluation. An additional 12 patients had objectively stable disease whereas two had disease progression and another two patients were not evaluable.

Table 1. Objective response at three months in patients treated with leuprolide.

	Prior endocrine therapy	
	None	Orchiectomy or DES
Complete response	0	0
Partial response	14 (46%)	0
Stabilization	12 (40%)	2 (17%)
Progression	2 (7%)	10 (83%)
Not evaluable	2 (7%)	0
Total	30	12

The duration of response in these patients remains to be defined. However, fifteen of these patients (50%) remain on study and are continuing with daily leuprolide injections. These patients have maintained evidence of disease remission for a median of 16 months with a range of 9 to 25 months. Ten patients who initially had evidence of disease response subsequently have developed progression and have been discontinued from the study. These patients remained in remission for a median of 12 months before progression. There have been three patients who died of other causes during the period of follow-up and while on study at 12, 13 and 16 months.

An additional 12 patients at the University of Utah have been treated with leuprolide after developing disease progression following an initial endocrine-induced remission with orchiectomy or DES. Previous evidence suggests that endocrine treatments generally are not additive in patients with prostatic cancer and our experience supports this. Of the 12 patients entered on the study, ten developed evidence of disease progression within three months or had died of prostatic cancer. Only one patient who had received prior endocrine therapy remained on leuprolide for longer than six months.

4. TREATMENT SIDE EFFECTS

Concurrent with the initial rise in androgen levels, three of our previously untreated patients (10%) had modestly increased bone pain in the first week of treatment. However, all three of these patients had a good symptomatic response by two weeks and went on to show objective evidence of disease response. There have been no other manifestations of a so-called 'disease flare' in any of the patients at the University of Utah treated with leuprolide.

Leuprolide has been an extremely well tolerated drug with no major adverse effects. In particular, there have been no thromboembolic or cardiovascular complications attributed to the drug. In addition, no patient has developed drug-related gynecomastia. Twenty-three of the previously untreated patients (77%) experienced vasomotor hot flashes. They fluctuated in severity and duration but clearly were more profound than the hot flashes seen occasionally in patients after orchiectomy. The reasons for this are uncertain and the ability to decrease or suppress hot flashes using low dose estrogens was not tested in our patients. Leuprolide was given as a daily, self-administered subcutaneous injection of 1 cc. Although there were occasional reports of irritation at the injection site, there were no problems with patient compliance or acceptance of this mode of administration.

Thirteen of our patients were sexually active prior to starting therapy with leuprolide. Of these, only three (23%) remained potent at 9, 11 and 14 months of treatment. Ten patients (77%) developed impotence and decreased libido a mean of six months after starting therapy with leuprolide.

5. DISCUSSION

Based upon these results, LHRH analogs such as leuprolide have been shown consistently to cause an initial transient rise in gonadotropins and testosterone followed by a profound, sustained suppression. These observed endocrine effects have predicated the use of such agents in patients with prostatic cancer.

The clinical responses which have been seen appear to be equivalent to those achieved with alternative hormonal manipulation, in particular DES or orchiectomy [8]. Although the duration of response in patients treated with LHRH analogs remains to be defined, preliminary evidence suggests that it will also be similar to that seen with orchiectomy or DES. Considering this, the role of LHRH analogs in treatment of carcinoma of the prostate is dependent upon improved patient acceptance and fewer side effects.

Clearly, LHRH analogs have been shown to be safe and without major adverse reactions. There have been no apparent drug-related thromboembolic or cardiovascular complications. In addition, painful gynecomastia which is frequently seen with estrogen administration is avoided. Furthermore, other side effects sometimes seen with estrogen administration such as edema, salt retention and nausea and vomiting have not been observed with LHRH analogs.

On the other hand, LHRH analogs appear to offer no substantial benefit in terms of preservation of sexual activity. The majority of our patients who had been sexually active prior to study entry developed decreased libido and erectile impotence. In addition, decreased sexual function was seen in a group of young men treated with a similar drug used to suppress spermatogenesis [9]. Although some patients retain their potency for a prolonged time after orchiectomy or DES administration, most have decreased libido and impotence concurrent with androgen suppression [10]. Therefore, a similar effect on sexual function may be anticipated with LHRH analogs.

Vasomotor hot flashes were the only side effects which occurred with any regularity in our patients. There was considerable variability in the severity of symptoms but sweating and flushing occurred as often as every hour in some patients. The mechanism behind the increased incidence of hot flashes in these patients compared to those receiving alternative endocrine treatment is uncertain. In addition, the ability to suppress or diminish hot flashes in these patients using low dose estrogens was not tested.

The potential significance of the 'disease flare' which may occur during the first week of study deserves further comment. Testosterone levels rise to 150–180% of basal concentrations during the first week of treatment with LHRH analogs. However, by two weeks, they have been suppressed consistently to below baseline and are at castrate levels by four weeks. A potential concern has been that this transient rise will result in a similar stimulation of disease activity in patients. Actually, this has been a very minor clinical problem in our patients. Although three patients did have a very mild increase in bone pain within the first week, no other evidence of a 'disease flare' was observed. As mentioned by Dr Trachtenberg, anti-androgens or, perhaps, short-term treatment with estrogens may block testosterone stimulation by LHRH analogs. At any rate, although it does not appear to present a problem in the majority of patients, the potential for a disease flare within the first week of treatment with LHRH analogs is a concern in patients with impending neurologic compromise or in those in whom a rapid symptomatic response is imperative.

In previously untreated patients with metastatic carcinoma of the prostate, the clinical effects of LHRH analogs appear to be equivalent to alternative endocrine treatments. In patients who can accept castration, the rapid suppression of serum testosterone and the ease and simplicity of orchiectomy continue to represent significant advantages. Previously, most patients who refused orchiectomy have been treated with estrogens. However, considering the lack of significant side effects found in this study, LHRH analogs may prove to be the preferred form of initial endocrine therapy for selected patients with metastatic carcinoma of the prostate.

REFERENCES

1. Huggins C, Hodges CV: Studies of prostatic cancer. I. The effect of castration, estrogen, and androgen injections on serum phosphatases in metastatic carcinoma of the prostate. Cancer Res 1:293, 1941.
2. Symes EK, Milroy E: An experimental approach to the optimum estrogen dosage in prostatic carcinoma. Br J Urol 50:562, 1978.

3. Byar DP: The Vetran's Administration cooperative urological research group's studies of cancer of the prostate. Cancer 32:116, 1973.
4. Alfthan O, Gholsti LR: Prevention of gynecomastia by local roentgen irradiation in estrogen treated prostatic cancer. Scand J Urol Nephrol 3:183, 1969.
5. Rivier C, Rivier J, Vale W: Chronic effects of [D-Trp6,Pro9-Net] luteinizing hormone releasing factor or reproductive processes in the male rat. Endocrinology 105:1191, 1979.
6. Labrie F, Cusan L, Sequin C, Belanger A, Pelletier G, Reves J, Kelly PA, Lemay A, Raynaud JP: Antifertility effects of LHRH agonists in the male rat and inhibition of testicular steroidogenesis in man. Int J Fertil 25:157, 1980.
7. Schmidt JD, Johnson DE, Scott WW, Gibbons RP, Prout GR, Murphy GP: Chemotherapy of advanced cancer. Evaluation of response parameters. Urology 7:602, 1976.
8. Walsh PC: Physiologic basis for hormonal therapy in carcinoma of the prostate. Urol Clin North Al 2:125, 1975.
9. Linde R, Doelle GC, Alexander N et al.: Reversible inhibition of testicular steroidogenesis and spermatogenesis by a potent gonadotropin-releasing hormone agonist in normal men. N Engl J Med 305:663, 1981.
10. Ellis WJ, Grayhack JT: Sexual function in aging males after orchiectomy and estrogen therapy. J Urol 89:895, 1963.

13. Nuclear Magnetic Resonance (NMR) Imaging in Urologic Oncology

RICHARD D. WILLIAMS and HEDVIG HRICAK

1. INTRODUCTION

The development of nuclear magnetic resonance (NMR) imaging is among the most recent advances in diagnostic modalities designed to peer non-invasively into the functioning human in order to distinguish abnormal from normal anatomy. The enthusiasm attending the clinical emergence of NMR imaging is based on NMR's unique ability to provide both precise anatomical detail displayed in multiple planar projections and the simultaneous delivery of physiologic and chemical information without harm to the subject. Such an approach may provide a window into the physiologic and biochemical abnormalities underlying disease processes, thus permitting predictive insights into these processes.

Herein we briefly review the history of NMR and the physical concepts central to the understanding of NMR imaging. The basic hardware and methods required to produce medical NMR images are described and the actual and potential advantages, as well as the possible risks, of medical NMR imaging are discussed. Finally, a limited overview of the current state of the art with respect to anatomical areas of interest to the urologic oncologist is presented.

2. HISTORY

The physical principles of NMR were first described in 1946 by Bloch [1] and Purcell and co-workers [2]. Since then NMR spectroscopy has been used widely as an analytical tool to determine the conformation of organic molecules and to monitor experimental metabolic reactions. The original discovery was of sufficient impact to gain Bloch and Purcell a jointly awarded Nobel Prize for Physics in 1952.

T. L. Ratliff and W. J. Catalona (eds), Urologic Oncology. ISBN 0-89838-628-4.
© *1984. Martinus Nijhoff Publishers, Boston. Printed in the Netherlands.*

Isolated living tissues were first studied by NMR spectroscopy in 1968 [3]. This was closely followed (1971) by the finding of substantial differences in NMR spectroscopy of benign and malignant tissues [4]. Lauterbur [5] in 1972 was the first to exploit NMR to produce cross-sectional tissue images in vitro. Demonstration of in vivo animal images in cross-section was reported in 1975 [6] and the first in vivo scans of humans were described in 1977 (a wrist) [7] and in 1978 (a head) [8]. Although the concept of body imaging for medical use existed already in the early 1970s, much of the success in adapting NMR for clinically useful images is owed to the development of the computers and software required for reconstruction of the 10^8 or more data bits necessary to produce computerized X-ray tomographic imaging (CT). Thus, despite a prolonged delay between conception and realization, the last 5 years have brought about clinically useful NMR imagers, first in Aberdeen and Nottingham in the United Kingdom, and now in the United States, with at least four commercial systems available. As is true with many medical scientific advances, NMR technology has preceded the practitioners' understanding of its physical principles. Consequently, the full impact of its utility awaits our gathering of information by careful clinical studies.

3. PHYSICAL PRINCIPLES

The concepts fundamental to the understanding of NMR imaging have been reviewed in detail in several recent reports [8–16]. These concepts are based on the presence of an abundant number of nucleons (atomic nuclei) with an odd atomic number (neutrons + protons = atomic number) in living tissues. Examples of naturally occurring isotopic species of atoms with odd atomic numbers are: C^{13}, O^{17}, FL^{19}, Na^{23}, P^{31}, and the most abundant in living tissues H^1. This natural abundance of hydrogen atoms (protons) is based on the ubiquity of water (which contains 2 protons) and lipids within living tissues. By virtue of its intrinsic property of spin or angular momentum, each species of nucleon with an uneven number of particles produces a small magnetic field around it. In general, these nucleons or atoms have a magnetic moment or magnetic force, the direction of which can be designated as a vector. An example is the proton seen in Figure 1. In undisturbed tissue at equilibrium the net magnetic moment of the atoms present is zero (Figure 2). This is true, although each has a separate minute magnetic moment, because they are in random thermal motion and therefore tend to cancel each other out.

However, if a group of atoms, for example protons, are placed in a static externally applied magnetic field, the magnetic moments of the protons will

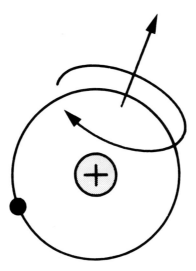

Figure 1. Hydrogen atom exhibiting an odd atomic number (1 proton) and intrinsic angular momentum resulting in a magnetic force vector.

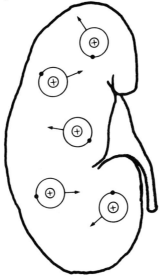

Figure 2. Random distribution of atoms in undisturbed tissue causes proton magnetic vectors to have a net magnetic moment of zero.

tend to align themselves in parallel along the direction of the field consistent with their lowest energy state, thereby reaching a new equilibrium (Figure 3). During alignment, not all of the proton vectors will lie in the same direction because of thermal motion within their environment. However, in general they will either be parallel or anti-parallel to the external magnetic field. Because just slightly more protons will line up parallel, the net vector

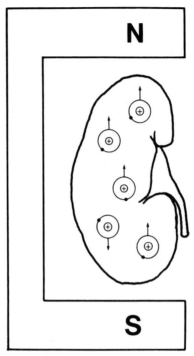

Figure 3. Within a strong external magnetic field the proton magnetic vectors will undergo alignment with the net magnetic moment directed toward the north pole of the magnet.

will be in the direction of the north pole of the external magnetic force. While in this new equilibrium state within the externally applied magnetic field, each proton continues to spin about its own axis and the axis of the magnetic field, much as a spinning top rotates around its own axis while simultaneously rotating around the vertical axis of the earth's gravitational field. The artificial spin angle induced by the external magnetic field is termed precession and the rate of precession is directly related to the strength of the applied magnetic force, but has a definite frequency (Larmor frequency) for each isotopic species within a specified magnetic field strength.

Units applied to magnetic field strengths are generally referred to as either Gauss (G) or Tesla (T). For example, the earth's gravitational field ranges around 0.6 G, whereas the field strengths used for medical NMR imaging range from 0.1 T to 1.5 T (1.0 T = 10 000 G). Thus, in a magnet with a field strength of 1.0 T, for example, the Larmor frequency of protons is 42.58 MHz.

Returning to the protons aligned in the magnetic field in Figure 3, if electromagnetic waves (another magnetic force) are applied at a right angle to the axis of the prior external field at exactly the protons' Larmor frequen-

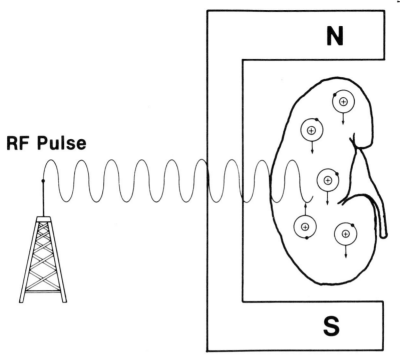

RF Pulse

Figure 4. Radiofrequency (RF) waves pulsed at right angles to the external magnetic field will cause a change in the alignment (precession) of the proton magnetic vectors within the tissue.

cy within the field, further precession occurs, which causes the net magnetic vector of the protons to shift to a new position or equilibrium state (Figure 4). It is important to note in this regard that for all isotopic atomic species useful for medical NMR imaging within the field strength 0.1–1.5 T the precession-inducing electromagnetic waves are in the radio frequency (RF) range. Further precession of the protons thus requires RF energy to be absorbed by the nuclei as their magnetic moments shift to the new position, which is a net higher energy state. Because the protons are still within a static magnetic field applied externally, when the RF pulse ceases, their magnetic moments will return to their prior lower energy state (i.e., resonate), thereby releasing the absorbed RF energy (Figure 5). This released energy will be emitted at exactly the same resonant frequency as that required to cause precession and can be detected by an RF wave monitor. It is precisely this measurable release of energy in the form of radio waves that accounts for the designation, 'NMR signal.' The NMR signal can be visualized as a decay curve that oscillates as it exponentially decreases, much as the swings of a compass needle oscillate about the north pole when released from an external magnetic field. The nature of this decay curve depends greatly on the atomic density (number of atoms) of a particular species

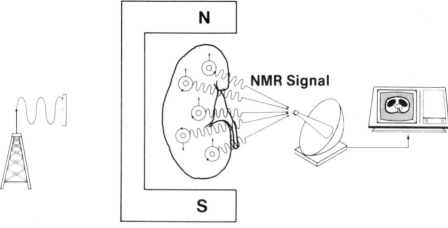

Figure 5. Cessation of the RF waves allows the proton magnetic vectors to realign (resonate) to their original position within the external magnetic field thereby releasing an RF signal which can be detected and processed to produce an image.

resonating within the sample as well as the local temperature, viscosity, and chemical environment.

In medical NMR imaging, we are less interested in the presence and number of H^1 atoms than in their relative position or spatial relationship within the tissue being examined. In order to provide this spatial information, it is necessary to vary the strength of the external magnetic field within the tissue sample. This is accomplished by introducing a separate electromagnetic force within the aperture of the external field so that a gradient in the field can be produced. Remembering that the Larmor or precessional frequency of each proton is directly related to and varies with the strength of the external magnetic field, it follows that, if the field strength can be slightly varied within a tissue sample, it will require different RF wave frequencies to excite or precess protons at different spatial points within the tissue. By electronically and differentially varying the field strength and RF pulse duration and frequency rapidly, the resultant NMR signals produced can be differentially received by an RF monitor. By virtue of sophisticated computer transformation and reconstruction, the NMR signals can be used to provide a proton density image depicting the relative position of the protons and their density, which can therefore reveal very subtle differences within and between tissues. In fact, these differences can be measured more precisely than is possible in CT imaging and should, therefore, produce images with greater anatomical discrimination. The fact that these subtle differences may relate physicochemical information as well, further raises the expectations of NMR imaging. It should be noted that it is exactly this variability in the field strength and, thus, excitation of selected nuclei at a given RF pulse frequency within the tissue, that can be used to develop images in almost any plane desired. This capability clearly offers a distinct advantage over CT imaging.

Thus far, we have only discussed proton density images; however, at least two other parameters are measurable and can be used to impart quite different information. These two parameters are based on measurement of proton precessional relaxation times. The relaxation of protons within a magnetic field of variable strength is not instantaneous but rather occurs over a time period characterized by time T_1; T_1 (or spin-latticed parameter) refers to the time required for proton precession to return to thermal equilibrium in a direction parallel to the external field with respect to the surrounding molecular environment after cessation of the RF pulse. This time can vary considerably: in solids at low temperatures, where random thermal motion is minimal, T_1 may be very long, i.e., hours. In pure liquids T_1 may be only a few seconds while in liquids containing proteins or blood it is even shorter. During image formation, RF pulses must be repetitively applied to result in appropriate data points. However, if the pulse repetition is too rapid, recovery of magnetization of the protons (realignment) cannot be established between pulses and, therefore, a weak NMR signal is produced. Therefore the time interval (TR) between successive RF pulses is important in determining the amount and nature of information obtained. Increasing TR can increase the intensity of the signal depending on T_1, but also increases the scanning time. The selection of TR for medical imaging can enhance contrast between tissues and can provide information about the nature of tissues.

The spin-spin relaxation time, T_2, refers to the NMR signal decay time which, owing to the inherent magnetic properties exerted by neighboring protons on each other, causes the transverse exponential decay to lose synchronization, i.e., some protons realign or relax faster than others. Therefore, T_2 or transverse magnetization is lost more rapidly than T_1 magnetization is regained; T_2 is in milliseconds while T_1 is usually in seconds. The time interval between an applied RF pulse and signal reception is given by the parameter TE. Contrast between tissues with different T_2 values changes with changes in TE. In solids, T_2 is short, in the microsecond range, but in liquids the internal fields are weaker and T_2 is longer.

Images then can be reconstructed that relate to proton density, T_1 relaxation times and T_2 relaxation times.

4. TECHNIQUES

Currently, multiple techniques such as spin echo (SE), inversion recovery (IR), saturation recovery (SR), and free inductive decay (FID), etc., are used to obtain NMR intensity images. Only SE and IR will be discussed as our experience at UCSF is limited to these pulse sequences. The spin echo technique is essentially an RF pulse of sufficient time to cause 90° precession of protons followed by a second pulse causing 180° precession.

The inversion recovery technique refers to an initial 180° RF pulse (reversal of magnetization), followed by a 90° pulse. This technique is used because it produces superb differentiation of tissues such as the grey matter and the white matter of the brain. However, the technique is almost entirely T_1-dependent and inversion recovery takes longer scanning time than does spin echo imaging.

Although a variety of techniques are available, it is obvious that by varying field strengths, appropriate pulse sequences, and RF wave frequency and intensity, the resultant NMR image can be made to reflect one or more of several NMR parameters inherent to the tissue being examined. Because the art is evolving, the precise combinations of the variables required to produce discriminating images in each clinical situation have not been determined. Yet, the technology is advancing rapidly: current evidence indicates that with appropriate selection of these variables, NMR images will have resolution superior to that of any currently known modality and will possibly permit isolation of parameters unique to disease states in specific anatomical locations.

5. INSTRUMENTATION

In general, the necessary components of an NMR imager are a magnet capable of imposing a strong uniform magnetic field; gradient coils that can internally alter the magnetic field depending on the imaging technique used; a transmitter to deliver RF waves to the subject; a receiver to gather NMR signals from the subject and deliver them to appropriate digitizing circuitry; and, finally, a computer capable of processing the information received into a spatial display (Figure 6).

Currently, two major approaches provide magnets of sufficient strength for medical NMR imaging. Because improvements in spatial resolution depend on relative differences in NMR signal intensity and, therefore, a high signal-to-noise ratio, it is evident that the higher the static magnetic field strength, the better the image produced. However, higher field strengths require higher frequency RF waves for proton excitation and at very high frequencies (greater than 15 MHz) the signals are attenuated. Therefore, design of NMR imagers has focused on producing images by magnets with as high a field strength as possible, allowing maximal signal detection in as rapid a time frame as possible.

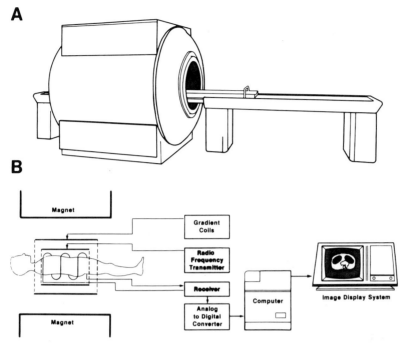

Figure 6. Typical design of a superconductive NMR imager; A. external view; B. cross-section schematic view showing the necessary components for image construction.

The air-core, resistive-coil, ambient-temperature electromagnet consists of four circular coils mounted side by side on a common central axis. The homogeneity of the field produced in this device, however, cannot be greater than a few parts in 10^5. Because the power requirements and thermal dissipation needs for this type of magnet are great, the maximal field strengths reachable are in the 1–2.0 kG range (0.2 T). Despite these limitations, resistive magnets can produce reasonably useful images and their cost is low (approximately $ 100 000).

The air-core superconductive magnet has the advantages of greater obtainable field strength (theoretically up to 14 T), superior homogeneity (1 part in 10^8) and increased stability. The basic magnet consists of filaments of a super-conductor (typically niobium-titanium in a surrounding copper matrix), which are super-cooled by being submerged in liquid helium and surrounded by a vacuum, a layer of liquid N_2, another vacuum, and finally an insulative layer. In this system, electricity is required to initiate the magnet but in the super-cooled environment ($-269\,°C$) the niobium-titanium filaments have almost no resistance and, therefore, conduct and maintain the current necessary to produce the magnetic field indefinitely. Consequently, the electrical power requirements of the magnet are minimal as compared to the power consumption of 20–50 kw for the resistive magnet. This may appear to be a cost advantage; yet the initial expense of a super-conductive magnet alone is ten times that of a resistive magnet and in combination with the cost of continuous supplies of liquid helium the power savings advantage is eliminated.

No general agreement has been reached as to which magnet is best for clinical NMR imaging. However, because super-conductive magnets produce a field stronger and more stable than that of resistive magnets, and because future imaging of nuclei other than protons will require a strong magnet, the super-conductive magnet is preferred.

6. ADVANTAGES AND DISADVANTAGES

The great potential of NMR imaging is that it may allow investigating human disease in physicochemical terms rather than the usual anatomico-pathologic terms. Proton imaging, because of the ubiquitous distribution of water and other proton-rich molecules such as lipids in living tissues, should allow detection of minor alterations in the relative concentration of protons in many disease states which should in turn profoundly change the NMR signal and lead, therefore, to significant advances in differential diagnosis. It had been hoped that NMR would be particularly helpful in discerning benign from malignant tissue as initially suggested by Damadian in 1971 [4], who reported that both T_1 and T_2 relaxation times are longer for malignant than for benign tissue. However, the overlap between relaxation times in tissues with a variety of pathologic states has made this finding less distinct [17, 18]. Indeed, as more becomes known about the various NMR scanning methods, a panel of pulse sequence parameters might be developed to permit an electronic differential diagnostic screen when pathologic abnormalities are suspected.

The specific advantages of NMR imaging over current conventional radiologic techniques are:

(a) Lack of ionizing radiation – unlike most other diagnostic probes, the NMR signal is a result of RF waves that are powerless to disrupt the molecules of living tissues.

(b) Lack of known harmful effects of magnetization in the power ranges utilized.

(c) Anatomic resolution comparable to unenhanced or enhanced CT in many organ sites.

(d) Minimal metal artifact – small objects such as surgical clips do not disrupt the images as with CT.

(e) Lack of bone interference – areas of the body where artifacts were produced by other modalities are now examined easily with NMR, i.e., posterior cranial fossa, and the pelvis.

(f) Blood flow measurement – during active blood flow the excited protons pass out of the field too rapidly to emit a detectable signal.

Despite what appear to be significant advantages to NMR imaging, consideration, of course, must be given to its possible risks and disadvantages:

(a) Claustrophobia – occurs in approximately 5% of patients.

(b) Relatively slow imaging time – although scan time has decreased as techniques improve, at present CT scanning is far more rapid.

(c) High initial cost of the magnet.

(d) Poor detection of bone and tissue calcium.

It is important with respect to potential toxicity to note that studies of NMR on cultured mammalian and human cells in vitro, completed under appropriately controlled conditions, have shown no tendency toward DNA breaks, sister chromatid exchanges, or inhibition of DNA synthesis [19, 20]. It has also been shown in bacterial cells and human lymphocytes exposed to NMR that DNA replication and repair are unaffected [20]. Studies on human volunteers following exposure to NMR for 90 minutes have revealed no short- or medium-term effects, even with multiple exposures; these studies also included specific examination of the personnel operating the apparatus [21]. On the basis of evidence available in 1981, the National Radiation Protection Board of the United Kingdom suggested that: static magnetic fields be limited to less than 2.5 T; variations in field strengths of 20 T per second be done for at least 10 msec; and pulsed RF waves be not greater than 15 MHz [22]. To date, experience with the scanner of the University of California, San Francisco (UCSF) in more than 800 patients indicates that at a field strength of 0.35 T and 15 MHz no toxicity has been observed in a variety of clinical conditions; thus, many of these restrictions have been reduced [23].

7. CURRENT CLINICAL STATE OF THE ART

NMR imaging has recently become a clinical reality and experience has accumulated rapidly over the past two years. For study of many organ systems NMR has already provided equivalence with or improvement over CT imaging, most notably for the head, spinal cord, pelvis, and extremities. Imaging of the thorax and abdomen has proven more difficult, partly owing to the damping of image quality caused by respiration, heart motion, and bowel peristalsis. Despite these limitations, NMR imaging has produced extremely informative images of intra-abdominal, retroperitoneal, and pelvic organs. Imaging of the genitourinary system has emerged as one of the ares of greatest potential benefit.

The NMR images have proven to be much more complex to interpret than CT images. This is due to many independent factors influencing the NMR signal intensity derived from the tissues examined. These factors include:

(a) Inherent tissue NMR characteristics – mobile proton density, relaxation parameters (T_1 and T_2), and bulk motion or flow, such as in urine or blood, occurring during imaging.

(b) Technique of imaging – RF pulse sequence (SE, IR, FID, SR), and timing between pulses and between pulse repetition.

(c) Magnetic field strength.

Even though these factors appear complex it is from the very complexity of NMR imaging techniques that its great potential is derived. Attention to controlled manipulation of the specific details of the imaging technique allows independent determination of a variety of separate NMR characteristics of the tissues under scrutiny. We have therefore not a single tissue characteristic (as for example with X-ray attenuation coefficients measured by CT imagers) but several different and independent tissue characteristics, each capable of providing useful information.

7.1 *NMR imaging technique*

The experience presented here was obtained on the UCSF NMR imager, a super-conducting electromagnet functioning at a field strength of 0.35 T (15 MHz) [23]. Images are produced by utilizing a selective irradiation technique with two-dimensional Fourier transformation.

A variety of imaging sequences can be used to create NMR images as previously discussed. The sequences chosen in our laboratory are spin echo (SE) and inversion recovery (IR) (Table 1). SE is accomplished using RF repetition intervals (TR) of 500 to 2000 msec and echo delay (TE) of both

Table 1. Imaging parameters at UCSF.

Pulse sequence type	TR msec	TI msec	TE msec	No. of sections	Time (min)
Spin echo	500		28/56	5	4.3
	1000		28/56	10	8.5
	1500		28/56	15	13
	2000		28/56	20	17
High resolution	2000		28/56	20	34
Inversion recovery	1000	420	28/56	5	4.3
	1800	277	28/56	9	15.4

28 and 56 msec. These parameters allow as many as 20 anatomic sections to be obtained simultaneously in approximately 17 minutes. IR is accomplished using repetition intervals of 1000 and 1800 msec with an inversion to recovery time (TI) of 420 and 277 msec, respectively, allowing up to 9 sections in 16 minutes. The choice of imaging sequences is of course important; were time of little consideration, we would choose to perform a multitude of sequences. Time limitations, however, have dictated that only 2–3 sequences be accomplished at any one setting to keep scanning time within 30–60 minutes. Further research is required to determine optimal pulse sequences or their combinations. Nonetheless, much has been done with the sequences outlined above.

In imaging the kidneys, pelvis, and retroperitoneum, we have used the following approach: the area of interest is probed, using two SE pulse sequences and one IR sequence. Depending upon the sequence chosen, as many as 15 anatomic sections can be simultaneously examined, without an increase in imaging time. Two SE sequences allow images of maximal spatial resolution to be obtained and provide quantitative T_1 and T_2 measurements and display of T_1 and T_2 cross-sectional maps of the anatomic regions of interest. The IR sequence emphasizes differences in T_1 values in the tissues examined. The imaging time necessitated by this technique totals approximately one hour. This includes patient positioning, coil tuning, operator software interaction, and actual data acquisition.

7.2 Kidney and ureter

7.2.1 *Normal anatomy.* On NMR imaging, fat, bone and blood are opposite in appearance to that seen on CT images. Adipose tissue and bone marrow appear white (high intensity signal), whereas flowing blood, gas, and cortical bone emit no NMR signal and thus appear black. Muscle and solid organs have medium intensity signal and densities. A representative normal NMR scan through the region of the kidneys is shown in Figure 7. On SE images, the renal hilum is a high intensity area due to hilar adipose tissue. The renal vasculature is seen as low intensity tubular structures within the hilar region. The pelviocalyceal system and the ureters are of low intensity related to the long T_1 and T_2 values of urine. Images obtained during diuresis have shown mild dilatation of the renal pelvis and calyces. The renal cortex can be distinguished easily from the medulla, the cortex having a higher intensity image than the medulla but lower than the renal sinus or perirenal fat. The medulla is a triangular low intensity area central to the cortex. The intensity and prominence of the medulla have been shown to be dependent upon the state of hydration [24]. An example of the exaggerated distinction between cortex and medulla apparent during forced diuresis is shown in Figure 8. Cortico-medullary distinction is enhanced on short interval pulse

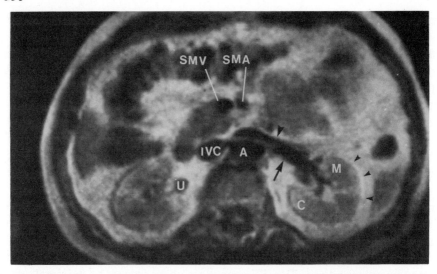

Figure 7. Normal kidney. Transaxial scan spin echo image at TR = 1000 msec, TE = 28 msec. Both right and left kidneys are well imaged. There is good differentiation between lower intensity medulla (M) and higher intensity renal cortex (C). Left renal artery (arrow) and vein (arrowhead) are seen traversing the renal hilum. The left renal vein is seen anterior to the aorta traversing toward the inferior vena cava (IVC). The aorta (A) shows arteriosclerotic changes along the right and posterior wall. Normal right ureter (U). There is low intensity line – Gerota's fascia (small arrows) seen separating peri from para-renal space. Note good display of superior mesenteric artery (SMA) and superior mesenteric vein (SMV) (reproduced with permission from Radiology, Hricak et al: NMR imaging of the kidney I[24]).

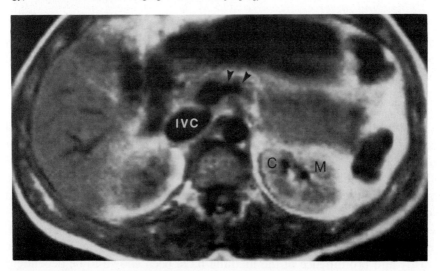

Figure 8. Hydration effect on the kidney of normal volunteer. Transaxial scan spin echo image at TR = 1000 msec, TE = 28 msec. The separation between the lower intensity swollen medulla (M) and higher intensity cortex (C) is well pronounced. Splenic portal confluence (arrows). Distention of the inferior vena cava (IVC).

sequences but is not readily apparent on longer interval sequences. Perirenal fat is seen as a high intensity area due to shorter T_1 and longer T_2 relaxation values. Gerota's fascia is readily visible as a low intensity line surrounding the perirenal space (Figure 7). On IR images, the renal cortex is significantly brighter than the medulla and differentiation between the two is more evident than on SE images. Perirenal and hilar fat remains intense owing to a short T_1. Urine remains dark because of its long T_1.

7.2.2 *Pathology.* Hydronephrosis is easily detectable by NMR, as is the dilated ureter (Figure 9). The distended ureter is differentiated from bowel, lymph nodes, and blood vessels by review of multiple SE intensity images and by noting the lumenal low intensity due to the presence of urine. On CT images, contrast enhancement is required to make this differentiation but is not always possible if urine is not being produced. Because fluid and fat have opposite NMR properties, peripelvic cysts and sinus lipomatosis are readily distinguished by NMR, whereas on CT partial volume averaging can result in ambiguity.

NMR promises to make a significant contribution in the diagnosis of renal parenchymal diseases. Renal volume calculation and parenchymal NMR characteristics can be assessed. The high degree of sensitivity of NMR to subtle changes in the composition of soft tissues suggests that monitoring the progression of medical renal disorders may be possible, perhaps limiting

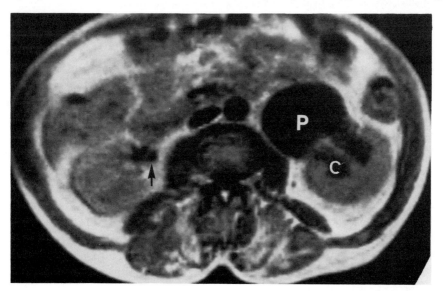

Figure 9. UPJ obstruction left kidney. Transaxial scan spin echo image at TR = 2000 msec, TE = 28 msec. The extra-renal pelvis (P) and the calyces (C) of the left kidney are dilated. Differentiation between cortex and medulla in the obstructive kidney is not possible. There is normal cortical medullary differentiation of the right kidney. Normal right ureter (arrow).

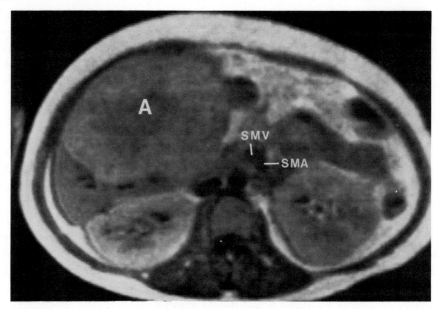

Figure 10. Glycogen storage disease. Transaxial scan spin echo image at TR = 1000, TE = 28 msec. There is an inhomogeneous intensity lesion in the liver representing liver adenoma (A). The superior mesenteric artery (SMA) and superior mesenteric vein (SMV) are displayed. Both kidneys are markedly enlarged and the intensity of the renal cortex is higher than normally seen. Biopsy-proven glycogen storage disease of the kidney.

the need for renal biopsy. In addition, because both acquired cystic disease and renal neoplasia are increased in patients with chronic renal failure, NMR imaging, obviating use of iodinated contrast material, may prove efficacious (Figures 10 and 11).

Our experience thus far suggests that the ability of NMR to differentiate solid from cystic renal lesions is accurate but not dissimilar to that of contrast enhanced CT (Figures 12 and 13) [25]. Renal cysts reveal homogeneous low intensity images with no internal structure. T_1 values of cysts are usually longer than 2 seconds and T_2 greater than 200 msec. Smooth interfaces with renal parenchyma are demonstrated but the cystic walls are not seen. Cystic margins next to perirenal fat, however, show an edge enhancement artifact seen as a low intensity line 1–2 mm wide, due to the widely divergent NMR intensities of fat and cyst fluid (Figures 12 and 13). Recently, hemorrhagic and infected cysts have been shown to have increased SE intensities as compared to simple cysts (Figure 14); this suggests that NMR can provide information about the chemical contents of cysts; thus, it may be valuable to evaluate patients in whom hemorrhagic or infected renal cysts are suspected.

Evaluation of the renal cell carcinomas studied by us and others to date

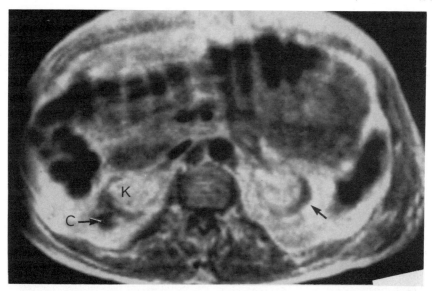

Figure 11. Chronic glomerulonephritis. Transaxial scan spin echo image at TR = 1000 msec, TE = 28 msec. Both kidneys are small. There is marked thinning of the renal parenchyma (arrow). There is a simple cyst (C) seen arising from the posterior aspect of the right kidney (K). There is an abundant amount of hilar adipose tissue.

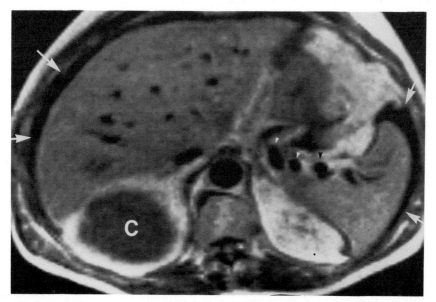

Figure 12. **Simple cyst right kidney.** Transaxial scan spin echo image at TR = 1000 msec, TE = 28 msec. There is a homogeneous low intensity lesion in the right renal bed. By T1 and T2 measurements this represents a simple renal cyst (C). There is ascites (small arrows) imaged with a low intensity signal seen surrounding the liver and spleen. Tortuous splenic artery (small arrowhead).

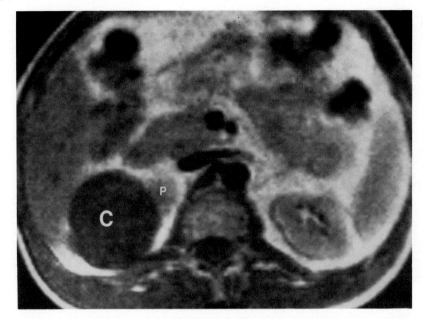

Figure 13. Simple cyst right kidney. Transaxial scan spin echo image at TR = 1000 msec, TE = 28 msec. The right renal cyst (C) is imaged with a homogeneous low intensity. There is a sharp demarcation at the normal renal parenchyma (P).

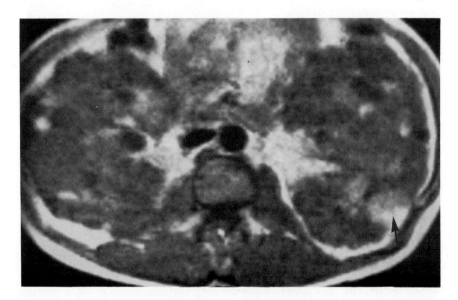

Figure 14. Polycystic kidney disease. Transaxial scan spin echo image at TR = 2000 msec, TE = 28 msec. Both kidneys are markedly enlarged and contain multiple various sized and various intensity cysts. Note high intensity cysts; the largest one at the posterior lateral aspect of the left kidney (arrow) represents an acutely hemorrhagic cyst.

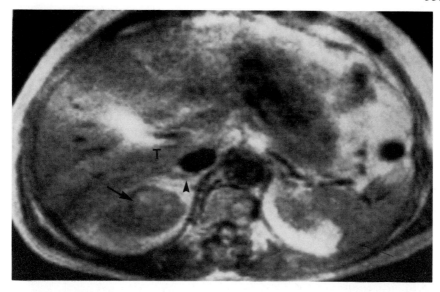

Figure 15. Renal cell carcinoma right kidney. Transaxial scan spin echo image at TR = 1000 msec, TE = 28 msec. There is an inhomogeneous, mainly high intensity lesion within the superior pole of the right kidney (T). The low intensity line (arrow) is seen interposed between the tumor and normal renal parenchyma representing tumor pseudo-capsule. Note normal right adrenal gland (arrowhead).

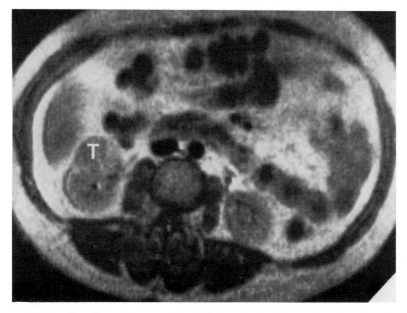

Figure 16. Renal cell carcinoma right kidney. Transaxial scan spin echo image at TR = 1000 msec, TE = 28 msec. There is a bulging contour along the anterior part of the right kidney. The tumor (T) is of inhomogeneous medium intensity.

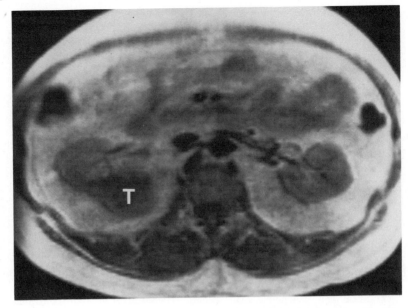

Figure 17. Renal cell carcinoma right kidney. Transaxial scan spin echo image at TR = 1000 msec, TE = 28 msec. There is an inhomogeneous but mainly lower intensity lesion (T) arising from the medial inferior aspect of the right kidney.

has shown a wide spectrum of NMR findings, with SE images showing a range from low intensity to very high intensity lesions (Figures 15, 16, 17) [25, 26]. A common feature, however, is a prolongation of the T_1 of the carcinomas relative to adjacent normal renal parenchyma, whereas the T_2 values are similar or increased relative to surrounding parenchyma. A low intensity line interposed between the tumor and the normal renal parenchyma was pathologically confirmed as a tumor pseudo-capsule in several of our cases (Figure 15). Staging of renal neoplasm by NMR is promising, but at this time only limited experience has been gained.

A potential drawback of NMR in the assessment of renal lesions is the indistinct definition of calcification, despite a variety of NMR imaging techniques. Calcifications have very low NMR intensity and are frequently not visualized. Even when seen, calcifications cannot always be readily differentiated from dense fibrous tissue because both have a similar low intensity signal. Whether this feature of NMR will prove to be a significant weakness remains to be seen.

Despite limited information at present, the expectation that further experience will reveal NMR to be of substantial value in defining renal parenchymal disease, detecting and categorizing renal masses, and perhaps staging renal neoplasms, appears justified.

7.3 *Adrenals*

7.3.1 *Normal anatomy.* The adrenal gland is a relatively homogeneous low intensity structure enveloped and clearly outlined by the high intensity periadrenal fat on NMR (Figures 15 and 18) [27]. In practice, the left adrenal has been visualized in all cases but the right in slightly fewer. The left adrenal is seen in the shape of an inverted 'V' or a triangle, whereas the right appears superiorly as a thin line extending from the inferior vena cava juxtaposed between the crus of the diaphragm and the medial aspect of the right lobe of the liver and inferiorly as a horizontal band posterior to the inferior vena cava. The characteristic periadrenal fat surrounding the left adrenal is constant, thus providing easy definition, whereas the fat surrounding the right is more variable, which explains its more problematic definition. In comparison to the liver, the adrenals tend to have a lower intensity on at least one of the four intensity images, particularly on the right. The T_1 and T_2 values are variable. Differentiation of the cortex and medulla appears possible, with the central portion of each gland of lower intensity than the outer rim. Subjectively, the central region has a longer T_1 and slightly shorter T_2 than the outer rim.

7.3.2 *Pathology.* To date five patients with known adrenal disease have been examined in the UCSF NMR scanner. Three patients had adrenal metastases, one had pheochromocytoma, and one congenital adrenal hyperplasia. In every case the lesions were clearly demonstrated by NMR. The metastases were visualized as masses with lower intensity than that of the

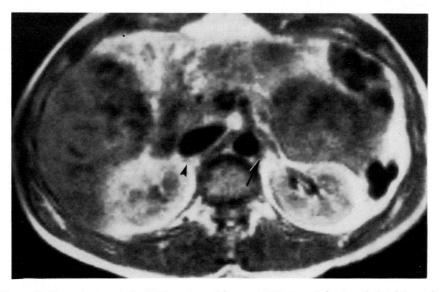

Figure 18. Normal adrenal gland. Note normal inverted 'V' shape left adrenal gland (arrow). The horizontal portion of the distal right adrenal gland (arrowhead) is seen as well.

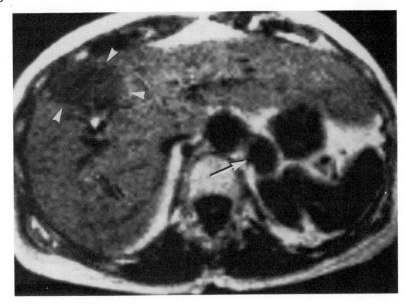

Figure 19. Adrenal and liver metastases secondary to colonic carcinoma. Transaxial inversion recovery image with TR = 1000 msec, TI = 422 msec. There is a low intensity lesion within the liver (arrowheads) representing liver metastases. There is also a low intensity lesion (arrow) in the left adrenal bed representing an adrenal metastatic lesion.

normal adrenal (Figure 19). The pheochromocytoma appeared as a non-homogeneous round mass with a low intensity rim and a higher intensity center which at gross pathologic examination was shown to be a blood-filled cystic area. The NMR of the patient with congenital adrenal hyperplasia revealed bilateral glandular enlargement. We interpret these early results as suggesting that NMR can match the ability of CT in demonstrating normal and pathologic adrenal anatomy. Because of their particular anatomic characteristics, the adrenals, with their surrounding fat, and the adjacent liver and large blood vessels, may eventually allow NMR to surpass CT in differential ability.

7.4 *Retroperitoneum*

To date, very little experience has been gained in NMR scanning of the retroperitoneum other than that previously described in relation to renal and adrenal anatomy [28–33]. Although a systematic approach to NMR scanning of the retroperitoneum has just been initiated at UCSF, we have recently seen one case of retroperitoneal sarcoma and three of retroperitoneal fibrosis [34]. The retroperitoneal leiomyosarcoma was extensive in the entire retroperitoneal space on the right and involved an occlusive tumor thrombus in the vena cava from below the renal vessels to the entrance of the main hepatic veins. The information obtained by NMR was similar to that from CT with regard to tumor volume and extent. However, on NMR, the tumor was clearly not involving the kidney or renal vein; contained a large high intensity central area found at surgery to be cystic degeneration of the tumor containing liquified hematoma; and the proximal extent of the thrombus similarly showed a cap of high intensity, which proved to be a clot on the leading edge of the tumor (Figure 20). These features were not appreciated by CT. In addition, collateral venous blood vessels coursing around the tumor contralaterally were accentuated on NMR imaging.

Retroperitoneal fibrosis appeared on NMR as an irregularly shaped mass. The NMR signal intensity was higher than for adjacent muscle but less than for the abundant local fat (Figure 21). T_1 values varied considerably but T_2 values were consistently low. The extent of involvement was easily determined by NMR and was particularly prominent on sagittal scans (Figure 22). Perhaps the most significant findings were in defining the relationship of the plaques to retroperitoneal vessels and the flow within them. Because of the lack of NMR signal from vessels with flowing blood, the perivascular component and consequent vessel narrowing were easily appreciated on NMR images (Figure 21). In addition, decreased or static blood flow was seen as a higher NMR signal intensity in the partially obstructed iliac veins, which could easily be differentiated from the pelvic ureters, particularly on images obtained using echo delay times of 56 msec. Although many of these findings can be seen on CT, contrast agents are required to obtain the differentiation seen on non-contrast NMR images. As yet, we have not imaged patients with a variety of metastatic and/or primary retroperitoneal lesions but, on the basis of our preliminary data, it seems probable that differing tissue types may be discriminated by NMR.

7.5 Liver

As with the retroperitoneum, experience in NMR imaging of the liver is in its early stages. Although there have been a few reports of comparisons of normal and pathologic hepatic states in the recent literature [35, 36] they, for the most part, used early generation methods and imagers and thus the information is not definitive. In these studies, the normal liver shows considerable soft tissue contrast, particularly on IR images. It is notable that on NMR the spleen, unlike on CT images, appears different than the liver, with a less intense NMR signal. The intrahepatic architecture is fairly uniform, the parenchyma showing medium intensity signals, whereas the ducts and vessels lack signal providing substantial contrast.

Primary liver tumors are clearly demonstrated on NMR, yet metastatic tumors appear to be better delineated owing to a T_1 markedly increased over that of either normal liver or primary tumors (Figures 10 and 19) [35].

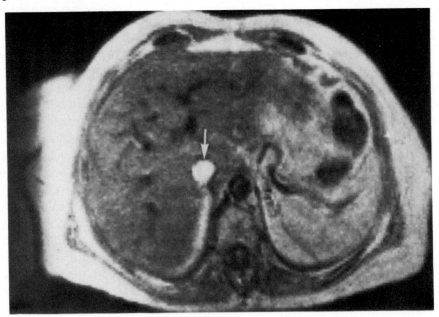

A. Transaxial scan through the upper abdomen. There is a high intensity signal within the inferior vena cava representing a blood clot (arrow).

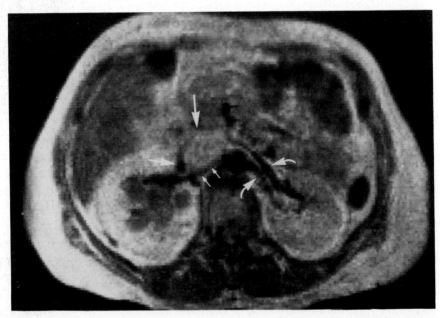

B. Scan obtained 5 cm caudally shows a medium intensity signal within the enlarged inferior vena cava. This represented the tumor extension. Note the normal right renal artery (small arrows) as well as the right renal vein (large arrow) curving around the inferior vena cava. Normal left renal artery and vein (curved arrows).

Figure 20. Leiomyosarcoma of the inferior vena cava.

In non-neoplastic hepatic parenchymal disease, changes in liver size, in homogeneous parenchyma, and irregular nodular margins seen on NMR are similar to those seen on CT. T_1 times, however, are prolonged, giving a dark appearance to the parenchyma [36]. One advantage of NMR appears to be in imaging the left lobe of the liver, where stomach artifact is a problem with CT [36].

7.6 Pelvis

The pelvis may well be the anatomic area where NMR imaging will find its most beneficial application. Initial expectations however for CT and ultrasound both exceeded the eventual sensitivity and specificity in diagnosis and staging of pelvic malignancies [37]. This is due in part to the relative lack of pelvic fat required for contrast in the case of CT and interference by pelvic bone with ultrasonographic study.

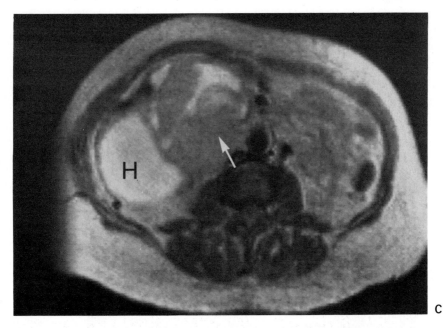

C

C. More caudally there is a large right retroperitoneal mass. The mass is inhomogeneous in intensity. It has a higher intensity area (H) representing hemorrhage. The tumor in the inferior vena cava (arrow) is continuous with the mass. Note the collateral vessels on the left.

Figure 20. Leiomyosarcoma of the inferior vena cava.

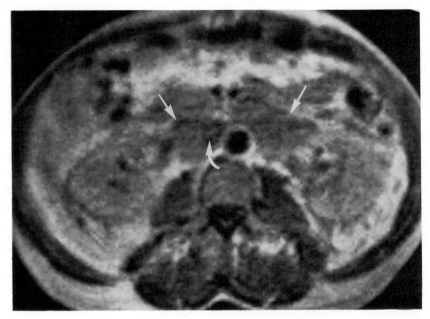

Figure 21. Retroperitoneal fibrosis. There are soft tissue plaques seen interposed between the aorta and superior mesenteric artery and vein (arrows). The inferior vena cava is seen with low intensity signal (curved arrow) indicating flow but the lumen of the cava is compressed.

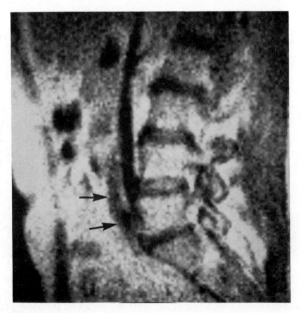

Figure 22. Sagittal scan retroperitoneal fibrosis. The aorta is clearly outlined. The aortic plaque is seen anterior to the distal portion of the aorta (arrows).

To date, studies in the UCSF imaging laboratory have been primarily confined to the male pelvis, with only recent information obtained from the female pelvis. We have studied five normal patients, five patients with primary bladder carcinoma, ten with benign prostatic hyperplasia, and nine with prostate carcinoma. For these patients, only SE images were obtained.

7.7 Bladder

7.7.1 *Normal anatomy.* The bladder routinely was distended with urine during scanning and therefore is easily demonstrated (Figure 23). The signal intensity of urine tends to be low, because of the longer T_1 and T_2 relaxation times [37]. As the pulse sequence interval increases, the second echo signal of urine is enhanced, owing to the prolonged T_2 time. The differentiation between bladder wall and urine is easily determined and wall thickness and irregularity are readily appreciated. Because perivesical adipose tissue has a higher intensity than bladder wall or pelvic muscle, the various tissue planes are discernible. The pelvic bones are easily distinguished by NMR; however, only the marrow is visualized as a high intensity area surrounded by cortical bone that emits almost no signal and is therefore of extremely low intensity (Figure 23). If the bladder is not distended, bowel loops can present considerable artifact at the dome of the bladder, but by analyzing several sections via a variety of pulse sequence intervals, the appropriate dis-

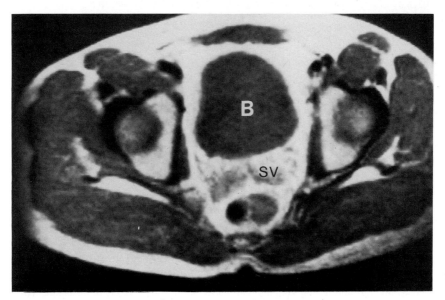

Figure 23. Normal male pelvis. Distended urinary bladder (B) is imaged with low intensity. Seminal vesicles (SV) are seen posterior to the bladder.

tinction can be made. It should also be noted that respiration has little effect on pelvic organs as imaged by NMR.

7.7.2 *Pathologic anatomy.* Bladder wall hypertrophy has a medium intensity NMR signal. Bladder carcinomas were demonstrated in all six patients examined. Exophytic tumors were particularly well seen and could be distinguished from normal bladder wall (Figure 24), due to a non-homogeneous appearance with a higher intensity signal. Depth of penetration of the neoplasms was best appreciated by combining axial and sagittal images (Figure 25). In contrast to these findings, CT allowed detection of tumor in only three patients. In one, a metastatic tumor to the bladder was more accurately defined on NMR than on CT, primarily because the mucosa was noted to be intact by NMR but not by CT, thus allowing exclusion of a primary bladder mucosal tumor. In general, NMR appears to be slightly better than CT in the diagnosis of bladder tumors, but it shows particular promise with respect to local staging.

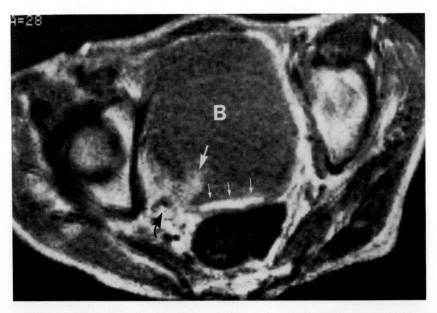

Figure 24. A. Transitional cell carcinoma of the bladder – axial scan. There is a high intensity lesion (arrows) seen protruding from the right lateral and posterior aspect of the bladder (B). The higher intensity signal is seen along the posterior wall of the bladder (small arrows). The same intensity signal is seen within the dilated right ureter (curved arrow).

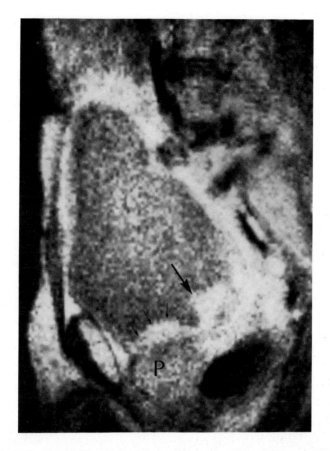

Figure 24. B. Sagittal scan showing the tumor (arrow) at the posterior aspect of the bladder. However also note the tumor extension along the bladder base (small arrows) which is much better appreciated on the sagittal image. Enlarged prostate gland (P). At surgery the transitional cell carcinoma was seen in the posterior aspect of the bladder as well as at the bladder base. The tumor was extending into the right ureter.

7.8 Prostate

7.8.1 *Normal anatomy.* The normal prostate reveals a homogeneous medium intensity signal. A thin rim of lower intensity corresponding to the surgical capsule can be demonstrated (Figure 26). Via the use of multiplanar images, contiguous structures, such as bladder base, rectum, and periprostatic fat in the space of Retzius are readily apparent (Figure 27). Superior to the prostate and posterior to the bladder, the seminal vesicles are clearly distinguished, embedded within the pelvic fat and surrounded by Denonvilliers' fascia (Figures 27 and 28). The seminal vesicles have a medium intensity signal, a short pulse sequence being used; this signal augments in intensity as the interval increases.

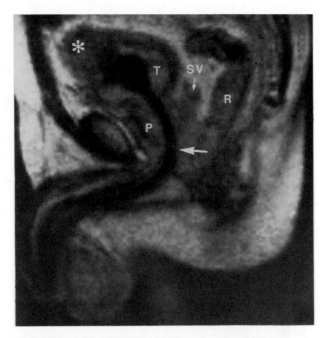

Figure 25. Transitional cell carcinoma of the bladder. Midline sagittal scan showing markedly thickened bladder wall with a higher intensity signal (T) from tumor along its inner surface. There is also a soft tissue mass at the bladder dome (asterisk) which corresponded to extension of the carcinoma in a urachal cyst. A Foley catheter (arrow) is present within the urethra. Enlarged prostate gland (P). Normal seminal vesicles (SV). Rectum (R).

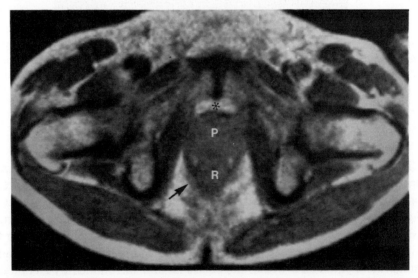

Figure 26. Normal pelvis – transaxial scan. The prostate gland (P) is imaged with medium intensity. There is a homogeneous distribution of the signal throughout the gland. Levator ani (arrow). Rectum (R). Adipose tissue in preprostatic area (asterisk).

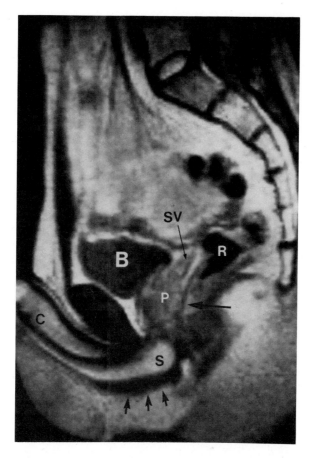

Figure 27. Male pelvis – sagittal scan. The prostate gland (P) is enlarged. There are at least two areas of intensity within it. These represent focal areas of prostatitis. Urinary bladder (B). Seminal vesicles (SV). Rectum (R). Denonvilliers' fascia (arrows) is clearly imaged as a low intensity line separating the prostate gland from the rectum. Corpus spongiosum (S). Corpora cavernosa (C). Bulbo-spongiosus muscles (arrowheads).

7.8.2 *Pathologic anatomy.* Benign prostatic hyperplasia appears as an increased volume of medium signal intensity, with a thick lower intensity rim surrounding it (Figure 29). Saggital scans obtained while a urethral catheter is in place are particularly striking (Figure 29). Prostatic carcinoma appears to show a higher intensity signal than normal or adenomatous tissue in the patients examined thus far, although images before transurethral prostatectomy or biopsy have not yet been adequately studied. In at least three cases of stage C disease, involvement of the seminal vesicles, confirmed by palpation and pathologic examination, was evident on NMR (Figure 30). In addition, the glands were non-homogeneous and distortion of the prostate

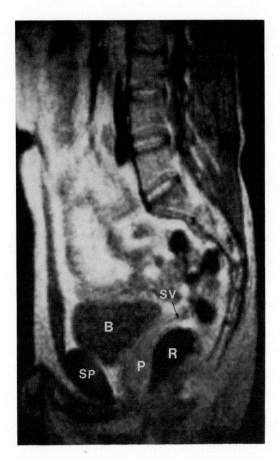

Figure 28. Male pelvis – sagittal scan. Urinary bladder (B). Prostate gland (P). Seminal vesicle (SV). Rectum (R). Symphysis pubis (SP).

contour and disruption of the lower intensity surgical capsule were seen (Figure 31). If these findings are confirmed by subsequent studies, NMR will emerge as the approach of choice in the diagnosis and local staging of prostatic neoplasms. In one patient who had a previous pelvic operation, metal surgical clips in the pelvis were seen as areas without NMR signal surrounded by a high intensity halo, but without streak artifacts as seen on CT (Figure 32).

In addition to the anatomic areas described above, limited examinations have revealed excellent display of the corpora cavernosa of the penis, the inguinal canal with demonstration of the vas deferens, patent spermatic vessels, and distinct images of the testes. Examples of pathology of these areas have yet to be imaged.

NMR of the pelvis appears to have resolving power exceeding that of CT, either with or without contrast enhancement. In particular, staging of neo-

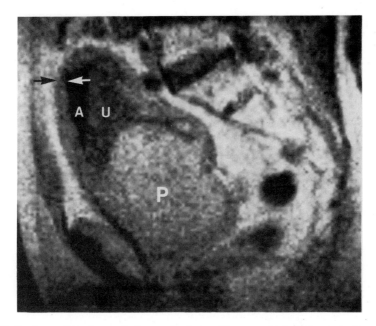

Figure 29. Benign nodular hyperplasia – sagittal scan. Prostate gland (P) is markedly enlarged. Note the nodularity along the intravesical and the posterior part of the prostate gland while the anterior surface retains its straight concave configuration. The wall of the urinary bladder is thickened (arrows). As a Foley catheter is present there is an air (A) – urine (U) level within the bladder.

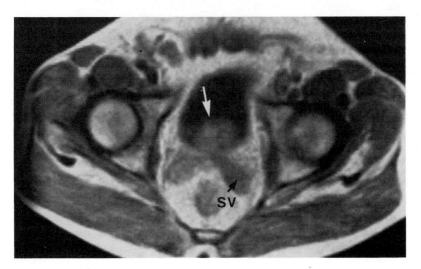

Figure 30. Prostatic carcinoma stage C. The intravesical portion of the prostate is enlarged. There is a high intensity area within the gland representing prostatic carcinoma (arrow). There is a difference in the intensity of the seminal vesicles (SV) with the right seminal vesicle being more voluminous and higher in intensity. At surgery there was extension of the prostatic carcinoma into the right seminal vesicle.

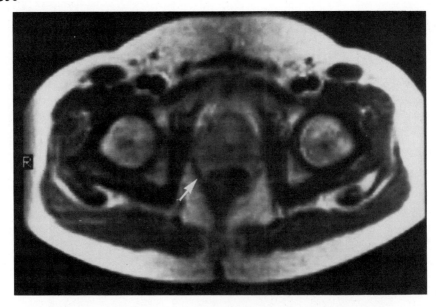

A

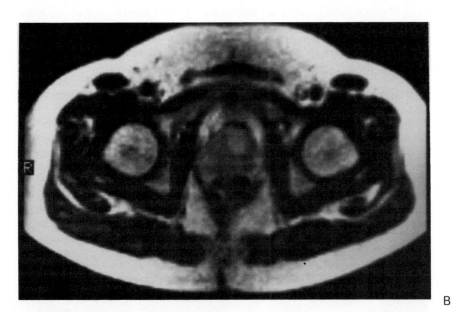

B

Figure 31. Clinical stage C prostatic carcinoma.
A. Transaxial scan, TR = 1000 msec, TE = 28 msec. The prostate gland is enlarged and of inhomogeneous intensity. While the right levator ani (arrow) is clearly imaged, there is involvement of the prostatic carcinoma towards the left levator sling.
B. The findings are better appreciated when the image is obtained with longer TE values, TE = 56 msec. There is definite extension of the malignant tissue into the periprostatic area on the left.

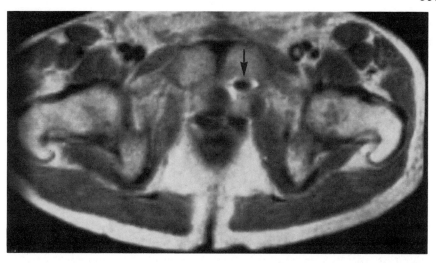

Figure 32. Surgical clip – transaxial image following radical prostatectomy. The surgical clips (arrow) are imaged as an area without signal surrounded by a high intensity halo. There are no artifacts secondary to metallic clips seen nor is the image distorted.

plasms is enhanced by the ability to examine the pelvis in at least two planes. Currently, the major obstacle appears to be the inability to depict pelvic lymph nodes clearly. As scanning techniques improve, however, this problem may be solved.

8. FUTURE PERSPECTIVES

The potential of NMR body imaging should be, in our view, enthusiastically optimistic. Thus far, the science is in its infancy. Nevertheless, for many organ sites, the images produced by early generation NMR scanners already are equal in anatomical resolution to those produced by current generation CT scanners; furthermore, these images are superior to enhanced CT in other organs, most notably the brian, retroperitoneum, and pelvis. With the advent of improved pulse sequencing techniques perhaps specific for organs or disease states, the art should rapidly advance. In the near future, it should be possible to obtain blood and urine flow measurements quantitatively, to determine presence of, and volume of, muscle ischemia or infarction, and to extend NMR imaging to other atoms such as P^{31} or FL^{19}, which may allow specific physiologic information to be gained.

It is a matter of conjecture whether current magnetic resonance imagers will be capable also to do spectroscopy. Switching from one mode to the other could in the future be made practical, but this probably will not occur for some time. It is extremely likely, on the basis of present experience, to expect rather full use of NMR imagers particularly in view of the many present clinical indications. Switching to spectroscopy even if it were almost instantaneous is therefore not to be expected in a busy clinical setting. Future systems in which this may be possible will be developed only if spectroscopy, on the basis of future research, justifies the large expenditures in creating such devices.

Similar and related questions also involve imagers with higher strength magnetic fields of 1.5 to 2.0 T. Research is needed to show that higher strength fields have clinical advantages over the lower field strength 0.35–0.6 T images to justify the added expense in purchase price, siting, and operation. There will in the future be a need for imaging of other elements, yet this will also need to be of proven value to expect public investment in imagers with rapidly changing magnetic field strengths.

Thus, the push button imager changing from one field strength to another with automatically removable gradient coils to allow instant spectroscopy in any tissue cube is possible and will be available when the need for it justifies the immense expense.

The same, however, may not be true for artificial intelligence computers which, with push button speed, will provide the right technique, right pulse sequences and planes when all the data from history, physical and laboratory diagnosis are provided.

Perhaps one of the more exciting developments in NMR imaging is the concept of using contrast agents to enhance the anatomic information now available. These agents are paramagnetic and thus shorten the T_1 and T_2 relaxation times [38–40]. Indeed, manganese chloride has been shown to reduce NMR signal intensity from zones of myocardial infarction in isolated perfused canine hearts [39]; oral ferric chloride has been used successfully for bowel intraluminal enhancement; and inhaled 100% oxygen has been used as an intra-cardiac blood enhancer in human volunteers. Recently, nitroxide-stable free radicals have been used effectively in animals as an intravenous urographic contrast agent [41].

The ultimate role of clinical NMR imaging and spectroscopy will require considerable further research to delineate the precise conditions required to produce optimal information; however, at present the utility of NMR imaging of the urinary tract is already of proven benefit.

REFERENCES

1. Bloch F: Nuclear induction. Phys Rev 70:460-473, 1946.
2. Purcell EM, Torrey HC, Pound RV: Physics Res 69:37, 1946.
3. Jackson JA, Langhan WH: Rev Scientif Instr 39:510, 1968.
4. Damadian R: Tumor detection by nuclear magnetic resonance. Science 171:1151-1153, 1971.

5. Lauterbur PC: Image formation by induced local interactions. Nature (London) 242:190-191, 1973.

6. Lauterbur PC: Magnetic resonance zeugmatography. Pure Appl Chem 2:40, 1975.

7. Hinshaw WS, Bottomley PA, Holland GN: Radiographic thin sectioning image of the human wrist by nuclear magnetic resonance. Nature 270:722, 1977.

8. Pykett IL, Newhouse JH, Buonanno FS, Brady TJ, Goldman MR, Kistler JP, Pohost GM: Principles of nuclear magnetic resonance imaging. Radiology 143:157-168, 1982.

9. Pykett IL: NMR imaging in medicine. Scientif Am 246:78-88, 1982.

10. Oldendorf WH: NMR imaging: Its potential clinical impact. Hospital Practice, 17(9):114-128, 1982.

11. Brownell GL, Budinger TF, Lauterbur PC, McGeer PL: Positron tomography and nuclear magnetic resonance imaging. Science 215:619-629, 1982.

12. James AE, Partain CL, Holland GN, Gore JC, Rollo FD, Harms SE, Price RR: Nuclear magnetic resonance imaging: The current state. Am J Roentgenol 138:201-210, 1981.

13. Bradley WG, Tosteson H: Basic physics of NMR. In: Nuclear Magnetic Resonance Imaging in Medicine, Kaufman L, Crooks LE, Margulis AR (eds). New York: Igaku-Shoin Medical Publishers, Inc. Chapter 2, pp 11-29, 1981.

14. NMR – An Introduction. General Electric Company Technical Manual, 1981.

15. Loeffler W, Oppelt A: Physical principles of NMR tomography. Eur J Radiol 1:338-344, 1981.

16. Partain CL, Price RR, Rollo FD, James AE (eds): Nuclear Magnetic Resonance (NMR) Imaging. Philadelphia: Saunders, 1983.

17. Hollis DP, Economou JS, Parks LC, Eggleston JC, Saryan LA, Czeisler JL: Nuclear magnetic resonance studies of several experimental and human malignant tumors. Cancer Res 33:2156-2160, 1973.

18. Eggleston JC, Saryan LA, Hollis DP: Nuclear magnetic resonance investigation of human neoplastic and abnormal non-neoplastic tissues. Cancer Res 35:1326-1332, 1975.

19. Wolff S, Crooks LE, Brown P, Ricci H, Painter RB: Tests for DNA and chromosomal damage induced by nuclear magnetic resonance imaging. Radiology 136:707-710, 1980.

20. Schwartz J, Crooks LE: NMR imaging produces no observable mutations or cytotoxicity in mammalian cells. Am J Roentgenol 139:583-585, 1982.

21. National Radiologic Protection Board: Exposure to nuclear magnetic resonance clinical imaging. Radiology XLVII:258-260, 1981.

22. Davis PL, Crooks L, Arakawa M, McRee R, Kaufman L, Margulis AR: Potential hazards in NMR imaging: Heating effects of changing magnetic fields and RF fields on small metallic implants. Am J Roentgenol 137:857-860, 1981.

23. Crooks L, Arakawa MA, Hoenninger J, Watts J, McRee R, Kaufman L, Davis CL, Margulis AR, Degroot J: Nuclear magnetic resonance whole-body imaging operating at 3.5 KGauss. Radiology 143:169-174, 1982.

24. Hricak H, Crooks L, Sheldon P, Kaufman L: NMR imaging of the kidney. Radiology 146:425-432, 1983.

25. Hricak H, Williams RD, Moon KL, Moss AA, Alpers C, Crooks LE, Kaufman L: NMR imaging of the kidney: Part II, Renal masses. Radiology 147:765-772, 1983.

26. Alfidi RJ, Hoaga JR, Yousef SJ et al.: Preliminary experimental results in humans and animals with a superconducting whole-body nuclear magnetic resonance scanner. Radiology 143:175-181, 1982.

27. Moon KL, Hricak H, Crooks LE, Gooding CA, Moss AA, Engelstad BL, Kaufman L: Nuclear magnetic resonance imaging of the adrenal gland: A preliminary report. Radiology 147:155-160, 1983.

28. Young IR, Bailes DR, Burl M, Collins AG, Smith DT, McDonnell MJ, Orr JS, Banks LM,

Bydder GM, Greenspan RH, Steiner RE: Initial clinical evaluation of a whole-body nuclear magnetic resonance (NMR) tomograph. J Comp Ass Tomogr 6:1-18, 1982.

29. Hadley DM, Nichols DM, Smith FW: Nuclear magnetic resonance tomographic imaging in xanthogranulomatous pyelonephritis. J Urol 127:301-303, 1982.

30. Pollett JE, Smith FW, Mallard JR, Ah-See AK, Reid A: Whole body nuclear magnetic resonance imaging: The first report of its use in surgical practice. Br J Surg 68:498-494, 1981.

31. Newhouse JH: Urinary tract imaging by nuclear magnetic resonance. Urol Radiol 4:171-175, 1982.

32. Smith FW, Hutchinson JM, Mallard JR, Reid A, Johnson G, Redpath TW, Seldie D: Renal cyst or tumor? Differentiation by whole body nuclear magnetic resonance imaging. Diagnostic Imaging 50:61, 1981.

33. Smith FW, Reid A, Hutchinson J, Mallard JR: Nuclear magnetic resonance imaging of the pancreas. Radiology 142:677-680, 1982.

34. Hricak H, Higgins CB, Williams RD: NMR imaging in retroperitoneal fibrosis. Am J Roentgenol 141:35-38, 1983.

35. Doyle FH, Pennock JM, Banks LM, McDonnell MJ, Bydder GM, Steiner RE, Young JR, Clarke GJ, Pasmore T, Gilderdale DJ: Nuclear magnetic resonance imaging of the liver: Initial experience. Am J Roentgenol 138:193-200, 1982.

36. Smith FW, Mallard JR, Reid A, Hutchinson JMS: Nuclear magnetic resonance tomographic imaging in liver disease. Lancet 1:963-966, 1981.

37. Hricak H, Williams RD, Spring DB, Moon KL, Hedgcock MW, Watson RA, Crooks L: Anatomy and pathology of the male pelvis as by magnetic resonance imaging. Am J Roentgenol 141:1101-1110, 1983.

38. Davis PL, Crooks LE, Margulis AR, Kaufman L: Nuclear magnetic resonance imaging: Current capabilities. West J Med 137:290-293, 1982.

39. Brady TJ, Goldman MR, Pykett IL, Buonanno FS, Kistler JD, Newhouse J, Hinshaw WS, Pohost GM: Proton nuclear magnetic resonance imaging of regionally ischemic canine hearts: Effect of paramagnetic proton signal enhancement. Radiology 144:343-347, 1982.

40. Young IR, Clarke GJ, Boiles DR, Pennock JM, Doyle FH, Bydder GM: Enhancement of relaxation rate with paramagnetic contrast agents in NMR imaging. J Com Tomogr 5:543-547, 1981.

41. Brasch RC, London DA, Wesbey GE, Tozer TN, Nitrecki DE, Williams RD, Doemeny J, Tuck LD, Lallemand DP: Nuclear magnetic resonance urography enhanced by a paramagnetic nitroxide contrast agent: Preliminary report. Radiology 147:773-779, 1983.

Editorial Comment

JEFFREY H. NEWHOUSE

1. INTRODUCTION

As Drs Williams and Hricak have pointed out, NMR imaging in the urinary tract as elsewhere has generated a great deal of excitement and anticipation with its introduction. Indeed, progress is so rapid in this field that it is dangerous to try to speculate about what the future holds: by the time the speculations are printed, they are likely already to have been proven or disproven. Nevertheless, it is worthwhile to try to predict the role that NMR imaging will play, after all, it is just such predictions which will guide clinical research. In this editorial, then, I will try to amplify the concept of the information contained in an NMR scan, and to guess what application of this information ultimately will provide.

2. PHYSICAL ISSUES

Drs Williams and Hricak have neatly described some of the ways in which NMR scanners operate to produce images. There are certainly other ways to create NMR images – for example, the parameter which is used to determine its site of origin may be phase, as well as frequency information – but this is of less importance to the clinician than to the designers of NMR equipment. What *is* important to clinicians is a clear understanding of the information content in the image regarding the anatomy, pathology and physiology of the body parts which are depicted, and it may be worthwhile to add to this information.

It has become common to state that NMR images may reveal 'chemistry' whereas other imaging techniques reveal 'only anatomy'. Indeed, NMR images have the capacity to reveal some chemical and physiologic information, but it is not really true that they have a monopoly upon this possibility. Radiographs, for example, may show changing amounts of calcium in bone, increases in fat in hepatic tissue, rapid movement of water across pulmonary alveolar membranes and gross alterations in glomerular filtration rate, which are, after all, 'biochemical' or 'physiologic' functions. What is true about NMR is that it shows *different* kinds of physiologic or biochemical information from radiographs and CT, along with very similar kinds of anatomic information. We will deal first with the anatomy, then with the biochemical and physiologic tissue alterations, which NMR is able to depict.

As has been clearly pointed out in the original article, NMR images are constructed as planar tomograms (not that there is any great necessity to limit the images to this form; 3-dimensional representations of anatomy by NMR are relatively easy to construct). NMR tomograms are more akin to CT tomograms than to radiographic tomograms in that the planes depicted by the image contain *no* contribution from adjacent tissue planes. Therefore, NMR images obtained in a transverse, or trans-axial planes, bear a great resemblance to the usual CT image: the spatial relationships of the anatomy displayed are identical. But, as has also been pointed out in the previous article, the planes may be oriented in any direction desired. Conversely, in CT, planes other than the transverse can be obtained only by reconstructing sagittal or coronal planes from a series of transverse planes (which markedly degrades the spatial resolution in the resultant dimensions) or, in a few anatomic regions, by stuffing the patient into the CT gantry in highly contorted, and usually uncomfortable, positions. Luckily, most experienced radiologists are capable of recreating in their imaginations a fairly good 3-dimensional conception of anatomy when they are presented with a series of parallel 2-dimensional tomographic images, so that restriction of CT images to the transverse plane has not been perceived as a tremendous handicap. Yet, upon reflection, it is clear that there are a few anatomic regions in which the ability to produce sagittal or coronal images are of tremendous value in urologic oncology. For example, it is often difficult with standard CT to distinguish a small polar lesion in the kidneys from normal parenchyma. It is difficult, if not impossible, to find a small mural lesion on the dome of the bladder, and extremely difficult to measure the depth of invasion of a lesion either on the dome or the base of this organ. NMR, therefore, ought to be more useful than CT both in staging and in detection of certain neoplasms of the bladder and kidneys. Still, the gross morphologic information provided by NMR scanning is very similar to that provided by CT scanning, and in projecting the future uses of the two techniques, it is probably accurate that in many clinical situations either imaging technique could be used to acquire the necessary information.

Since it is possible to perform NMR imaging in a way that information is collected from a 3-dimensional volume at once, with the possibility of constructing 3-dimensional images, it is theoretically easier to measure volumes of structures or tissues of a particular kind by NMR imaging than it is by CT or ultrasound. After all, in the latter two techniques, volumes must be calculated by measuring areas in successive planes and summing them, which is both tedious and subject to technical error. But since entire 3-dimensional volumes can be scanned at once with NMR, volume measurements of tissues of a particular kind may be done by computer, ultimately with great accuracy.

In all of the techniques for diagnostic imaging in use prior to the advent of NMR, it is true that the images produced constitute anatomic maps of variations in one parameter. For radiographs and CT, the parameter is X-ray attenuation of tissue, in ultrasound, it is amplitude of echos returned by tissue and in scintigraphic images it is the amount of gamma radiation emitted by the tissues. And although other information may be inferred indirectly from these parameters, for each technique, the parameter is single. Therefore, for imaging physicians, it became a convenient shorthand to describe the images in terms of their local density variations: an area in a radiograph might be said to be 'dense' as, for example, in describing bone; an area of a sonogram might be said to be 'dense' as, for example, in describing a region of fat. Since in all images of a particular technique the gray scale meant the same thing from examination to examination, it makes sense to describe the images in terms of density: everyone knows what the term means. But the situation is quite different in NMR imaging. The density of a region of the image – the place it occupies upon the gray scale is usually a function of *several* parameters. As has been pointed out, these are proton density, spin-lattice relaxation (T_1) and spin-spin relaxation (T_2); in addition, tissue motion, such as blood flow, may affect the gray scale of an image. To make things more complicated, there is no standard way of arranging the contribution of each of these factors to the overall gray scale, so that in one image a certain tissue may appear particularly bright with respect to others, whereas in an image obtained in a slightly different way, the same tissue may appear darker than others. Therefore, it is insufficient merely to state that a particular portion of tissue is light or dark in an NMR image; it must also be stated exactly what pulse sequence was used. Unless the pulse sequence is unknown, it is impossible to determine from the brightness of a particular region on the image the individual contributions of proton density, T_1 and T_2 to that portion of the image. And since it is precisely these characteristics that vary from tissue to tissue, if there is to be any hope of specific tissue differentiation by NMR proton imaging, at least an estimate of the contribution of each of these parameters must be obtainable from the image. In general, saturation recovery (two or more pulses) and inversion recovery (a 180° pulse followed by a 90° pulse) sequences can be made to highlight T_1 differences among tissues, whereas the variations on the spin echo pulse sequence (a 90° pulse followed by one or more 180° pulses) can be made to highlight T_2 differences.

In general (at least with the exceptions of cortical bone and fatty tissue), water content of human tissues does not vary a great deal from tissue to tissue, and the overall proton concentration is not greatly different from tissue to tissue even when fat is included. Therefore, at least in proton NMR images, distinction among tissues is largely made on the basis of differences in T_1 and T_2 relaxation times.

The specific characteristics of tissue which determine T_1 and T_2 are by no means entirely worked out, and are beyond the scope of this discussion. In general, they have to do with the interaction of individual nuclei with their neighboring ones. As a very general rule, within the range of relaxation times encountered in human tissue, it seems to be true that the more free water is added to tissue, the longer the relaxation times become. As a result, tissue which has become edematous, inflamed or malignant tends to have a prolonged relaxation time when compared to its normal state.

Research is being pursued along two lines: that intended to discover what precise factors lead to alteration in relaxation times in tissue, and empiric investigation into the specific relaxation times of particular tissues in particular physiologic and pathologic states. The latter will determine the possibilities and limitations of specifically identifying and discriminating among diseased states in man by NMR scanning, and will probably constitute a region of particularly intense investigation over the next several years.

In the accompanying paper, it is stated that areas of flowing blood often appear to emit no measurable signal because the protons in the blood which are emitting the signal move out of the plane being imaged before their signal is detected. Indeed, motion of the signal-emitting protons between the time they are excited by an RF pulse and the time the signal is detected is an important phenomenon, and may manifest itself not only by absence of signal, but by signal enhancement. This latter effect is probably due to the fact that within an image plane, the strength of the signal emitted is in part determined by the rate at which the magnetism parallel to the external field is able to grow after it has been lessened or abolished by a previous RF pulse. Blood entering the imaged plane may contain protons whose magnetization has not been altered at all by previous RF pulses, and therefore which can be made to emit a larger signal than the other proton within the plane, so that moving blood appears as a particularly bright signal. The alteration in brightness depends upon the speed of flow, and promises to be useful in measuring the specific velocity, and hence volume flow, of blood in identified vessels. The accuracy of such measurements remain to be determined, however, at least in part because the alterations in signal intensity from flowing blood are caused not only by the motion of the blood into or out of the imaged plane, but by alterations in the degree to which a spin echo has its intensity altered even by motion within the plane. Nevertheless, some degree of accuracy in measurement of blood flow will undoubtedly be possible.

NMR spectroscopy has been briefly alluded to in the original manuscript. It has been pointed out that since, at a given magnetic field, each nucleus absorbs and emits NMR energy at specific a frequency, specific elements, in addition to hydrogen, might be sought for and have their concentrations measured. But NMR spectroscopy ultimately holds the promise of providing much more information, indeed, the field has been a very active one for decades, and as a result of extensive experimentation by biochemists, knowledge regarding NMR spectroscopy is advanced. In particular, not only may specific nuclei be sought, but specific compounds may be identified as well. Such nuclei in these compounds have their ambient magnetic fields created not only by the external magnet but by the magnetic fields of adjacent subatomic species, identical nuclei occupying different positions in a molecule will emit signals of slightly different frequencies. These frequencies can be distinguished, so that the different concentrations of individual compounds, as well as individual elements, may be measured by virtue of strength of signals at specific frequencies.

In view of these facts, a number of possibilities for further development of in vivo NMR have appeared. First of all, it is possible to have an NMR imager receive signals from nuclei other than protons, so that images which consist of maps of local concentrations of other nuclei, are possible. Indeed, preliminary images showing distribution of sodium, in the kidney and elsewhere, have already been made in our laboratory. And so-called 'chemical shift' images are possible as well. In these, images are made from signals of a frequency so carefully defined that the images reveal the distribution of individual compounds or classes of compounds, rather than of individual elements. These images have been recently created using hydrogen as a substrate, and successfully distinguishing the distribution of water from the distribution of lipids (whether this will be useful for hydrogen remains to be seen; it is certainly technically easier to distinguish water and lipids on proton scans by virtues of their different relaxation times rather than by their different resonant frequencies). Of much greater importance would be chemical shift imaging of elements like phosphorus, the level of individual compounds of which (like ATP) are of extreme importance in the investigation of ischemic disease.

In general, it is true that chemical shift images, and images of nuclei other than protons, produce images of much poorer spatial resolution than those of protons, since other elements are not as abundant in tissue and the signal to noise ratio for these elements is lower. But even at relatively low spatial resolution images may provide important biochemical information. In general, there is a trade-off between spatial resolution and specificity of spectroscopic information: the more the technique uses a particular frequency peak, the more other information is discarded, and the more difficult it is to create an image with high spatial resolution. But the compromise may be worthwhile even at extremes: an 'image' of such poor spatial resolution that it essentially consists only of a single large voxel may yield important information if the location of the voxel can be accurately determined within the body. At this extreme, in vivo NMR spectroscopy can be performed with the greatest biochemical information at the expense of spatial resolution.

The foregoing discussion has involved imaging of tissue without regard to artificial manipulation of its NMR characteristics. But there is a class of compounds exhibiting a quality known as paramagnetism which are capable of altering the relaxation times of other species with which they are in close contact. Paramagnetic agents may be administered in solution and shorten the relaxation times of tissues within which they are distributed. This effect alters the intensity of the NMR image seen in the tissue, so that paramagnetics are roughly analogous to soluble contrast agents in radiographic studies. As the original manuscript mentioned, certain metallic ions have already been shown to be effective in this regard as have simple organic molecules whose distribution and excretion have been found to be similar to those of iodinated intravascular radiographic contrast agents.

The field of developing paramagnetic agents has tremendous potential. Since paramagnetic molecules are sufficiently active to be detected by NMR imaging in quite low concentrations, they are as amenable to being incorporated in as wide a variety of diagnostic pharmaceuticals as are radionuclides used in scintigraphic imaging. Combining the use of paramagnetic molecules designed with great tissue, pharmacologic and physiologic specificity with the high spatial resolution offered by proton NMR imaging raises the possibility of developing a diagnostic science which combines many of the best features of emission scintigraphy and transmission X-ray computed tomography.

3. CLINICAL ISSUES

What may all of this mean with regard to the future applications of NMR imaging in urologic oncology? The accompanying manuscript has outlined the findings encountered so far in patients with urologic neoplasms, and has pointed out quite correctly that a great deal more research needs to be done before all of the possibilities are explored. Therefore what follows must largely be speculation, but the predictions can be based upon well-known characteristics of urologic neoplastic disease and upon the capacities of NMR imaging, and are likely, at least in general, to be correct.

NMR imaging may well play an important role in screening for the presence of urologic neoplasms. In the kidney, its anatomic accuracy and capacity to make images in multiple planes should make it quite useful in depicting the gross morphologic abnormalities that renal carcinomas produce. Insufficient experience exists to date to determine the efficacy of NMR imaging in the differentiation of renal masses. It will almost certainly be true that the distinction between carcinomas and angiomyolipomas may be easily made by NMR, since the NMR characteristics of fatty tissue are already known to be quite different from that of tissues with smaller amounts of lipid. It may be true that the NMR characteristics of tumors such as oncocytomas, which may be treated differently from carcinomas, may be sufficiently different to allow preoperative distinction.

In the prostate, as has been pointed out, NMR imaging ought to be more sensitive and specific than any imaging technique available to date. Unlike radiographs and CT, which cannot distinguish among different kinds of prostatic tissue, and unlike ultrasound, which is very non-specific in its depiction of focal prostatic abnormalities, NMR may make clear distinction between normal prostatic tissue, prostatic carcinoma and benign hypertrophy. Since, if the examination is limited to the prostate, it can be accomplished relatively fast, it may well be inexpensive enough for fairly large-scale screening. Within the testis, where the differential diagnosis between malignant and non-malignant sources of testicular enlargement, pain or masses, and the differentiation among the various kinds of testicular tumors are still not extremely accurate, NMR imaging may prove to be of great value. In addition to accurate morphology, the T_1 and T_2 characteristics, along with potential changes in NMR appearance which could be elicited by the administration of paramagnetics, promise to increase the specificity of diagnosis.

NMR may also be of great value in the staging of urinary tract tumors. In renal carcinoma, where the morphologic extent of bulky tumor is one of the most important features in staging, NMR clearly should be helpful. In the staging of transitional cell carcinomas, especially within the bladder, NMR will undoubtedly provide improvements in preoperative staging of tumors (as has been pointed out in the accompanying manuscript) since it can distinguish between tumor and bladder walls; since CT cannot do this, and the efficacy of ultrasound in this regard has not yet been proven, NMR will probably prove to be of important value. With regard to tumors of the prostate, it may turn out that details of anatomy of the prostatic capsule may be sufficiently demonstrable by NMR that crossing of the capsule by tumor, as opposed merely to enlargement of the entire gland, may be visible. Finally, retroperitoneal metastasis from testicular tumors ought also to be clearly seen by NMR imaging.

All of these factors concern either the formation of distant large metastasis or local invasion by tumors. With the continued development of tumor-specific antigens, and the possibility of combining them with paramagnetic agents, metastatic deposits which are too small to be seen morphologically may be detectable by local alterations in relaxation times after administration of the paramagnetics. If this turns out to be the case, a great advance in preoperative evaluation of tumor extent will have been made.

Changes in proton NMR characteristics of tumor tissue attendant upon chemotherapy and radiotherapy may turn out to be visible on NMR images. If so, the response of neoplasms to therapy can be monitored much more accurately and earlier in the stage of therapy than has been hitherto possible. The change in tumor volume, which underlies a great deal of the current evaluation of response to therapy, will probably turn out to be a much later event than immediate tissue changes. If this is the case, trials of therapy in individual patients will undoubtedly be capable to being performed with much greater specificity and rapiditiy than has been hitherto possible.

The role of NMR imaging using nuclei other than protons, or even the role of in vivo NMR spectroscopy without high resolution images, must be an even more speculative field in urologic oncology. NMR images using sodium as a substrate are now capable of revealing the overall sodium concentration of regions of tissue; since with cellular damage, there tends to be an influx of sodium into the intracellular spece with an overall increase of sodium in the affected region of tissue, it may be that tumor cell damage caused by therapeutic agents might be visible almost immediately. In vivo spectroscopy of phosphorus compounds has already been shown to be possible; it is only a short technical step before specific regions of tissue within the body (possibly within tumors) may be identified for spectroscopy, so that changes in high energy phosphorus levels attendant upon tumor therapy may be quickly demonstrated as well.

To date, the major vessels supplying tumors, especially in the kidney, have been demonstrable only by arteriographic techniques. CT imaging is able to outline only the major renal arteries and veins, and, on occasion, very large collaterals; intravenous arteriography by digital subtraction method has to date been able to find small vessels. But NMR imaging of vessels is relatively easy (as long as there is blood flowing within their lumens); therefore, the preoperative use of NMR proton imaging to outline vessels which will be encountered in surgery may turn out to be useful.

With regard to the postoperative period, no method currently exists for locating small deposits of recurrent tumors and distinguishing them from local benign postoperative changes. Proton NMR imaging may well turn out to be able to distinguish between recurrent tumor and scar tissue, and may be useful in this regard.

Subject index

Acid phosphatase
  lysosomal, 91
  as tumor marker, 112-114
Actinomycin D, 256, 257
Adrenal cancer
  neuroblastomas, 124-125, 285
  NMR imaging of, 337-338
  pheochromocytomas, 124-125, 337-338
  tumor markers in, 124-126
Adriamycin
  action of, 52-53
  in combination therapy, 54-55, 56-57, 63-
    65, 78
  in disseminated testicular cancer, 257, 258
  in prostatic cancer, 54-59, 63-65, 78
  as single agent, 58-59
AFP. See Alpha-fetoprotein (AFP)
Agar assay, double-layer soft, 94-104, 108-
  109
Agar gel electrophoresis, 41
Alkaline phosphatase, 130, 199
Alpha-fetoprotein (AFP)
  as surgical contraindication, 261-262
  as tumor marker, 126-128, 197, 199, 260
Aminoglutethimide, 70-71
Ammonium sulfate precipitation, 40-41
Androgen receptors
  levels in prostatic cancer, 20-28
  measurement of, 18-20, 39-45
  vs. non-receptor steroid binding proteins,
    42-43
  in stromal-epithelial interactions, 28-33
  temperature effect on, 18. 43
Angiogenesis
  capillary stimulation in, 10
  defined, 1
  inhibition of, 8-11, 15
  lymphocytes in, 14
  macrophages in, 14

mechanism of, 2-5
techniques for studying, 14
tumor detection based on, 5-8, 14-15
tumor vs. normal, 15
Anti-androgens, 69-70
Antibody, as tumor marker, 119
Antigens
  blood group, 18-19
  carcinoembryonic, 120
  embryonic, 192-196
  fetal, 192-196, 291
  HLA. See HLA antigens
  Ia, 280, 287
  prostate, 114-115
  resistance, 281
  stage-specific, 193, 194
  tumor-associated, 195-196
Avascular phase, 1-2

Bacillus Calmette-Guerin. See BCG therapy
BCG therapy
  for carcinoma in situ, 177-179, 186
  vs. chemotherapy, 176-177
  clinical trials of, 170-176
  cyclophosphamide and, 175-176
  dosage in, 181-182
  historical background of, 169-170
  vs. interferon, 245
  in invasive transitional cell carcinoma, 187
  maintenance schedules for, 186
  mechanism of action of, 186-187
  mode of administration in, 181, 185-186
  oral, 174-175
  patient selection for, 172, 182
  for recurrent superficial bladder tumor, 170-
    177
  for residual bladder tumor, 179-181
  side effects of, 171, 175, 176-177
  toxicity of, 181-182, 185